# Lessons in Cookery

*Hand-book of the National Training
School for Cookery*

*by*

Rose Owen Cole
Thomas King Chambers
Eliza Ann Youmans

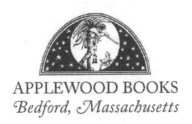

APPLEWOOD BOOKS
*Bedford, Massachusetts*

*Lessons in Cookery*

was originally published in

1879

ISBN: 978-1-4290-1205-8

Thank you for purchasing an Applewood book.
Applewood reprints America's lively classics—
books from the past that are still of interest
to the modern reader.
For a free copy of
a catalog of our
bestselling
books,
write
to us at:
Applewood Books
Box 365
Bedford, MA 01730
or visit us on the web at:
For cookbooks: foodsville.com
For our complete catalog: awb.com

**Prepared for publishing by HP**

# LESSONS IN COOKERY.

## HAND–BOOK

### OF THE

## NATIONAL TRAINING SCHOOL FOR COOKERY

### (SOUTH KENSINGTON, LONDON).

TO WHICH IS ADDED

## THE PRINCIPLES OF DIET IN HEALTH AND DISEASE.

### By THOMAS K. CHAMBERS, M.D.

EDITED BY

### ELIZA A. YOUMANS.

NEW YORK:

D. APPLETON AND COMPANY,

549 AND 551 BROADWAY.

1879.

# PREFACE TO THE AMERICAN EDITION.

THE present work on cookery appeared in England under the title of "The Official Hand-Book of the National Training School for Cookery," and it contains the lessons on the preparation of food which were practised in that institution. It has been reprinted in this country with some slight revision, for the use of American families, because of its superior merits as a cook-book to be consulted in the ordinary way, and also because it is the plainest, simplest, and most perfect guide to *self-education in the kitchen* that has yet appeared. In this respect it represents a very marked advance in an important domestic art hitherto much neglected.

A glance at its contents will show the ground it covers, and how fully it meets the general wants. The dishes for which it provides have been selected with an unusual degree of care and judgment. They have been chosen to meet the needs of well-to-do families, and also those of more moderate means, who must observe a strict economy. Provision is made for an ample and varied diet, and for meals of a simple and frugal character. Receipts are given for an excellent variety of soups, for cooking many kinds of fish in different ways, for the preparation of meats, poultry, game, and vegetables, and for a choice selection of entrées, soufflés, puddings, jellies, and creams. Besides the courses of a well-ordered dinner, there are directions for making rolls, biscuits, bread, and numerous dishes for breakfast and tea, together with a most valuable set of directions how to prepare food for the sick. The aim has been to meet the wants of the great mass of people who are not rich enough to abandon their kitchen to the management of professional cooks, and who must keep a careful eye to expense. But while the costly refinements of artistic and decorative cookery are avoided, there has been a constant reference to the simple requirements of good taste in the preparation of food for the table.

But the especial merit of this volume, and the character by which it stands alone among cook-books, is the superior method it offers of teaching the art of practical cookery. It is at this vital point that all our current cook-books break down; they make no provision for getting a knowledge of this subject in any systematic way. So much in them is vague, so much taken for granted, and so much is loose, careless, and misleading in their receipts, that they are good for nothing to teach beginners, good for nothing as guides to successful practice, and only of use to those who already know enough to supply their deficiencies and protect themselves against their errors. In fact, the hand-book required to teach cookery effectually cannot be made by any single person in the usual manner, but it must be itself a product of such teaching.

The present volume originated in this way, and embodies a tried and successful method of making good practical cooks. The lessons given in the following pages came from a training kitchen for pupils of all grades, and the directions of its receipts are so minute, explicit, distinct, and complete, that they may be followed with ease by every person of common-sense who has the slightest desire to learn. They are the results of long and careful practice in teaching beginners how to cook, and have grown out of exercises often repeated with a view of making them as perfect as possible. It is commonly regarded as a good thing in a cook-book that its compiler has tested some of its receipts and points out the troubles and failures likely to occur in early trials. But the completeness of the instructions in this work was attained through the stupidities, blunders, mistakes, questionings, and difficulties of hundreds of learners of all capacities, doing the work over and over again under the critical direction of intelligent, practical teachers, who were bent upon finding out the best method of doing each thing, and the best method of teaching others how to do it. Not a single item necessary to perfect the required process is omitted. The steps are separated, and given in numerical order, so as to enforce attention to one thing at a time, and the right thing at the right time, while the precautions against mistakes are so careful that even the dullest can hardly go wrong. Each receipt in the volume is not only the formula for a dish, but it is also a lesson in a practical process, so that in the preparation of every article of food something is gained toward greater proficiency in the art of cooking well.

A few words in regard to the origin of the school in which it was produced will still further illustrate the character of this work. A vigorous movement has been made in England to elevate this branch of domestic economy by establishing schools for training pupils in the art of cookery. These schools have grown immediately out of the need of greater general economy among the working classes, as it was seen that the high prices of provisions were seriously aggravated by not knowing how to make the most of them in their kitchen preparation. The attention of the managers of the South Kensington Museum of Arts in West London was several years ago drawn to the subject; and feeling that something required to be done, they established public lectures on the preparation of food with platform demonstrations of various culinary operations. But it was quickly found that mere exposition and illustration, though not without use, were wholly inadequate to the object in view; because a cooking school, to be thorough, must provide for practice. Lecturing, and explaining to pupils, and barely showing them how things are done, is sure to fail because cookery, like music, can only be learned by actually doing it. As well undertake to teach the piano by talking and exhibiting its capabilities as to teach a person how to make a dish properly by only listening and looking on. Provision had therefore to be made for forming classes to do themselves what they at first only saw others do.

But this task was by no means an easy one. There were no pre-existing plans to follow; qualified teachers and suitable text-books were wanting; it was an expensive form of education; the public thought it a doubtful innovation; and educational authorities discouraged it. But the parties interested decided that the time had come for a systematic and persistent effort. They felt their way cautiously, and in 1874 organized classes for graded courses of practice. The object was to give women the best possible instruction in practical cookery, and for this purpose the school was open to all. But to make its work most largely useful, it was constituted as a Normal School for training teachers to go out and establish other cooking schools in different parts of the country. This has been since done with the most encouraging success, so that there are

, already a large number of cooking schools in England connected with the National or Common School system.

As no cook-book to be found was worth anything to aid the practical instruction proposed, the teachers had to take this matter in hand at the outset. They began by drawing up a careful set of directions to be followed by the learners in doing their work. For each lesson in all the grades each pupil was furnished with a printed sheet of these directions, stating the ingredients of each dish to be prepared, the quantities and separate cost of these ingredients, what was to be done first, what next, and so on through the whole series of operations, nothing being assumed as known, and all the minute steps being indicated in the order that was found best. These guides were necessarily imperfect at first, and were subject to constant revision and extension as experience suggested corrections; in fact, they embodied the progress of the school in the successful attainment of its object. At each new printing the improvements that had been made were incorporated, and only after years of trial were these guides to practice at length combined and issued in a book-form. The lessons or receipts of this volume were all slowly elaborated in this painstaking manner, and the mode of working proved perfectly successful with the pupils. It was easy and pleasant, yet careful and thorough, and secured a rapid and gratifying proficiency.[1]

In saying that the South Kensington Cooking School has been successful, I speak from direct knowledge of it. I was a pupil there for several weeks, and carefully observed its operations. The classes showed the most extraordinary mental and social diversity. There were cultivated ladies, the daughters of country gentlemen, old housekeepers, servants, cooks, and colored girls from South Africa, together with a large proportion of intelligent young women who were preparing to become teachers. They worked together with a harmony and good feeling that, I confess, somewhat surprised me, but

---

[1] The honor of contributing chiefly toward the establishment of this school and superintending its development is due to Sir Henry Cole, the able director and master mind of the South Kensington Museum. By his firm purpose and excellent judgment a novel experiment, surrounded by many difficulties, became a recognized success and a great national benefit. The "Lessons" were gradually brought into shape by the teachers, under the supervision of the accomplished daughter of Sir Henry Cole, whose initials (R. O. C.) were appended to them as revised for use in the school, and are also subscribed to the English Preface of this work.

they were all closely occupied and thoroughly interested in a common object. There were teachers to provide materials, to plan the daily work, to direct operations, and to be consulted when necessary; but the admirable method adopted left each learner to go through her task with but a small amount of assistance. Indeed, the completeness of the directions in hand seemed to assure the success of every pupil from the start. There was, of course, a difference in dexterity, and in facility of work previously acquired; but raw beginners went on so well that they were astonished at what they found themselves able to do.

American ladies when looking over these lessons are apt to smile at their extreme simplicity and triviality, but it must be remembered that the difference between good and bad cookery is very much a matter of attention to trifles. Slight mistakes, small omissions, little things done at the wrong time, spoil dishes. The excellence of these lessons consists in their faithfulness in regard to minutiæ, and the habits they enforce of attention to trifling particulars. They make no claim to literary merit. The receipts are homely, direct, and meant only to be easily and distinctly understood. They are full of repetitions, because processes are constantly repeated, and it was necessary that the directions in each receipt should be full and complete. They are not enticing reading, because they were made to work by. The book, in fact, belongs in the kitchen where cookery is done; and it is now republished because its success there has been demonstrated. Many hundred persons totally ignorant of the subject have become efficient and capable cooks by pursuing the mode of practice here adopted—by going through these lessons— and the same results can be obtained by pursuing the same method anywhere. American housekeepers who have any real interest in home improvement, and are willing to take a little pains to instruct their daughters or their servants in the art of cooking well, will find the volume an adequate and invaluable help toward the attainment of this object. It will prove a useful text-book in the cooking schools and young ladies' cooking clubs that are springing up in this country, and classes could be advantageously formed, by its help, for kitchen practice in every female seminary.

In revising these lessons but very slight changes have been made, and those only of form. The prices of articles, an important feature in the original work, and essential in the cooking school, have been omitted, as they do not apply in this country; and American prices have not been substituted because they vary so much in different localities. As the lessons were furnished on separate sheets for daily use in the school, they all took the form of the following example, and have been modified in the manner shown by referring to the same lesson on page 180 of the present volume:

---

### MAYONNAISE SAUCE.

*Average cost of Mayonnaise Sauce (about half a pint).*

INGREDIENTS.

| | *d* |
|---|---|
| 2 eggs.................................................. | 2 |
| Salt and pepper................................... | |
| 1 teaspoonful of French vinegar................. | 1 |
| 1 teaspoonful of mustard.... ................... | |
| 1 teaspoonful of tarragon vinegar............... | 1½ |
| 1 gill of salad oil................................. | 6 |
| | 10½ |

*Time required, about 10 minutes.*

---

Now we will show you how to make *Mayonnaise Sauce.*

1. We take *two eggs* and put the *yolks* in one basin and the *whites* (which will not be wanted) into another basin.

2. We take a wooden spoon and just stir the *yolks* enough to break them.

3. We add to them *a saltspoonful of salt* and *half a saltspoonful of pepper* and *a tablespoonful of French vinegar.*

4. We take a bottle of *salad oil*, and, putting our thumb half over the top, pour in, drop by drop, the *oil*, stirring well with a whisk the whole time; *a gill of oil* will be sufficient.

N. B.—We might add *a teaspoonful of ready-made mustard or tarragon vinegar* if liked, stirring it in smoothly.

5. The *sauce* is now ready for use.

Now it is finished.

---

It has been suggested that the volume ought to be *Americanized* by omitting some of the English receipts that are but little used in this country, and substituting others for special American dishes.

But this suggestion involves a total misconception of the character of the work, which is valuable solely on account of the qualities it derives from the experience of the Training School. As American dishes are not used in England, there were of course no "lessons" in their preparation. Common receipts would be out of place in the following pages, and receipts for American dishes could not be properly introduced until they had been assimilated to the plan and peculiarities of the work. There are many hundred good English receipts that will be sought in vain in the volume; and those who refer to it to find the last new things in American cookery will of course be disappointed. It is not a receipt-book, but a book to show how to use and improve receipts; or, as stated in the English preface, it is not a dictionary of reference, but rather a grammar of processes. Its merit is that it offers an improved mode of kitchen practice; and, as the principles and conditions of good cookery are everywhere the same, all that is characteristic of the volume is just as applicable and valuable in this country as in England.

As the subject of cookery is in close relations with that of diet, I have aimed to increase the usefulness of the present work by appending a valuable essay upon "Diet in Health and Disease," the latest that has appeared, and by an eminent living authority on dietetical questions. Dr. Chambers is the author of various able works on the uses and effects of food, and in this article, which he recently contributed to the new edition of the "Encyclopædia Britannica," he has summed up in an admirable manner the leading facts and principles of modern dietetical science. Hints derived from this essay will often be found of much service in directing housekeepers as to what it is best to cook, and in the composition of meals in various circumstances, with reference to occupation, enjoyment, and health.

E. A. Y.

New York, *August*, 1878.

# PREFACE TO THE ENGLISH EDITION.

I. THIS work has been written to explain in an easy way the first principles of good Cookery, and in the form of lessons is especially addressed to those who wish to carry them into practice. It has been the aim of the writer to leave no detail, however small, vaguely stated. It is taken for granted that the learner has no knowledge on the subject. The loose expressions, such as "a pinch," "a little," found in all cookery books, are therefore avoided, and precise quantities are given.

II. The work is not to be regarded as an exhaustive cookery book with numerous recipes. It aims to be rather a grammar than a dictionary.

III. The lessons give a sufficient number of examples of cookery illustrating many degrees of cost: thus the rich may have a dish of curried rabbit for 3s. 8d., and the poor may have a dish of curried tripe for 10¾d.

IV. The work has been used and tested in the National Training School for Cookery since 1875, and the instructors now employed in local schools throughout the country have been taught and practised by means of these lessons.

V. It has been found that it is most convenient to practise the lesson with the instructions in sight close at hand. An edition of each lesson has been printed on separate sheets of thick paper, for the use of students and teachers, which may be obtained at the National Training School for Cookery, or at any of the local schools.

VI. The writer requests that the notice of any errors and omissions which are inevitable in a work of this kind may be communicated to R. O. C., at the National Training School for Cookery, Exhibition Road, London, S. W.

R. O. C.

*July,* 1877.

# CONTENTS.

## CHAPTER V.

## CHAPTER VI.

## CHAPTER VII.

## CHAPTER VIII.

## CHAPTER IX.

## CHAPTER X.

## CHAPTER XI.

## CHAPTER XII.

## CHAPTER XIII.

## CHAPTER XIV.

## CHAPTER XV.

## CHAPTER XXIII.

# LESSONS IN COOKERY.

## CHAPTER I.

### ON CLEANING RANGES, STOVES, AND KITCHEN UTENSILS.

#### LESSON FIRST.

##### TO CLEAN A KITCHEN RANGE OR STOVE.

**1.** Dump the grate, and, with the poker, carefully remove the clinkers that adhere to the fire-brick.

**2.** Shovel into a scuttle the ashes, clinkers, and cinders or partially-burned coal.

> N. B.—These should be sifted. Throw away the ashes and clinkers, but save the cinders, to use in kindling fires.

**3.** Take a brush or wing, and sweep down all the soot from the flues and oven.

> N. B.—This should be done every day, when bituminous coal is burned; but if anthracite coal is used, the flues will not need cleaning oftener than once in two weeks.[1] Wood-stoves should be cleaned as often as once a week.

---

[1] Directions for keeping ranges and stoves in order are usually furnished by the dealer; and as they vary with the construction, they may be appealed to for more specific instructions.

**4.** Mix some stove-polish in an earthen dish, with enough water to make it into a smooth liquid.

**5.** Dip the blacking-brush in the mixture, and cover with it the whole of the range, working from the top downward.

**6.** When the blacking is dry, rub it all over with a dry brush.

**7.** Then take another brush and polish the range all over, so as to make it quite bright.

**8.** Now sweep the soot and dust from the stove and the hearth.

**9.** Steel handles and bolts may be polished by rubbing with emery-paper, but brass handles and bolts should be polished with both brick-dust and a leather.

**10.** To clean the slate or limestone hearth in front of the range, get a flannel and a pail of hot water; put in it some soda, and wash the hearth all over.

**11.** Then wring the flannel out in hot water and smooth the hearth over, rubbing lightly all in one direction.

**12.** Black-lead and polish the inside of the fender in the same way as you did the range, and brighten the rim of it with emery-paper.

### TO KINDLE A FIRE.

**1.** Place a few sifted cinders at the bottom of the grate.

**2.** Then put in some crumpled paper and arrange sticks over it, laying them across each other. For kindling anthracite coal, hard wood should be added. Charcoal is sometimes used in place of wood, and is better, when it can be afforded.

**3.** Place a few cinders above the wood, and light the paper at the bottom.

**4.** When the wood is well on fire, put on a small quantity of coal, and wait till it is thoroughly heated and beginning to burn before more is added.

---

## LESSON SECOND.

### TO CLEAN A GAS-STOVE.

**1.** Lift out the *rest* at the top.

**2.** Wash the top of the stove and the *rest* with a flannel dipped in hot water and soda, so as to remove all grease and dirt; then wring out the flannel, and partially dry the top of the stove.

**3.** Now cover with stove-blacking, and polish in the same way as the kitchen range.

> N. B.—Be careful not to stop up the gas-holes with the stove-polish.

**4.** Sweep away the soot and dust, and put the *rest* back over the stove.

---

## LESSON THIRD.

### TO CLEAN AN IRON SAUCEPAN.

**1.** Wash the saucepan well in hot water and soda.

> N. B.—All the black should be removed from the outside and bottom.

**2.** Soap the palm of one hand, or a brush, and rub the inside of the saucepan.

> N. B.—In washing any greasy utensil, it is best, if possible, to use the hand instead of a flannel, as the latter retains the grease, and so keeps putting the grease on again, instead of rubbing it off.

**3.** Mix some sand and powdered soda together, and then dip the soaped hand or brush into it, and rub the inside of the saucepan until it is quite clean and bright.

**4.** Now rinse it in water and dry it with a cloth.

**5.** Clean the lid in the same way.

> N. B.—A white enameled stewpan is cleansed in the same way. Great care should be taken to remove all the stains off the white enamel inside.

> N. B.—Salt might be mixed with the sand, and used to remove the stains from the enamel.

---

### LESSON FOURTH.

#### TO CLEAN A COPPER STEWPAN.

**1.** Mix some sand and salt together on a plate—half the quantity of salt to that of sand.

**2.** Wash the stewpan well in hot water and soda.

**3.** Soap the hand, or a brush, dip it in the salt and sand, and rub the inside of the pan until all stains are removed and it has become clean and bright.

**4.** Rinse it out well in the water, dry the inside quickly, and then turn over the pan and clean the copper outside.

**5.** Rub it in the same way with a soaped hand, or a brush dipped in sand and salt.

> N. B.—If there are many stains on it, an old half lemon, or vinegar, might be used to remove them.

> N. B.—Only the copper part should be cleaned with lemon or vinegar.

**6.** Now rinse it again thoroughly, and dry it quickly with a cloth.

# CHAPTER II.

## *ROASTING, BOILING, BAKING, FRYING.*

---

LESSON FIRST.

ROASTING.

To Roast Meat at an open range:

**1.** Take your joint—say a leg of mutton.

**2.** See that it is quite clean, and, if necessary, scrape it with a knife, and wipe it over with a clean cloth.

> N.B.—As a rule, meat should not be washed in water, as it takes some of the goodness out. If meat has been kept some time, and is not quite fresh, then you might wash it with a little vinegar and water, but it must be well wiped afterward.

**3.** With a sharp knife cut off the *knuckle-bone* from the *leg* of *mutton*.

> N.B.—Put aside the knuckle-bone. It can be used with beef for beef-tea, or be put in the stock-pot; or the trimmings and one pint of water will make gravy for your joint when done, allowing it to boil while the joint is roasting.

**4.** Trim off the *piece* of *flank*, and remove the thick piece of skin from the part where the leg joins the loin.

(These trimmings must be put aside, as they can be used for other purposes.)

5. Now *weigh* the *leg* of *mutton*, so as to find out how long it will take to roast it, as a quarter of an hour is allowed for each pound-weight, and one quarter of an hour besides.

N. B.—When you have a joint without bone, such as *rolled ribs of beef* or *topside of beef*, allow twenty minutes to each pound, as it is all solid meat.

6. Take the *leg* of *mutton*, which weighs say *seven pounds*, and will therefore require *two hours* to roast.

7. Put the tin oven [1] in front of the fire.

8. See that the dripping-pan is in the oven with the dripping-ladle.

9. Take the *hook* of the oven, or of the roasting-jack, if you have one, and pass it through the *knuckle-end* of the leg.

10. Wind up the jack with the key before you put the joint on, so as to make it twist the meat round.

11. Put the joint close to the fire for the *first five minutes*.

12. After that time, draw it a little back, or it will cook too quickly, and become burnt and dried.

N. B.—Meat that is frozen must be placed some way from the fire at first, and then drawn gradually toward it, as it must thaw slowly, or it may become tough.

[1] In this country, tin ovens placed before the fire take the place of the English screen and roasting-jack. These ovens are made in various ways, but they all have a door at the back for basting, a hook in the centre from which the meat is suspended, and a dripping-pan in the bottom. A French roasting-jack may take the place of the simple hook, and with this you may proceed with the roasting according to the directions given above. There are stoves and ranges so made that tin ovens for roasting can be securely fastened to the front, and taken away when not in use.

**13.** Baste the joint every *five* minutes with the drippings that run from it into the pan, using the dripping-ladle.

**14.** Let it roast for *two hours*, as its weight is seven pounds.

**15.** Just before you dish up the joint, you must sprinkle about a saltspoonful of salt over, and then baste it well.

**16.** Warm a large dish.

**17.** Take the hook of the jack and place the joint on the hot dish, and draw out the hook.

**18.** Pour about a gill of hot stock into the dish. (This makes the gravy, and when the joint is cut, the juices from the meat will add to it.)

**19.** Cut a piece of demy-paper like a fringe, and put it round the end of the knuckle-bone.

> N. B.—The dripping in the pan should be poured into a basin, and when it is cold, there will be under the crust of dripping a good gravy. When the dripping is required for use, it must be carefully removed from the top of the gravy and clarified (*see* Lesson on " Frying "). Nearly all joints can be roasted in this way. Attention should be paid to the rules given above for joints of meat without bone.

---

## LESSON SECOND.
### BOILING.

To Boil *Meat:*

**1.** Give attention to the *fire*, and build it up gradually with small pieces of *coal*, so as to make it burn clear and bright.

**2.** You must not have a smoky *fire* for boiling, or the *meat* will get smoked. Start with a good *fire*, and keep it up by adding occasionally small *coal*, and so prevent smoke as much as possible.

> N. B.—You do not require such a clear, bright fire as for roasting.

2

**3.** Take a saucepan sufficiently large to hold the *joint* to be cooked.

**4.** Fill the saucepan almost full of *cold water*, and put it on the fire to warm.

> N. B.—*Salt* should always be added to the *water* in the saucepan to make the *water* taste, unless the *meat* to be cooked is already *salted*, in which case it should be omitted.

**5.** Now take the *joint*, say, for example, a piece of the *silver-side of beef, salted*.

**6.** See that it is quite clean, and, if necessary, scrape it with a knife, and wipe it over with a clean cloth.

> N. B.—*Meat* should not, as a rule, be washed in *water*, as it takes some of the goodness out. *Meat* that has been kept some time, and is not quite fresh, might be washed with *vinegar and water*, but it must be well wiped afterward.
>
> N. B.—*Salt meat* must not be washed with *vinegar and water*, but only with *salt and water*.

**7.** Now weigh the piece of *salt beef*, so as to find out how long it will take to boil, as *ten minutes* are allowed for each *pound of meat*.

> N. B.—This rule refers to the boiling of all meat except *pork*, which requires *fifteen minutes* to each *pound of meat*.
>
> A.—In boiling *fresh meat* to be eaten, the *joint* should be first plunged into *boiling water*, in order that the albumen on the outside of the joint may become hardened, and so prevent the escape of the *juices of the meat*.
>
> B.—The temperature of the water should then be lowered gradually (by adding a small quantity of cold water and drawing the saucepan to the side of the fire), and the *meat* allowed to simmer gently, or it will become tough.
>
> C.—In boiling *meat* for the purpose of making *soup*, the *meat* should be put into *cold water*, in order to extract all the goodness from it.
>
> D.—The water should be brought gradually to boiling point, then moved to the side of the fire, and left to simmer gently for some length of time.

N. B.—*Salt meat* must be put into *warm water*, so as to extract a little of the *salt* before the pores of the skin are closed up. If the *meat* were put into *boiling water*, the pores of the skin would be closed, and the meat would be hardened by the *salt* not being allowed to escape.

**8.** When the water in the saucepan is warm, take the *beef*, which weighs say *eight pounds* (it will therefore take about *one hour and twenty minutes*), and put it in the saucepan. There should be only just enough water to cover the joint.

**9.** Let the water just boil up, and then move the saucepan to the side of the fire, and let it simmer gently for the remainder of the time.

**10.** As soon as the water comes to the boil, you must take a large spoon and *skim* it carefully.

N. B.—The *scum* should be skimmed off directly it rises, or it will boil down again in the *meat* and spoil it. *Scum* is the *impurity* which rises from the *meat*.

N. B.—Be very careful not to let the *meat* boil, or it will be *hardened* and *tough*.

**11.** When the *meat* is sufficiently cooked, take it carefully out of the saucepan, and put it on a hot dish for serving. Pour about *a gill* of the *liquor* (in which it was boiled) round the *joint*. (This makes the *gravy*, and when the *joint* is cut, the *juices* from the *meat* will add to it.)

N. B.—The *liquor* from *boiled meat* can always be used for different purposes, and should therefore never be thrown away, but poured into a clean basin and put aside to cool. The *fat* should be carefully removed from the top of the *liquor* while it is cold, before being used. *Salt liquor* is often used for making *pea-soup*.

### BAKING MEAT, BREAD, PASTRY, ETC.

To Bake Meat:

**1.** You must have a good fire, and keep it up, adding by degrees small pieces of coal, as the oven is required to be very hot.

> N. B.—If it is a close range with which you are dealing, you should pull out the damper placed over the oven, in order to draw all the heat of the fire toward the oven. The ventilator [1] of the oven should be closed.

> N. B.—In kitchen stoves there is usually either a handle at the top of the oven, to be pulled out for opening the ventilator, or a slide-ventilator at the bottom.

**2.** Test the heat of the oven by the thermometer, which is fixed in the door of the oven. The heat should rise to 240° Fahr.

**3.** See that the joint is clean, as directed in the Lesson on "Roasting," Note 2. Weigh it, to find out how long it will take to bake, as ten minutes are allowed for each pound of weight.

> N. B.—When you have a joint without bone, you must allow about fifteen minutes to each pound of weight, as it is solid meat.

**4.** Take the hot-water tin on which the stand for the meat is placed, lift up the upper tin or tray, and fill the

---

[1] As a rule, American ranges and stoves are not supplied with a separate arrangement for ventilating the ovens. The heat is usually controlled by opening and closing the damper in front of the fire. Ability to manage a range or stove in this respect comes only with experience. But in all our generally-approved ranges and stoves a competent cook can obtain well-baked meat, such as is described in this lesson, by making the oven very hot at first, and after a little, partially or wholly closing the damper, to lessen combustion.

under tin half full of warm water; then fit on the upper tin.

> N. B.—In one corner of the upper tin is a small hole for the escape of steam. The water must only just reach this hole, and not come into it.
>
> N. B.—The *water* is placed in the *tin* to prevent the *tin* and the *meat* from getting burnt, and so causing a disagreeable smell.

**5.** Place the *stand* on the *hot-water tin*, to raise the *joint* and prevent it from standing in its own *dripping*, which would sodden and spoil the *meat*.

**6.** Now take the *joint*, which weighs say *seven pounds* (it will, therefore, take *one hour and ten minutes to bake*), and put it on the *stand*. Dredge *flour* over it.

**7.** Put the *tin*, with the *meat*, in the *oven*. The *oven* should be kept *very hot* for the first *five minutes*, in order to form a brown crust on the outside of the joint, to keep in the juices of the meat; after that time the ventilator of the oven should be opened, so as to allow the steam to escape, or the meat would get soddened.

> N. B.—Meat that is frozen must be gradually warmed to thaw it, before shutting it up in the hot oven, or it will be tough.

**8.** Baste the joint every fifteen minutes with the drippings that run from the meat into the pan, using the dripping-ladle.

> N. B.—Joints that are not very fat must be even more frequently basted, or they will burn. If there is not enough dripping from the meat, a little extra dripping should be put in the pan.
>
> N. B.—Joints that have no fat should be covered with a piece of whity-brown paper which has been spread with butter or dripping; it will prevent the meat catching too quickly.

**9.** Turn the joint over occasionally, as the upper side will brown quicker than the under.

N. B.—Potatoes, washed and peeled, or a small suet or dripping and flour pudding (*see* " Puddings," Lesson 28), or a Yorkshire pudding (*see* "Puddings," Lesson 29), might be baked under the meat ; but they should be put in only half an hour before the meat is finished.

**10.** Just before you dish up the joint, sprinkle a salt-spoonful of salt over it, and then baste it well.

**11.** Serve the joint on a hot dish (as described in the Lesson on " Roasting," Note 18), and act with regard to the dripping according to N. B. after Note 19.

N. B.—Pastry or bread, etc., should not be baked in the oven at the same time as the meat, for the steam would prevent their baking properly. For baking small patties or tartlets made of puff-paste, the heat of the oven should rise to 300° Fahr. For meat-pies, tarts, etc., the heat should rise to 280°, and be reduced, after a quarter of an hour, to 220°.

———

## LESSON FOURTH.

### FRYING, AND THE CLARIFYING OF BUTTER, FAT, AND DRIPPING.

The principles of Frying :

**1.** You must have a clear, bright fire.

N. B.—Be very careful it is not smoky.

**2.** Be careful that the utensil used is very clean ; for if there is anything sticking at the bottom of the pan, it will quickly catch or burn, and so spoil the contents.

**3.** Clarify all *fat* (*not lard*), *dripping*, and *butter* before using them, to remove the impurities from the former, and the buttermilk and other watery substance from the latter.

N. B.—*Fat* need not be clarified more than once. After using it, always pour it off carefully in a basin, and, when it is cold, remove the sediment from the bottom of the cake of *fat*. *Butter* must be clarified each time it is used, to remove all watery substances.

**4.** You must have the *fat* very hot; good frying depends on the *fat* being properly heated.

**5.** You should test the heat of the *fat* by a frimometer, if possible. The heat should rise to 345° Fahr. for ordinary frying, and 400° for *whitebait*.

> N. B.—If there is no frimometer, the heat of the *fat* may be tested by the look—as *fat* gets quite still and begins to smoke when it is very hot—or by throwing in a small piece of *crumb of bread;* and if it fries directly a light brown, the *fat* is ready for use.

**6.** Use a deep pan, with plenty of *fat*, so that anything put in may be entirely covered.

**7.** You can fry *bacon* in its own *fat;* it only requires watching and turning till it is done (*see* Lesson on "Liver and Bacon," from Note 1 to Note 5).

**8.** You may fry *chops* or *steaks*, or *slices of meat*, in an *ounce* of either *clarified dripping* or *butter*.

**9.** Melt the *fat* first, but it does not require to be heated.

**10.** Be watchful, when the *meat* is frying, not to allow it to burn; you should turn it over occasionally.

> N. B.—If there is a gridiron, it is much better to broil *chops* and *steaks*, as it prevents their being greasy (*see* Lesson on a "Broiled Steak"). For frying *Fish, see* "Fish," Lessons Nos. 3, 6, 7, and 13. For frying *Meat, Rissoles, Potatoes*, etc., *see* "Cooked Meat," Lessons Nos. 2 and 6; "Australian Meat," Lesson No. 8; "Entrées," Lessons Nos. 4 and 11; and "Vegetables," Lessons Nos. 3 and 4.

To render down or clarify *fat :*

**1.** Take any scraps of *cooked* or *uncooked fat*, and cut them up in small pieces.

**2.** Put the pieces in an old but clean saucepan, and pour in just enough *cold water* to cover them.

**3.** Put the saucepan on the fire, and keep it boiling;

it will take about *an hour*. The lid should be off the
saucepan.

**4.** Stir the *fat* occasionally, to prevent it from burning,
or sticking to the bottom of the saucepan.

**5.** When the *water* has evaporated, and the pieces of
*fat* are cooked, pour the melted *fat* through an old sieve
into a basin, and, when cold, it can be used for all frying
purposes, instead of *lard*.

To clarify *dripping :*

**1.** Put the *dripping* in the saucepan, and put it on the
fire to boil.

**2.** When it boils, pour it into a basin, in which there
should be *half a pint of cold water.*

**3.** When the *dripping* is cold, take a knife and cut
round the edge, so as to take out the *cake or dripping.*

4 Scrape off all the sediment that will be found on the
bottom of the *cake*, and wipe it dry with a cloth.

To clarify *butter :*

**1.** Put the quantity of *butter* required for present use
in a small saucepan, and put it on the fire and let it boil.

**2.** When the *butter* has boiled, take a spoon and remove the *white scum* from the top.

**3.** Then pour the clear *butter* carefully into the pan for
use, as below the *butter* will be a little more *watery substance.*

# CHAPTER III.

## *THE RE-COOKING OF MEAT.*

### HASHED MEAT.[1]

**Ingredients.**—One pound of scraps of cold meat. Two small onions. One-half a turnip. One bunch of herbs.[2] About a tablespoonful of flour. One dessertspoonful of mushroom catsup. Sippets of bread. Salt and pepper. Half an ounce of butter.

*Time required, about two hours ; or, if the stock for the gravy is already made, then only half an hour.*

To Hash Cold Meat:

**1.** Take any remains of *cold meat*, cut off all the meat from the bone, and cut it into thin slices.

**2.** Chop the bone in pieces, and put them into a saucepan.

**3.** Peel *one onion*, and cut it in quarters.

[1] The food called " Hash " in this country is more like the English minced meat (*see* Lesson No. 7, on " Re-cooked Meat ").

[2] This means a small handful of parsley, a sprig of thyme or marjoram, one or both, and one bay-leaf. The parsley should be washed, the dried herbs placed in the midst of it, and the ends of the parsley should be folded around them, making a bunch about three inches long. Tie with a string, and trim away any leaves that might break off if left. This is known among cooks as a " bouquet garni," or " faggot."

4. Wash and scrape *one carrot*, and cut it in quarters.

5. Peel *half a turnip*, and cut it in half.

6. Wash a *sprig of parsley*, and dry it on a cloth.

7. Take *one bay-leaf*, one sprig of marjoram and thyme, and the parsley, and tie them tightly together with a piece of string.

8. Put the *herbs* and *vegetables* into the saucepan with the bones, and cover them with cold water.

9. Put the saucepan on the fire, and, when it boils, add *pepper* and *salt*, according to taste.

10. Now put the lid on, and move the saucepan to the side of the fire, to stew gently for *one hour, or one hour and a half;* watch it, and skim it occasionally.

11. Take a *small onion*, peel it, and cut it in slices.

12. Put *half an ounce of butter* into a frying-pan.

13. Put the pan on the fire, and, when the *butter* is melted, add the *sliced onion*, and let it fry a nice brown.

14. Shake the pan occasionally, to prevent the slices of *onion* from sticking to the bottom of the pan and burning.

15. When the *onion* is sufficiently browned, strain off the *butter*, and put the *onion* on to a plate.

16. When the *bones* have stewed long enough, strain off the liquor into a basin.

17. Wash out the saucepan, and pour back the liquor.

18. Put a *tablespoonful of flour* into a small basin.

19. Add a *tablespoonful* of the *liquor* to the *flour*, and stir it into a smooth *paste*.

20. Stir this *paste* gradually into the *liquor* in the saucepan.

21. Add the *browned onion* and a *dessertspoonful of mushroom catsup*.

**22.** Put the saucepan on the fire, and stir the *sauce* until it boils and thickens.

**23.** Let it boil for *two or three minutes*, until the *flour* is cooked.

> N. B.—Be careful to stir the sauce smoothly while it boils, or it will be lumpy.

**24.** Then move the saucepan to the side of the fire, and, when it is off the boil, lay in the pieces of *meat*, to warm through.

> N. B.—Do not let the sauce boil while the meat is in it, or the meat will get hard and tough.

**25.** Cut a *thin slice of bread* into square pieces.

**26.** Cut these square pieces in half, cornerwise, making the pieces into triangles.

**27.** Put one *ounce* of *clarified dripping* (*see* Lesson on "Frying") in a frying-pan, to melt.

**28.** When the dripping is quite hot, put in the *sippets of bread*, and let them fry a light brown.

**29.** Turn them, so that they will get browned on each side.

**30.** Put a piece of kitchen-paper [1] on a plate, and, when the *sippets* are fried, turn them on to the paper to drain off the grease.

> N. B.—If liked, the bread could be toasted before the fire, instead of fried; in which case it should be cut into sippets after it is toasted.

**31.** For serving, put the *slices* of *meat* on a hot dish in the centre, strain the *sauce* over them, and put the *sippets of bread* round the edge of the dish.

---

[1] Kitchen-paper is unsized white paper, such as is used for wall-paper. It is common in English kitchens, and very convenient for many purposes.

LESSON SECOND.

MEAT FRITTERS.

**Ingredients.**—Slices of cold meat. Six ounces of flour. One tablespoon-ful of salad oil. Two eggs. Dripping for frying.

*Time required, about half an hour (and one hour for the batter to rise).*

To make "Meat Fritters"—i. e., meat fried in batter:

1. Put six *ounces* of *flour* and *half a salt-spoonful* of *salt* into a basin.

2. Add a *tablespoonful* of *salad oil*, and mix the *flour* into a smooth paste.

> N. B.—Be careful that the oil is sweet. One ounce of melted butter can be used instead.

3. Now stir in smoothly, by degrees, *half a pint* of *tepid water*. Be careful that there are no lumps.

4. Break *two eggs ;* put the *whites* on a plate. (The *yolks* should be put in a cup, as they will not be required for present use.)

5. Sprinkle a *quarter of a salt-spoonful of salt* over the *whites of the eggs*, and whip them to a stiff froth with a knife.

6. Stir the whipped *whites of the eggs* lightly into the *batter*.

> N. B.—In winter, clean snow might be used in the batter, instead of the whites of eggs.

> N. B.—This batter might be made without the whites of eggs, in which case it should be mixed with half a pint of beer, instead of the water; but the batter made with beer will not rise as much as when eggs are used.

> N. B.—The beer will not taste after the batter is fried.

**7.** Stand the *batter* aside *for one hour* to rise, or until required for *frying ;* but it should not stand longer than *two hours.*

**8.** Put *half a pound of clarified dripping* (*see* Lesson on " Frying ") into a saucepan, and put it on the fire to heat.

**9.** Take some *cold meat,* and cut it up into thin slices.

> N. B.—Cold boiled or roast pork, or boiled bacon, is very nice fried in batter.

**10.** When the *batter* has risen, and the *fritters* are required for use, stir the *batter* lightly with a spoon, so as to be sure that there are no lumps settled at the bottom.

**11.** When the *dripping* is quite hot and smoking, take the *slices of meat,* dip them in the *batter* so as to quite cover them, and then drop them into the *hot fat.*

> N. B.—Do not put in too many slices at a time, as they should not touch each other.

**12.** Turn them over, so that they will fry to a nice brown on both sides.

**13.** Put a piece of *kitchen-paper* on a plate.

**14.** As the *fritters* are fried, take them carefully out of the fat with a *perforated spoon,* and put them on the paper, to drain off the grease.

> N. B.—Be careful to skim the fat from time to time, or the little loose pieces of batter will burn, and spoil the fat.

> N. B.—Slices of apple or orange can be fried in this batter in the same way, only that the batter should be sweetened, and sugar sprinkled over the fritters when they are fried.

> N. B.—Fish can be fried in batter the same way, only that the batter is usually made with beer, instead of white of egg.

**15.** For serving, turn the *fritters* on to a hot dish.

## LESSON THIRD.

### GOBLET PIE.

**Ingredients.**—Any scraps of cold meat. Two tablespoonfuls of chopped suet, two of moist sugar, two of currants, two of plums, and two of chopped apples. A quarter of a pound of flour. A quarter of a tea-spoonful of baking-powder. One ounce of dripping.

*Time required, about three-quarters of an hour.*

To make " Goblet Pie ":

**1.** Take any scraps of *cold meat* (even the smallest scraps, that would not do for anything else), put them on a board,[1] and chop them up as finely as possible. (There should be about *two tablespoonfuls* of *chopped meat.*)

**2.** Take about *two ounces of suet*, put it on a board, cut away the *skin*, and chop it up very finely. (There should be about *two tablespoonfuls.*)

**3.** Peel *two small apples*, cut out the core, and chop them up finely. (There should be about two tablespoon-fuls.)

**4.** Take *two tablespoonfuls* of *plums*, stone them, and chop them in small pieces.

**5.** Wash *two tablespoonfuls* of *currants*, dry them in a cloth, and pick them over.

**6.** Put all these *ingredients* into a basin with *two table-spoonfuls of moist sugar*, and mix them all well together with a spoon.

---

[1] When only small quantities of things are to be made fine, it is very convenient to place them upon a board, and, taking a sharp knife, hold down the free end of the blade with the left hand, and chop by moving the handle rapidly up and down with the right hand. Some cooks chop in this way upon the table, but a board is preferable.

7. Turn the mixture into a small pie-dish.

8. Put a *quarter of a pound of flour* into a basin, and mix into it a few grains of *salt,* and a *quarter of a tea-spoonful of baking-powder.*

9. Take *one ounce of clarified dripping,* and rub it well and lightly into the *flour* with your hands, until it resembles *sifted bread-crumbs.*

10. Add to it sufficient water to mix it into a stiff *paste.*

11. Flour a board, and turn the *paste* out on it.

12. Take a rolling-pin, flour it, and roll out the *paste* to the shape of the pie-dish, only a little larger, and to about a *quarter of an inch* in thickness.

13. Wet the edge of the pie-dish with *water.*

14. Take a knife, dip it in *flour,* and cut a strip of the *paste* the width of the edge of the pie-dish, and place it round the edge of the dish.

15. Cut this strip of *paste* from round the edge of the *paste,* leaving the *centre* piece rather larger than the top of the pie-dish.

16. Wet the edge of the *paste* with *water.*

17. Take the remaining piece of *paste* and place it over the pie-dish, pressing the edges together with your thumb.

N. B.—Be very careful not to break the *paste.*

18. Take a knife, dip it in *flour,* and trim off all the rough edges of the *paste* round the edge of the dish.

19. Take a knife, and with the back of the blade make little notches in the edge of the *paste,* pressing the *paste* firmly with your thumb, to keep it in its proper place.

20. Make a little hole with the knife in the *centre* of the *pie,* to let the *steam* out while the *pie* is baking.

21. Put the *pie* into the oven (the heat should rise to 220°), to bake for *half an hour.*

LESSON FOURTH.

CURRY.

**Ingredients.**—Scraps of cold meat.  Two ounces of clarified dripping, or butter.  Two apples.  One onion.  One dessertspoonful of curry-powder. Salt.

*Time required, about three-quarters of an hour.*

To make a " Curry " :

**1.** Put *two ounces of clarified dripping*, or *butter*, into a saucepan, and put it on the fire to heat.

**2.** Take *one onion*, peel it, put it on a board, and chop it up as finely as possible.

**3.** When the *dripping* is quite hot, put in the *chopped onion* to brown.  Be careful it does not burn.

**4.** Shake the saucepan occasionally, to prevent the *onion* from sticking to the bottom.

**5.** Take the *cold meat* and cut it up into small pieces.

**6.** Peel *one small apple*, take out the core, and chop it up very finely on a board.

**7.** When the *onion* is sufficiently brown, strain it off, and pour the *dripping* back into the saucepan.

N. B.—Put the browned onion on a plate.

**8.** Now put the pieces of *cold meat* into the saucepan, and let them brown on both sides.

**9.** Add *one dessertspoonful of curry-powder*, the *chopped apple*, and a little *salt*, according to taste.

**10.** Now pour in *half a pint of cold water*, and put back the *browned onion*.

N. B.—If the onion had been left in while the meat was browning, it would have got burnt.

**11.** Stir smoothly and carefully until it boils, and then move it to the side of the fire, to simmer for *half an hour*.

**12.** The lid should be off the saucepan, as the *sauce* is to reduce.[1]

**13.** For serving, we take the *meat* out of the saucepan, and put it on a hot dish and pour the *sauce* over it.

N. B.—*Boiled rice* should be served with the *Curry* (*see* "Vegetables," Lesson 13).

---

### LESSON FIFTH.

### SHEPHERD'S PIE.

**Ingredients.**—Scraps of cold meat. One small onion. Pepper and salt. One and a half pound of potatoes. One ounce of butter. One-half a gill of milk.

*Time required, about an hour and a half.*

To make "Shepherd's Pie":

**1.** Take *one and a half pound of potatoes*, wash them, and boil them as described (*see* "Vegetables," Lesson No. 1).

N. B.—This quantity of potato will cover a quart pie-dish.

N. B.—Any remains of cold potatoes should be used, instead of boiling fresh ones.

**2.** Put *one ounce of butter* and *half a gill* of *milk* into a saucepan, and put it on the fire to boil.

**3.** Put the *boiled potatoes* into another saucepan, and mash them up with a fork or spoon.

**4.** When the *milk* boils, pour it into the *mashed potatoes*, and stir them into a smooth paste.

**5.** Put the saucepan on the fire, and let the *potatoes* just boil. Be careful they do not burn.

**6.** Take any *scraps of cold meat*, cut them in small pieces, and put them in a pie-dish in layers.

---

[1] To reduce a sauce, is to boil it down to the requisite thickness.

**7.** If there is not much *fat* with the *meat*, mix with it a few slices of *pork-fat*.

**8.** Take *one small onion*, peel it, and chop it up as finely as possible on a board.

**9.** Sprinkle each layer of *meat* with plenty of *pepper and salt*, and a little of the *chopped onion*.

**10.** Fill the dish half full of *cold water*.

> N. B.—If there is any cold gravy, it would, of course, be better than the water.

> N. B.—The pie-dish should be quite full of meat, and rather heaped in the centre, so as to raise the crust of potato.

**11.** Take the *mashed potato* and put it over the top of the *meat*, smoothing it over neatly with a knife.

**12.** Take a fork, and mark all over the top of the *potato*.

> N. B.—If liked, the mashed *potato* might be mixed with half its weight of flour into a dough, to make a more substantial crust; it must then be rolled out with a rolling-pin, like pastry.

**13.** Put the pie-dish into the oven, or into a tin oven in front of the fire, for *half an hour*, to brown the crust of *potato* and warm the *meat* through.

---

### LESSON SIXTH.

#### FRIED RISSOLES.

**Ingredients.**—Scraps of cold meat, two ounces. Two tablespoonfuls of chopped suet; two of bread-crumbs; two of chopped parsley. One tablespoonful of chopped marjoram and thyme. Two eggs. Crumb of bread. Salt and pepper. Use of dripping for frying. (This quantity makes about eight.)

*Time required, about half an hour.*

To make " Rissoles " with cold meat:

**1.** Put about *half a pound* of *clarified dripping* into a saucepan, and put it on the fire to heat.

**2.** Take some *scraps* of *cold meat*, and chop them up as finely as possible on a board. When chopped, there should be about *two tablespoonfuls*.

**3.** Cut away the skin from *two ounces* of *suet*, put it on a board, and chop it up as finely as possible. There should be two tablespoonfuls.

**4.** Grate some *crumbs* of *bread* on to a piece of paper.

> N. B.—More than *two tablespoonfuls* of *bread-crumbs* will be required, as the rissoles should be dipped in *bread-crumbs* before they are fried.

**5.** Wash *two* or *three sprigs* of *parsley*, and dry it in a cloth.

**6.** Chop it up finely on a board. There should be *two tablespoonfuls*.

**7.** Take a *sprig* of *marjoram* and a *sprig* of *thyme*, take away the stalks, and rub the leaves through a strainer, or chop them up finely on a board.

> N. B.—The *stalks* of the *herbs* are bitter to the taste, and can therefore only be used for flavoring, and not for eating.

**8.** Put the *meat*, *suet*, and *two tablespoonfuls* of *bread-crumbs*, into a basin, and mix them together.

**9.** Now add the *herbs* and a *teaspoonful* of *salt*.

> N. B.—If liked, a little chopped *onion*, or chopped *lemon-peel*, might be added.

**10.** Break *one egg* into the basin, and mix all together lightly.

**11.** Take a board, flour it, and turn the *mixture* on to it.

**12.** Flour your hands, to prevent the *mixture* from sticking.

**13.** Form the *mixture* into little balls, and sprinkle a little *flour* over them.

**14.** Break an *egg* on to a plate, and beat it very slightly with a knife.

**15.** Put the *balls* into the *egg*, and egg them well all over.

**16.** Now put them into the *bread-crumbs*, and cover them well, but not too thickly.

N. B.—Be careful to finger them as little as possible.

**17.** Put the *rissoles* into a frying-basket, a few at a time, as they must not touch each other.

**18.** When the *fat* in the saucepan is quite hot and smoking, put in the frying-basket, and let the *rissoles* fry a pale brown.

**19.** If there is not sufficient *fat* to cover the *rissoles*, shake the basket occasionally, that they may get fried on all sides alike.

N. B.—If there is no frying-basket, put the *rissoles* into the *fat* with a spoon, and then turn them over, so as to get them equally browned.

**20.** Put a piece of kitchen-paper on a plate.

**21.** When the *rissoles* are fried, turn them carefully on to the paper to drain off the *grease*.

**22.** For serving, put them on a hot dish.

---

## LESSON SEVENTH.

### MINCED MEAT.

**Ingredients.**—Scraps of cold meat. One tablespoonful of mushroom catsup. Pepper and salt. Half a pound of rice, or one pound of potatoes.

*Time required to cook the potatoes, half an hour; to cook the mince, five minutes.*

To make a " Mince " of cold meat:

**1.** If the *mince* is served with rice, *see* Lesson on

"Rice"; or if with *mashed potatoes, see* "Vegetables," Lesson No. 2.

**2.** Put any *scraps* of *cold meat* on a board, and mince them up with a sharp knife.

**3.** Put the *minced meat* into a saucepan, with about a *tablespoonful* (or enough to moisten the mince) of mushroom catsup, or some gravy, and season it with *pepper* and *salt* to taste.

**4.** Put the saucepan on the fire, to let the *mince* just warm through.

**5.** Stir it occasionally, to prevent the *meat* from sticking to the bottom of the saucepan.

**6.** For serving, turn the mince on to a hot dish, with a border of boiled rice or mashed potato.

# CHAPTER IV.

## *ENTREES.*

---

### LESSON FIRST.

#### CURRY.

**Ingredients.**—One rabbit or chicken. Half an ounce of coriander seed. Two cloves of garlic. One dessertspoonful of turmeric. Eight berries of red pepper. Two inches of the stick of cinnamon. Six cardamomums. A small piece of green ginger, the size of a chestnut. Five small onions. Salt. Three ounces of fresh butter. Half a pint of cream or good milk. The juice of half a lemon.

*Time required, about two hours.*

To make *Curry:*

1. Take a *rabbit* (which has been skinned and properly prepared for cooking), and put it on a board.

2. Cut it up in the same way as for carving, taking care that the pieces are nearly all of one size.

> N. B.—*Chicken, veal,* and *other meats* would serve the purpose for curry as well as rabbit.

3. Take *a quarter of an ounce of coriander seed,* put it into the mortar, and pound it very finely with a pestle.

4. Take the pounded seed out of the mortar, and put it on a piece of paper. We must scrape out the mortar, so that none be lost.

**5.** Take *two cloves of garlic*, peel them with a sharp knife, and place them in the mortar.

**6.** Also put into the mortar *a dessertspoonful of turmeric.*

**7.** Add *eight berries of red pepper* and *one inch* of the *stick of cinnamon.*

**8.** Put in *four cardamomums.*

**9.** Take a piece of *green ginger* about the size of a chestnut, and slice it very thin.

**10.** Take *three small onions,* and peel off the two outer skins.

**11.** Divide the onions into quarters, and place them and the sliced ginger in the mortar.

**12.** Pound up all these spices and the onions as fine as possible with the pestle.

**13.** Now add to them the pounded *coriander seed,* and mix them all up together.

**14.** Turn this pounded mixture out of the mortar into a half-pint basin.

**15.** Take a *teacupful* of *cold water* and rinse out the mortar, and then pour the water on to the pounded mixture in the basin.

**16.** Take the pieces of *rabbit* and wash them in cold water.

**17.** Take them out of the cold water and place them on a sieve to drain.

**18.** Take a stewpan, and put in it *three ounces of fresh butter.*

**19.** Put the stewpan on the fire to melt the butter.

N. B.—Be careful that it does not burn.

**20.** Take *two small onions* and peel off the two outer skins.

**21.** Divide the *onions* in half down the centre, and cut them up so that the slices are in half-circles.

**22.** Put these sliced onions into the melted butter, add also *two cardamomums*, and let them fry a pale brown.

**23.** Then take the onions carefully out of the stewpan with a slice, and place them on a piece of whity-brown paper, to drain off the grease.

**24.** Now take the basin of spices, and add as much cold water as will make the basin three parts full.

**25.** Add to the basin of spices a small *dessertspoonful* of *salt*.

**26.** Now pour all the contents of the basin into the melted butter in the stewpan, to cook for about *twenty minutes*, stirring well all the time with a wooden spoon.

> N.B.—To test when the spices are sufficiently cooked, you should smell them, and if they are quite done, no particular spice should predominate.

**27.** Now place the pieces of rabbit in the stewpan to brown.

**28.** Turn them occasionally, so that they will get brown on all sides.

**29.** Now pour into the stewpan a teacupful of cold water, to make the meat tender.

**30.** Put the lid on the stewpan, and let it all cook steadily for about an hour.

**31.** Watch it carefully, and stir it perpetually.

> N.B.—A good deal of stirring is required.

**32.** Add, by degrees, a teacupful of cold water, to wash down the bits of spice which will stick to the sides of the stewpan.

**33.** Also add, by degrees, *half a pint of cream* or good milk (*water* might even be used instead), and mix it well together with a wooden spoon.

> N. B.—You must be careful that no pieces of meat, or spices, stick to the bottom of the pan.

**34.** Now take half the *fried onions*, chop them up finely, and add them to the *curry*.

**35.** Then put into the mortar *five coriander seeds* and *one inch of the stick of cinnamon*, and pound them well together with a pestle.

**36.** When the rabbit is quite done, take the pieces out with a fork, arrange them nicely on a hot dish, and pour the gravy round.

**37.** Then sprinkle over the rabbit the remainder of the fried onions, and the pounded cinnamon and coriander seeds.

**38.** Take a fresh lemon, cut it in *half*, and squeeze all the juice of it through a strainer over the rabbit.

> N. B.—*Boiled rice* should be served with the above *Curry* (*see* Lesson on "Rice").

---

## LESSON SECOND.

### QUENELLES OF VEAL.

**Ingredients.**—One pound of the fillet of veal. Two ounces of butter. Two and three-quarters ounces of flour. Three-fourths of a pint of second white stock. Two eggs. One dozen button mushrooms. One gill of cream. One teaspoonful of lemon-juice. Salt.

*Time required, about three-quarters of an hour.*

To make *Quenelles of Veal:*

**1.** Put *one ounce of butter* and *two ounces of flour* into a stewpan, and mix them well together with a wooden spoon.

3

**2.** Add one gill of second *white stock*. (*See* Lesson on " Stock.")

**3.** Put the stewpan on the fire, and stir well until it boils and thickens, and leaves the sides of the stewpan.

**4.** Now pour this mixture, or *panada* (as it is called), on to a plate.

**5.** Stand the plate aside to cool.

**6.** Take one pound of the *fillet of veal* and put it on a board.

**7.** Take a sharp knife, cut away all the skin and fat, and cut up the *meat* into small pieces.

**8.** Put these pieces of *veal* into a mortar, and pound them well with the pestle.

**9.** Place a wire sieve over a plate; take this pounded *meat* and pass it through the sieve, rubbing it with a wooden spoon.

**10.** When the *panada* on the plate is cold, put half of it and one egg in the mortar, and pound it to a cream.

**11.** Then add half the *meat*, and *salt* and *pepper* to taste, and pound all well together with the pestle.

**12.** Put into the mortar the remainder of the *panada*, and break in another egg, and add the rest of the *meat*.

**13.** Pound these well together again with the pestle.

**14.** Turn the mixture from the mortar into a basin.

**15.** Take a sauté-pan and butter it inside.

**16.** Take a dessertspoon and fill it with the mixture, shaping it to the form of an oval with a knife, which you must dip occasionally into hot water, to prevent the mixture from sticking.

**17.** Take another dessertspoon and dip it into boiling water.

**18.** Scoop the *quenelle* from the first spoon into the second spoon, and put it into the sauté-pan, and continue doing this till you have used up all the mixture.

**19.** Now make the sauce to be served with the *quenelles*.

**20.** Take a stewpan, and put in half an ounce of butter and half an ounce of flour.

**21.** Put the stewpan on the fire, and mix them together with a wooden spoon.

**22.** Take *one dozen* of *button mushrooms*, cut off the ends of the stalks, and wash them well in cold water.

**23.** Take them out of the water, put them upon a board, and peel them carefully with a sharp knife.

**24.** Pour *half a pint* of second white stock into the mixture in the stewpan, and add the mushroom peelings for flavoring.

**25.** Stir well until it boils and thickens.

**26.** Stand the stewpan by the side of the fire, with the lid half on, and let it boil for a *quarter of an hour*.

**27.** Then take a spoon, and skim off all the *butter* from the top of the *sauce*.

**28.** Now stir into the *sauce one gill* of *cream*, and stand the stewpan aside to keep warm, until required for use.

**29.** Take the peeled *mushrooms* and put them in a stewpan, with a piece of butter the size of a chestnut.

**30.** Squeeze over them a *teaspoonful of lemon-juice*, and pour in *one tablespoonful of cold water*.

**31.** Put the stewpan on the fire, and just bring them to the boil.

**32.** Now pour boiling water carefully into the sauté-pan, enough to cover the *quenelles*.

> N. B.—Be careful to pour the water very gently into the sauté-pan, or the quenelles will be spoiled.

**33.** Put the sauté-pan on the fire, to poach the *quenelles* for ten minutes.

> N. B.—Watch them, and occasionally turn them carefully with a spoon.

**34.** When the *quenelles* are done, lift them out of the water, and lay them on a cloth to drain off the water.

**35.** For serving, arrange them tastily in a circle on a hot dish.

**36.** Fill in the centre of the dish with the *boiled mushrooms*.

> N. B.—Peas (*see* " Vegetables," Lesson No. 9), or spinach (*see* "Vegetables," Lesson No. 8), may be served with them instead, according to taste.

**37.** Take the stewpan off the fire, and pour the sauce through a strainer over the *quenelles*.

---

### LESSON THIRD.

#### BRAISED FILLETS OF BEEF.

**Ingredients.**—One pound of fillet of beef. A piece of the fat of bacon. A bouquet garni of parsley, thyme, and bay-leaf. Two young carrots. One onion, and one-fourth of a stick of celery. A pint of good stock.

*Time required (the stock should be made the day before), about one hour and a half.*

To Lard and Braise *Fillets of Beef :*

**1.** Take one pound of fillet of beef (cut from the under-cut of the sirloin), and put it on a board.

**2.** Take a sharp knife, and cut the beef into small round *fillets*, to about the size of the top of a coffee-cup, and about three-quarters of an inch in thickness, and trim them neatly.

**3.** Take a strip of the *fat of bacon* (nearest the rind is best, as it is harder), about *one inch* wide.

**4.** Take a sharp knife, and cut up this piece of *bacon* into little strips, *an inch* long and *one-eighth of an inch* in width and thickness.

**5.** Take each *fillet*, and hold it in a clean cloth.

**6.** Take a larding-needle, with a little strip of *bacon* in it, and lard each *fillet* neatly in regular rows, until one side of the *fillet* is entirely covered with strips of *bacon*.

**7.** When you have larded all the fillets, lay them carefully in a clean sauté-pan.

**8.** Add a *bouquet garni*, consisting of a little *parsley*, *thyme*, and a *bay-leaf*, all tied neatly and tightly together.

**9.** Take *two young carrots*, scrape them clean with a knife, and cut them in halves.

**10.** Take an *onion* and peel it carefully.

**11.** Add these vegetables, and a quarter of a stick of celery, to the *fillets* in the sauté-pan.

**12.** Now pour in a *pint* of good *stock*, put the sauté-pan on the fire, and baste the *fillets* continually.

N. B.—The stock must not cover the meat.

**13.** Take a piece of kitchen-paper, and cut a round to the size of the sauté-pan and butter it.

**14.** As soon as the stock boils, lay this round of paper on the fillets in the sauté-pan.

N. B.—This paper is to prevent the meat browning too quickly.

**15.** Lift the paper every now and then, when you require to baste the fillets.

**16.** Put the sauté-pan into a very hot oven, to brown the *fillets*.

**17.** Let the pint of stock reduce to a half-glaze, which will take about half an hour.

**18.** Watch it, frequently raise the paper, and baste the fillets with the stock.

N. B.—If the fillets are not brown enough, take a salamander [1] and heat it in the fire.

---

[1] A salamander is a tile-shaped piece of iron, which can be lifted by a handle, like the cover of a stove.

**19.** Hold the salamander over the fillets, to brown them a nice color.

**20.** For serving, take the fillets carefully out of the sauté-pan, and arrange them on a hot dish in a circle, on a border of mashed potatoes. (*See* " Vegetables," Lesson No. 2.)

> N. B.—You must stand this dish on the hot plate, or near the fire, to keep warm, until the sauce is ready.

**21.** Put the sauté-pan on the fire, and let the sauce reduce to a half-glaze.

**22.** Then strain the glaze round the meat.

> N. B.—The centre of the dish may be filled in with mixed vegetables— i. e., peas and beans, which should be cut in the shape of dice, carrots and turnips, cut with a cutter to the size of the peas.

---

### LESSON FOURTH.

#### MUTTON CUTLETS.

**Ingredients.**—Three pounds of the best end of the neck of mutton. Bread-crumbs. One egg. Salt and pepper. Three ounces of clarified butter.

*Time required, about three-quarters of an hour.*

To Fry *Mutton Cutlets :*

**1.** Take *three pounds* of the best end of the *neck* of *mutton*, and put it on a board.

**2.** Take a saw and saw off the end of the *rib-bone*, leaving the *cutlet-bone three inches* in length.

**3.** Saw off the *chine-bone*, which lies at the back of the cutlets.

**4.** Joint each *cutlet* with the chopper.

**5.** Take a sharp knife, and cut off each *cutlet* close to the bone.

6. Take a cutlet-bat, wet it, and beat each *cutlet* to about *half an inch* in thickness.

7. Trim the *cutlet* round, leaving about half an inch of the *rib-bone* bare.

8. Form the cutlets to a good shape.

> N. B.—The trimmings of the cutlets should be put aside, as the fat may be clarified and used as dripping.

9. Take a wire sieve and stand it over a piece of paper.

10. Take some *crumb of bread* and rub it through the sieve.

11. Take one egg and beat it on a plate with a knife.

12. Season the cutlets on both sides with pepper and salt.

13. Lay them in the egg, and egg them well all over with a brush.

14. Then put them in the bread-crumbs, and cover them well.

> N. B.—Be careful to finger them as little as possible, and lift them by the bare bone.

15. Take a sauté-pan, and pour in it one ounce of melted clarified butter or lard, or clarified dripping.

16. Now lay in the cutlets, with the bones to the centre of the sauté-pan.

17. Pour over them two more ounces of melted clarified butter or fat.

18. Now put the sauté-pan on a very quick fire for about seven minutes.

19. Watch and turn the cutlets when they have become a light-brown, so as to fry them the same color on both sides.

20. Place a piece of whity-brown paper on a plate.

21. When the cutlets are done, take them carefully out

with a fork, and lay them on the paper on the plate, to drain off the grease.

N. B.—Be careful to stick the fork into the fat, and not into the meat, or the gravy will run out.

22. For serving, arrange them nicely in a dish, in a circle, one leaning over the other. The centre may be filled with any *vegetable*, according to taste.

---

### LESSON FIFTH.

#### CHAUD FROID OF CHICKEN.

**Ingredients.**—One chicken. One half-pint of white sauce. One gill of cream. Two tablespoonfuls of aspic jelly. Chopped pieces of aspic jelly. Mixed vegetables. One gill of mayonnaise sauce.

*Time required, about one hour and three-quarters.*

To make *Chaud Froid of Chicken:*

1. Put *half a pint* of *white sauce* (*see* " Sauces," Lesson No. 1) in a stewpan.

2. Put the stewpan on the fire to boil, and stir well with a wooden spoon, till the sauce is reduced to one gill.

3. Then add one gill of cream, and stir again, until it just boils.

4. Take a tammy sieve and stand it over a basin.

5. Take the stewpan off the fire, and pass the contents through the sieve into the basin.

6. When it is all passed through into the basin, stir in *two tablespoonfuls* of *aspic jelly* (*see* " Jelly," Lesson No. 2).

N. B.—This aspic jelly should be made with chicken as well as veal.

7. Take a cold roast chicken (*see* " Trussing a Fowl for Roasting "), and put it on a board.

N. B.—The chicken must be young, as the flesh should be as white as possible.

**8.** Cut it up in the same way as for carving, taking care that the pieces are all of one size. Remove the skin, and neatly trim each piece.

**9.** Dip these pieces of chicken in the sauce, covering them well over.

**10.** Stand a drainer over a dish.

**11.** Place the pieces of *chicken* on the drainer, and let them remain until the *sauce* is set over each piece.

**12.** For serving, arrange the pieces of chicken on chopped *aspic jelly* (*see* "Jelly," Lesson No. 2), in a circle on a dish.

**13.** The centre should be filled in with mixed vegetables—i. e., cooked *potato*, *carrot*, and *beet-root*, stamped out with a vegetable-cutter; cooked French peas, cut to the shape of dice; and green peas—all mixed together, with two tablespoonfuls of *mayonnaise sauce*. (*See* "Sauces," Lesson No. 3.)

---

### LESSON SIXTH.

#### VEAL CUTLETS.

**Ingredients.**—Three pounds of the best end of the neck of veal. Savory thyme. The rind of half a lemon. One bunch of parsley. One ounce of butter. One teaspoonful of lemon-juice. One egg. Pepper and salt. Bread-crumbs. One-half pound of bacon for rolls.

*Time required, about one-half hour.*

To Broil *Veal Cutlets:*

**1.** Take three *pounds* of the best end of the *neck of veal*, or *veal cutlet*, and put it on a board.

**2.** Take a saw and saw off the end of the rib-bone, leaving the *cutlet-bone three inches* in length.

**3.** Saw off the *chine-bone*, which lies at the back of the *cutlets.*

**4.** Joint each *cutlet* with the chopper.

**5.** Take a sharp knife and cut off each *cutlet* close to the bone, so as to get an extra *cutlet* between each bone.

**6.** Take a cutlet-bat and beat each *cutlet* to about half an inch in thickness.

**7.** Trim the cutlet round, leaving about *half an inch* of the rib-bone bare.

**8.** Form the cutlets to a good shape.

> N. B.—The trimmings of the cutlets should be put aside, as the fat
> may be clarified, and used for dripping.

**9.** Take a little *savory thyme*, put it on a board, and chop it up very fine. (The thyme, when chopped, should fill a salt-spoon.)

**10.** Take *half a lemon* and peel it very thin.

**11.** Chop this *lemon-rind* up very fine.

**12.** Wash a small bunch of parsley in cold water, and dry it in a cloth.

**13.** Chop up this parsley very fine on a board.

**14.** Put *one ounce* of *butter* on a kitchen-plate, and put it in the oven to melt.

**15.** When the butter is melted, add a tablespoonful of lemon-juice, and the chopped *thyme, lemon-rind,* and *parsley.*

**16.** Add *one egg*, and pepper and salt to taste, and beat all up together with a knife.

**17.** Take a wire sieve and stand it over a piece of paper.

**18.** Rub some crumb of bread through the sieve.

**19.** Dip each cutlet into the plate, and cover it all over with the mixture.

**20.** Then put it in the *bread-crumbs*, and cover it well.

N. B.—You should finger them as little as possible.

**21.** Take a gridiron and hold it to the fire to warm.

**22.** Arrange the *cutlets* on the gridiron.

**23.** Place the gridiron in front of a bright fire, but not too near, or the *bread-crumbs* will burn before the *cutlets* are sufficiently cooked.

**24.** Then let them broil for about ten minutes, and when they have become a pale brown on one side, turn the gridiron, so as to brown them on both sides alike.

**25.** For serving, arrange the cutlets on a wall of mashed potatoes (*see* "Vegetables," Lesson No. 2), in a circle on a hot dish, one leaning over the other; the centre may be filled in with rolls of bacon (*see* below), and with a thick brown sauce (*see* "Sauces," Lesson No. 2).

For *Rolls of Bacon:*

**1.** Cut some *thin slices of bacon*, about *two inches* wide and about four inches in length.

**2.** Roll up these strips of bacon.

**3.** Take a skewer and run it through the centre of each roll of bacon.

**4.** Place this skewer, with the bacon, on a tin, and put it in the oven for *six minutes*.

**5.** For serving, take the rolls of bacon off the skewer, and arrange them in the centre of the cutlets, as described above.

LESSON SEVENTH.

FRICASSEE OF CHICKEN.

**Ingredients.**—One young chicken. One small carrot. One-half an onion. One stick of celery. Two or three sprigs of parsley. One sprig of thyme. One bay-leaf. Two cloves. Six pepper-corns. One blade of mace. One and a half pint of second white stock. One ounce of butter. One and a half ounce of flour. Two dozen of button mushrooms. Fried bread. One gill of cream.

*Time required, about one hour and a half.*

To make a *Fricassee of Chicken :*

**1.** Take a young *chicken,* clean it, draw it (*see* " Trussing a Fowl for Roasting," from Note 1 to Note 12), and skin it.

**2.** Cut the *chicken* into joints, and put them into a basin of cold water for about *ten minutes.*

**3.** After that time, take the pieces of *chicken* out of the water and dry them in a clean cloth.

**4.** Take *one small carrot,* wash and scrape it clean, and cut it into slices.

**5.** Take *half an onion* and peel it.

**6.** Take *one stick of celery* and *two or three sprigs of parsley,* and wash them in cold water.

**7.** Put these vegetables into a stewpan.

**8.** Add to them *one sprig of thyme, one bay-leaf, two cloves, six pepper-corns,* and *one blade of mace.*

**9.** Now put in the pieces of *chicken,* and add one pint and a half of *second white stock.*

**10.** Put the stewpan on the fire to boil gently for about half an hour.

**11.** When the pieces of *chicken* are quite done, take them out of the stewpan, wash them in a basin of cold water, and dry them in a cloth.

**12.** Strain the stock from the stewpan into the basin.

**13.** Take two dozen *button mushrooms*, cut off the ends of the stalks, wash them in cold water, and peel them.

**14.** Take the peeled *mushrooms*, and put them into the stewpan, with a piece of *butter* the size of a chestnut.

**15.** Squeeze over them a *teaspoonful* of *lemon-juice*, and pour in a *tablespoonful* of *cold water*.

**16.** Put the stewpan on the fire, and just bring them to the boil.

**17.** Then take the stewpan off the fire and turn them on to a plate.

**18.** Wash out the stewpan, and then put in it one ounce of butter.

**19.** Put the stewpan on the fire to melt the butter.

**20.** Then add *one and a half ounces* of *flour* to the *butter*, stirring it well with a wooden spoon.

**21.** Now remove all the *grease* from the *chicken stock*, and add it and the trimmings of the *mushrooms* to the stewpan, and stir well until it boils.

**22.** Move the stewpan to the side of the fire, and let it boil gently for twenty minutes. The cover of the stewpan should be half on.

**23.** After that time, take a spoon and carefully skim off all the butter that will have risen to the top of the *sauce*.

**24.** Now put the stewpan over the fire to boil, and let the sauce reduce to about one pint, and then add *one gill of cream*.

**25.** Take the pieces of *chicken* and put them in another stewpan, with the two dozen button mushrooms.

**26.** When the sauce is sufficiently reduced, strain it over the chicken.

**27.** Then stand the stewpan in a saucepan of hot water over the fire, until the chicken is quite hot.

**28.** For serving, arrange the fricassee of chicken on a hot dish, with fried bread (as described in " Vegetables," Lesson No. 7, Note 13 to Note 17).

FOR COLD CHICKEN.

**Ingredients.**—Some cold chicken, say half of one. One-half a carrot. One-fourth of an onion. One-half a stick of celery. A bouquet garni of parsley, thyme, and bay-leaf. One gill of cream. One clove. Three pepper-corns. One-half a blade of mace. One pint of good white stock. One-half an ounce of butter. One ounce of flour. One dozen button mushrooms. Fried bread. Salt.

*Time required, about forty minutes.*

To make a *Fricassee of Cold Chicken :*

**1.** Take some cold roast or boiled chicken.

**2.** Cut away all the meat from the bone, and cut it up into neat pieces.

**3.** Put one pint of good white stock (*see* Lesson on " Stock ") and the chicken-bones into a stewpan.

**4.** Wash half a carrot, scrape it, and cut it into slices.

**5.** Peel a quarter of an onion.

**6.** Wash half a stick of celery in cold water.

**7.** Put these vegetables into the stewpan.

**8.** Add to them a bouquet garni (consisting of a little parsley, one sprig of thyme, and one bay-leaf, tied tightly together), one clove, three pepper-corns, and half a blade of mace.

**9.** Put the stewpan on the fire, and let it boil for *twenty minutes.*

**10.** After that time, strain the stock into a basin.

**11.** Take one dozen button mushrooms, cut off the ends of the stalks, wash them in cold water, and peel them.

**12.** Take the peeled mushrooms and put them in a stewpan, with a piece of butter the size of a chestnut.

**13.** Squeeze over them a teaspoonful of lemon-juice, and pour in a tablespoonful of cold water.

**14.** Put the stewpan on the fire, and just bring them to the boil.

**15.** Then take the stewpan off the fire, and turn them on to a plate.

**16.** Put *half an ounce* of *butter* into a stewpan.

**17.** Put the stewpan on the fire. When the *butter* is melted, put in *one ounce of flour*, stirring it well with a wooden spoon.

**18.** Now add the *chicken stock* and the *mushroom-peelings*, and stir the *sauce* well until it boils.

**19.** Let it boil for *ten minutes*, to cook the *flour*.

**20.** After that time, add *one gill of cream*, and *salt* to taste.

**21.** Put the pieces of *chicken* and the *button mushrooms* into another stewpan.

**22.** Strain the *sauce* over the *chicken*, and then stand the stewpan in a saucepan of hot water over the fire, until the *chicken* is quite hot.

**23.** For serving, arrange the *fricassee of chicken* on a hot dish, with some *fried bread* (as described in "Vegetables," Lesson No. 8, Note 13 to Note 17) put round the edge.

---

### LESSON EIGHTH.

#### BEEF OLIVES.

**Ingredients.**—One pound and a half of beef or rump steak, or the fillet of beef. Two ounces of beef-suet. Three ounces of bread-crumbs. One teaspoonful of chopped parsley. One-fourth of a teaspoonful of chopped thyme and marjoram. A little grated lemon-rind and nutmeg. Salt and pepper. One egg. One pint of brown sauce or stock.

*Time required, about one hour.*

To make *Beef Olives :*

**1.** Take one pound and a half of *beef* or *rump steak*, or the *fillet of beef*, and put it on a board.

**2.** Cut the beef in slices about *half an inch* in thickness and *four inches* in length, and beat them out with a wet cutlet-bat.

N. B.—You should be careful that all the slices are of the same size.

**3.** Take the trimmings that remain, chop them up very fine, and put them in a basin.

**4.** Take two ounces of *beef-suet*, and put it on a board.

**5.** Cut away all the skin, and chop the suet up very fine.

**6.** Stand a wire sieve over a piece of paper.

**7.** Rub some *crumb* of *bread* through the sieve. (There should be *three ounces* of *bread-crumbs*.)

**8.** Take a little parsley, and chop it fine. (There should be one teaspoonful of chopped parsley.)

**9.** Take a little thyme and marjoram, and chop them fine. (There should be about a quarter of a teaspoonful of chopped thyme and marjoram.)

**10.** Add all these things (i. e., suet, bread-crumbs, parsley, thyme, and marjoram) to the chopped beef in the basin.

**11.** Grate half a teaspoonful of *lemon-rind* and *nutmeg* into the basin.

**12.** Season it with plenty of *pepper* and *salt*, add *one egg*, and mix all well together with a wooden spoon.

**13.** Take this mixture out of the basin, and form it into pieces the shape and size of a cork.

**14.** Roll up each slice of beef, placing a piece of *stuffing* in the centre.

**15.** Tie each roll round with a piece of twine, to fasten it securely together.

**16.** Place these rolls in a stewpan, with about one pint of brown sauce (*see* "Sauces," Lesson No. 2), or good stock (*see* Lesson on "Stock".)

**17.** Put the stewpan on the fire, and let them stew gently for *three-quarters of an hour*.

**18.** For serving, arrange the beef olives on a hot dish in a circle, pouring the sauce round the edge. The centre may be filled in with *dressed spinach* (*see* "Vegetables," Lesson No. 7), or with mashed potatoes (*see* "Vegetables," Lesson No. 2).

---

### LESSON NINTH.

#### IRISH STEW.

**Ingredients.**—Three pounds of the best end of the neck of mutton, or the scrag end. One teaspoonful of salt. One salt-spoonful of pepper. One dozen of button onions, or two of moderate size. Six large potatoes.

*Time required, about two hours.*

To make an *Irish Stew :*

**1.** Take the best end of the *neck of mutton*, and cut and trim the *cutlets* in the same way as for "Haricot Mutton" (*see* "Entrées," Lesson No. 10, from Note 1 to Note 8).

**2.** Place the *cutlets* in a stewpan.

**3.** Sprinkle over them a *teaspoonful of salt* and a *salt-spoonful of pepper*, and pour in *one pint and a half of cold water*.

**4.** Put the stewpan on the fire, and, when it has come to the boil, skim it.

**5.** Now draw the stewpan to the side of the fire, and let it simmer gently for *one hour*.

**6.** Watch it and skim it occasionally, and remove all *fat*.

**7.** Wash *half a dozen potatoes*, scrub them, and peel them.

**8.** Cut these *potatoes* in halves.

**9.** Take *one dozen of button onions*, or two moderate-sized ones, and peel them carefully.

**10.** Add the *onions and potatoes* to the stew, and let it simmer for *one hour*.

**11.** After that time, take a fork and feel if the *vegetables* are quite tender.

**12.** For serving, arrange the *cutlets* in a circle on a hot dish, and pour the *sauce* round, with the *vegetables* in the centre.

> N. B.—The scrag end of the neck of mutton might be used instead of the best end, but care should be taken in cleansing it before use.

---

LESSON TENTH.

HARICOT MUTTON.

**Ingredients.**—Three pounds of the best end of the neck of mutton. One onion. Pepper and salt. One tablespoonful of flour. One pint of second stock. One carrot. One turnip. One dozen button onions.

*Time required, about an hour and a half.*

To make *Haricot Mutton:*

**1.** Take the best end of the *neck of mutton* and put it on a board.

**2.** Saw off the end of the *rib-bone*, leaving the *cutlet-bone three inches in length*.

**3.** Saw off the chine-bone, which lies at the back of the *cutlets*.

**4.** Joint each *cutlet* with a chopper.

**5.** Take a sharp knife and cut off each *cutlet*.

6. Beat each *cutlet* with a cutlet-bat to rather more than half an inch in thickness.

7. Trim the *cutlet* round, leaving about *half an inch* of the rib-bone bare.

8. Form the *cutlets* to a good shape.

N. B.—The trimmings of the cutlets should be put aside, as the fat may be clarified and used for dripping (*see* Lesson on " Frying ").

9. Take *one onion*, peel it, and cut it in slices.

10. Put the *onion* and the *cutlets* in a stewpan, with *two ounces of butter*.

11. Put the stewpan on a quick fire, to fry the *cutlets* a nice brown.

12. Watch and turn the *cutlets* when they have become a light-brown, so as to fry them the same color on both sides. Then remove them from the stewpan.

13. Pour off the *grease* from the stewpan, and leave the *onion*; then add *one tablespoonful of flour*, and pour in, by degrees, *one pint of second stock*, and stir well until it boils.

14. Strain this *sauce*, and return the *cutlets*, with the *sauce*, into the stewpan.

15. Wash *one carrot*, scrape it clean with a knife, and cut it in the shape of young carrots, or into fancy shapes, with a cutter.

16. Peel *two turnips*, and cut them in quarters.

17. Peel *one dozen button onions* very carefully, so as not to break them in pieces.

18. Put the stewpan on the fire, and let the *meat* stew gently for *half an hour;* then add the prepared *vegetables*, and let all simmer for *half an hour.*

19. After that time, take a fork and feel if the *vegetables* are quite tender.

**20.** For serving, arrange the *cutlets* in a circle on a hot dish, with the *vegetables* in the centre. Remove all *grease* from the *sauce,* and pour it round.

> . N. B.—The scrag end of the neck of mutton might be used instead of the best end, but care should be taken in cleansing it before use.

---

### LESSON ELEVENTH.

#### CROQUETTES OR RISSOLES OF CHICKEN.

**Ingredients.**—One-half a cold chicken. Two ounces of lean ham or bacon. Six mushrooms. One ounce of flour. One ounce of butter. Half a gill of cream. One gill of stock. Seasoning. The juice of half a lemon. One egg. Half a pound of bread-crumbs. If for Rissoles with paste, four ounces of flour and three ounces of butter.

*Time required, about one hour.*

To make *Croquettes* or *Rissoles of Chicken :*

**1.** Cut away all the *flesh* from the *bones* of *half a chicken* (either roasted or boiled), and put it on a board.

**2.** Remove the *skin,* and mince the *meat* very fine.

**3.** Wash and peel *six mushrooms* and mince them with *two ounces of lean ham,* and mix them with the *minced chicken.*

**4.** Put *one ounce of butter* in a stewpan, and place it over the fire.

**5.** When the butter is melted, stir in one ounce of flour, and mix it to a smooth paste.

**6.** Now add the *stock,* and stir again smoothly, until it boils and thickens.

**7.** Move the stewpan to the side of the fire, and stir in *half a gill of cream.*

**8.** Take *half a lemon* and squeeze the *juice* of it into the *sauce.*

> N. B.—Be careful not to let any *pips* fall in.

**9.** Season the *sauce* with *pepper and salt* according to taste, and, if liked, grate about *half a salt-spoonful of nutmeg* into it.

**10.** Now stir in the *minced chicken, ham,* and *mushrooms,* until all are well mixed together.

**11.** Take a plate, and turn the contents of the stewpan on to it.

**12.** Cut a piece of *kitchen-paper* to the size of the plate, *butter* it, and lay it on the top of the *mixture,* and stand the plate aside to cool.

**13.** When the *mixture is cold,* put *one pound and a half of lard,* or *clarified dripping,* in a deep stewpan, and put it on the fire to heat.

**14.** Rub some *crumb of bread* through a wire sieve on to a piece of paper.

**15.** If *rissoles* are required, put *four ounces of flour* on a board, and rub into it *three ounces of butter,* until both are thoroughly mixed and there are no lumps remaining.

**16.** Mix the *flour and butter* into a stiff, smooth *paste* with cold *water.*

**17.** Flour a rolling-pin, sprinkle some *flour* over the board, and roll the *paste* out into as thin a sheet as possible.

**18.** *Flour* your hands, dip a knife in *flour* (to prevent any sticking), and form the *chicken mixture* into any fancy shapes for croquettes, either in *balls* or long *rolls,* etc., or roll it in the *paste* for *rissoles.*

**19.** Break an *egg* on to a plate, and beat it up slightly with a knife.

**20.** Dip the *croquettes* or *rissoles* into the *egg,* and *egg* them well all over with a paste-brush.

**21.** Now roll them in the *bread-crumbs,* covering them well all over.

N. B.—You must be careful to cover them smoothly, and not too thickly.

**22.** Take a *frying-basket*, and arrange the *croquettes* or *rissoles* in it. Finger them as little as possible, and do not allow them to touch each other.

**23.** When the *fat* is quite hot and smoking, put in the *frying-basket* for *two minutes* or so, to fry them a *pale-yellow*.

**24.** Put a piece of *whity-brown paper* on a plate, and, as the *rissoles* are fried, turn them on to the paper to drain off the *grease*.

**25.** For serving, arrange them tastily on a hot dish, with fried *parsley* in the centre.

> N. B.—Cold veal or pheasant, etc., might be used for the rissoles and croquettes, instead of chicken, if preferred.

---

### LESSON TWELFTH.

#### CURRIED RABBIT.

**Ingredients.**—One rabbit, or one and a half pound of veal cutlet. One-fourth of a pound of butter. Two onions. One apple. Two tablespoon-fuls of curry powder. One pint of good stock. One gill of cream. One lemon. One-half a teaspoonful of salt.

*Time required, about two hours and a half.*

To make a *Curry* of *Rabbit* or *Veal:*

**1.** Put *a quarter of a pound of butter* into a stewpan, and put it on the fire to melt.

**2.** Peel *two onions*, put them on a board, and chop them up as finely as possible.

**3.** Put the *chopped onions* into the *melted butter*, and let them fry a light-brown.

> N. B.—You must be careful that they do not burn.

**4.** Take a *rabbit* (which has been skinned and properly prepared for cooking), wash it well, and dry it in a cloth.

**5.** Put the *rabbit* on a board and cut it up in pieces of equal size.

**6.** If *veal* is used, put it on a board and cut it into equal-sized pieces.

N. B.—If preferred, *chicken* can be used instead of *rabbit* or *veal.*

**7.** When the *onions* are fried, strain them from the *butter*.

**8.** Put the *butter* back into the stewpan.

**9.** Now put in the pieces of *meat*, put the stewpan over a quick fire, and let it fry for *ten minutes*.

**10.** Watch it, and turn the pieces of *meat* occasionally, so that they will be fried on both sides alike.

**11.** Peel an *apple*, cut out the core, and chop it up as finely as possible on a board.

**12.** When the *meat* is fried, add to it *two tablespoonfuls of curry powder* and *half a teaspoonful of salt*, and stir well over the fire for *five minutes*.

**13.** Then put in the *fried onions*, the *chopped apple*, and *one pint of good stock*.

**14.** Move the stewpan to the side of the fire, and let it simmer gently for *two hours*.

**15.** After that time, stir in *one gill of cream*.

**16.** Wipe a *lemon* clean with a cloth, and peel it as thinly as possible with a sharp knife. (The *peel* should be put aside, as it is not required for present use.)

**17.** Cut the *lemon* in half, and squeeze the *juice* of it through a strainer into the stewpan.

**18.** For serving, take the pieces of *meat* out of the stewpan, and arrange them nicely on a hot dish, and pour the *sauce* over the *meat*.

N. B.—Boiled rice should be served with the *curry.*

# CHAPTER V.

## *STEWS.*

### LESSON FIRST.

#### A-LA-MODE BEEF.

**Ingredients.**—One cow-heel. An ox-cheek. Three ounces of dripping. Three carrots. Six onions. One bunch of herbs (marjoram, thyme, parsley, and bay-leaf). Two tablespoonfuls of flour. Pepper and salt.

*Time required, three hours.*

To make *A-la-Mode Beef :*

**1.** Take a *dressed cow-heel* and wash it thoroughly in water.

**2.** Put the *cow-heel* on a board and cut off all the *flesh.* Cut the *flesh* into neat pieces.

**3.** Take an *ox-cheek* and wash it well in cold water.

N. B.—Be sure it is quite clean, and free from all impurities.

**4.** Put the *ox-cheek* on a board and rub it well with *salt.*

**5.** Then rub it quite dry in a clean cloth.

**6.** Put *three ounces of clarified dripping* into a large saucepan, and place it on the fire to melt.

**7.** Cut the *ox-cheek* up into neat pieces.

N. B.—Weigh the flesh of the *ox-cheek* and *cow-heel*, so as to know how much *water* should be added, as *one pint* is allowed to each *pound of meat*.

**8.** *Flour* each piece.

**9.** When the *dripping* is melted, put in the floured pieces of *ox-cheek*, and let them fry a nice brown.

**10.** Stir the *pieces* occasionally, and do not let them stick to the bottom of the saucepan.

**11.** Take *three carrots*, wash them, scrape them clean, and cut them in slices with a sharp knife.

**12.** Take *six onions*, peel them, and cut them in slices.

**13.** Take *a sprig or two of parsley*, wash it, and dry it in a cloth.

**14.** Take *one sprig of marjoram, thyme, one bay-leaf*, and the *parsley*, and tie them tightly together with a piece of string.

**15.** Put these *vegetables* and the *bunch of herbs* into the saucepan.

**16.** Pour in the proper quantity of *water*—namely, *one pint of water* to each *pound of meat*.

**17.** Put *two tablespoonfuls of flour* into a basin, and mix it into a smooth *paste* with cold water.

**18.** Now put the pieces of *cow-heel* into the saucepan, and plenty of *pepper and salt* to taste.

**19.** Stir the *paste* smoothly into the saucepan.

**20.** Put the lid on the saucepan, and, when it boils, move the saucepan to the side of the fire, and let it stew gently for *three hours*.

**21.** Watch it, and skim it very often.

N. B.—Be always careful to skim anything that is cooking directly the *scum* rises, or it will boil down again into the *meat*, and will spoil it. *Scum* is the impurity which rises from the *meat* or *vegetables*.

**22.** When the *stew* is finished, pour it into a large dish or a soup-tureen. It is then ready for serving.

N. B.—The *bones* of the *cow-heel* should be put into the *stock-pot*.

———

LESSON SECOND.

BRAZILIAN STEW.

**Ingredients.**—Four pounds of shin or sticking of beef. Two carrots. Two turnips. Four onions. A bunch of herbs (marjoram, thyme, and parsley). Pepper and salt. One gill of vinegar.

*Time required, about three hours and ten minutes.*

To make *Brazilian Stew* :

**1.** Take *four pounds* of the *shin of beef* or the *sticking of beef*, put it on a board, and cut all the meat off the bone.

**2.** Cut up the *meat* into neat pieces.

**3.** Dip each piece of *meat* into some *vinegar* in a basin.

N. B.—Putting meat into vinegar will make it tender, therefore any tough pieces may be used for this stew. The vinegar will not be tasted when the meat is cooked.

**4.** Wash *two carrots*, scrape them clean, and cut them into slices with a sharp knife.

**5.** Peel *two turnips* and *four onions*, and cut them in slices.

**6.** Put the pieces of *meat* into a saucepan, arranging them closely together.

**7.** Sprinkle some *pepper and salt* over the *meat*.

**8.** Now put in all the *vegetables*, and also add a *small bunch of herbs*—namely, a *sprig of marjoram*, *thyme*, and *parsley*, tied tightly together.

N. B.—Put no *water* in this stew; the vinegar draws out the juices of the meat, and makes plenty of gravy.

9. Shut down the lid tight; put the saucepan by the side of the fire, and let it simmer gently for at least *three hours.*

10. For serving, turn the *stew* on to a hot dish, or into a soup-tureen.

---

## IRISH STEW.

**Ingredients.—**Two pounds of potatoes. One pound of the scrag end of mutton. One pound of onions. Pepper and salt.

*Time required, about three hours.*

To make an *Irish Stew :*

1. Take *two pounds of potatoes* and wash them well in cold water.

2. Take a sharp knife, peel them, carefully cut out the eyes or any black specks about the *potatoes,* and cut them in slices.

3. Peel *one pound of onions,* and cut them in slices.

4. Take *one pound of the scrag end of the neck of mutton,* wash it in cold water, and scrape it clean with a knife.

5. Put the *meat* on a board, and cut it up in small pieces.

6. Take a large saucepan; put in a layer of *meat,* then a layer of *potatoes,* then a layer of *onions.*

7. Sprinkle a little *pepper and salt* over each layer for seasoning.

8. Continue to fill the saucepan in this way till there is no *meat* or *vegetables* left.

9. Pour in enough *cold water* to cover the bottom of the saucepan (about *half a pint*).

10. Put the saucepan on the fire, and when it has come

to the boil draw it to the side of the fire, and let it stew gently for from *one hour and a half to two hours.*

**11.** Watch it, and stir it occasionally, to prevent its catching.

**12.** For serving, turn the stew out on a hot dish.

> N. B.—If a larger quantity of *potato* is required in the *stew*, the extra quantity should be parboiled (*see* note below), and then cut in slices and added to the *stew*, *half an hour* before it is ready for serving. If all the *potatoes* were put in with the *meat* at first, so much water would be required that the stew would be spoiled.

> N. B.—For parboiling (or half-boiling) *potatoes*, wash them and peel them; put them in a saucepan, with enough *cold water* to cover them; put the saucepan on the fire, and let the *potatoes* boil for about *half an hour.*

---

### LESSON FOURTH.

#### STEWED BRISKET OF BEEF.

**Ingredients.**—Seven pounds of brisket of beef. Two carrots. One turnip. Two onions. One head of celery. One leek. Bouquet garni (i. e., sprig of thyme, marjoram, and bay-leaf). Six cloves. Twelve pepper-corns. Six allspice. One tablespoonful of salt.

*Time required, about four hours.*

To make *Stewed Brisket of Beef,* to be served cold:

**1.** Take *seven pounds of brisket of beef* (not very fat); see that it is quite clean, and, if necessary, scrape it with a knife and wipe it with a clean cloth, and then put it into a large saucepan.

**2.** Take *two carrots,* wash and scrape them clean, and cut them in halves.

**3.** Wash *one turnip* and *two onions,* and peel them, and cut the *turnip* in quarters.

**4.** Take *one leek* and *one head of celery*, wash them well in water, cut the long green leaves off the *leek*, and the green tops from the *celery*.

**5.** Add all these *vegetables* to the *meat* in the saucepan.

**6.** Add also a *bouquet garni* of *thyme*, *marjoram*, and a *bay-leaf*, tied tightly together, *six cloves*, *twelve peppercorns*, *six allspice*, *one tablespoonful of salt*, and *three quarts of cold water*.

**7.** Put the saucepan on the fire, and, when it comes to the boil, skim it well.

**8.** Then move the saucepan to the side of the fire, and let the contents simmer gently for *three hours*. Watch it, and skim it occasionally.

**9.** After that time, take the *meat* out of the saucepan and put it on a dish.

**10.** Take a knife and carefully remove the flat bones at the side of the *beef*.

**11.** Place the *beef* between two dishes, with some heavy weight on the top to press it.

**12.** Pour the *stock* through a strainer into a basin, and, when it is cold, remove every particle of *fat*.

**13.** Then pour the *stock* into a stewpan, and put it on the fire to boil, without the lid, so as to reduce the *stock* to a *glaze*, about a *gill*.

**14.** Now take the *beef*, and, with a paste-brush, cover the joint with the *glaze*, brushing it over several times, until all the *glaze* is used up; as soon as it is cold, and has set, the *beef* is ready for serving.

# CHAPTER VI.

## *TRIPE.*

LESSON FIRST.

CURRIED TRIPE.

**Ingredients.**—One pound of tripe.  One-quarter of a pound of rice.  One onion.  Flour, sugar, and curry-powder.

*Time required, about three hours.*

To make a *Curry of Tripe :*

1. Put *one pound of tripe* in a saucepan of cold water, and let it boil.  Take it at once out of the water.

N. B.—This is called "blanching."

2. After the *tripe* is blanched, scrape it with a knife, and thoroughly cleanse it.

3. Cut the *tripe* up into small pieces.

4. Take a saucepan and lay the pieces of *tripe* in it, and pour in enough *cold water* to cover it.

5. Take a *small onion* and peel it, and cut it partially through.

6. Put the *onion* into the saucepan of *tripe.*

7. Put the saucepan on the fire, and, when it boils, remove it to the side of the fire, and let it simmer for not less than *two hours and a half.*

**8.** After that time, try the *tripe* with a fork, and if it is sufficiently cooked, it will be very tender.

**9.** Take the saucepan off the fire, and stand it on a piece of paper on the table.

**10.** Take out the pieces of *tripe* with a fork, and put them on a dish.

**11.** Take a small saucepan, and put in it *one ounce of flour, one dessertspoonful of curry-powder*, and *half an ounce of dripping*, and mix them all well together with a wooden spoon.

**12.** Add enough *cold water* to make the above into a stiff *paste*.

**13.** Now pour in *half a pint of the liquor* in which the *tripe* was boiled.

**14.** Put the saucepan on the fire, and stir the mixture well until it boils and thickens. Do not let it get lumpy.

**15.** Stir in a *quarter of a teaspoonful of brown sugar*, and *salt* according to taste. Now stand the saucepan aside to get cool.

**16.** Take the *onion* which was boiled with the *tripe*, and cut it in shreds, and add it to the *sauce*.

**17.** When the *sauce* is a little cool, put in the pieces of *tripe*, and let them just warm through.

**18.** Take a dish and warm it, and pour the *tripe* and *sauce* on it, keeping it as much in the centre of the dish as possible.

**19.** Take a *teacupful of rice*, wash it well in two or three waters, and put it in a saucepan full of boiling water. Be sure the water is boiling. Add to it a *salt-spoonful of salt.*

N. B.—Rice should be boiled in plenty of water.

**20.** Let it boil from a *quarter of an hour to twenty minutes*. After that time, feel the *rice*, to see if it is soft.

**21.** When the *rice* is sufficiently cooked, strain it off, and pour *cold water* over it.

**22.** Then put the *rice* back into the empty saucepan, and stand the saucepan by the side of the fire, to dry the *rice*. The lid should be only half on the saucepan.

**23.** When the *rice* is quite dry, take it out of the saucepan, and arrange it round the *tripe*.

---

### TRIPE IN MILK.

**Ingredients.**—One pound of tripe. Three or four good-sized onions. One pint of milk. Seasoning and flour.

*Time required, about two hours and a half.*

To cook *Tripe in Milk:*

**1.** Put *one pound of tripe* in a saucepan of cold water, to boil up and blanch. When it boils, take it off the fire.

**2.** Then take it out of the water, scrape it, and cleanse it thoroughly.

**3.** Cut it up in small pieces on a board.

**4.** Peel *three or four good-sized onions*, and cut them partially through.

**5.** Put the *tripe* and *onions* into the saucepan, with *one pint* of *milk*.

**6.** Put the saucepan on the fire to boil.

**7.** When it boils, move it to the side of the fire, and let it simmer for not less than *two hours*.

**8.** Then try it with a fork, and, if sufficiently cooked, it will be very tender.

**9.** Take the saucepan off the fire, and stand it on a piece of paper on the table.

**10.** Take the *onions* out of the saucepan, and put them on a board and chop them fine.

**11.** Take the *tripe* out of the saucepan, and arrange it on a warm dish.

**12.** Stand the dish near the fire, to keep warm.

**13.** Take a *dessertspoonful of flour*, and mix it to a smooth *paste* with *cold milk*.

**14.** Stir, by degrees, the *paste* into the *hot milk*, and let it boil and thicken.

**15.** Now stir the *onion* into the *milk*, and let it warm through.

**16.** Season the *onion-sauce* according to taste, and pour it over the *tripe*.

------

LESSON THIRD.

TRIPE À LA COUTANCE.

**Ingredients.**—One pound of thin tripe. One-half a pound of bacon. One small carrot. Four mushrooms. One-half a large onion, or six small green ones. Bouquet garni. Two shallots and parsley. Two ounces of butter. One tablespoonful of Harvey sauce. One tablespoonful of mushroom catchup. One ounce of flour. One pint of stock. The juice of half a lemon. Salt and pepper.

*Time required, about two hours and a half.*

To cook *Tripe à la Coutance :*

**1.** Wash the *tripe* well in cold water.

**2.** Put the *tripe* in a stewpan, with cold water enough to cover it.

**3.** Put the stewpan on the fire, and bring it to the boil.

N. B.—This is to blanch the *tripe.*

**4.** Then take the *tripe* out of the stewpan, and dry it in a clean cloth.

**5.** Put the *tripe* on a board, and, with a sharp knife, cut it into *strips about two inches wide and four inches in length.*

> N. B.—Only the *thin part of the tripe* can be used for *Tripe à la Coutance.* If there are any *thick pieces*, they can be cooked with *milk and onions* (*see* "Tripe," Lesson No. 2).

**6.** Take the *half pound of bacon* and cut it into very thin slices, the same size as the *strips of tripe.*

**7.** Take *one peeled shallot* and *two or three sprigs of parsley*, and chop them fine on a board.

**8.** Lay one *slice of bacon* on each *strip of tripe*, sprinkle a little *chopped shallot and parsley* over each *slice of bacon*, roll them up together, and tie them firmly round with a piece of string.

**9.** Take the *carrot*, wash it, scrape it clean with a knife, and cut it in slices.

**10.** Take the *half onion* and the other *shallot*, peel them, and cut them in slices.

**11.** Take a *sprig of marjoram, thyme*, and a *bay-leaf*, and tie them tightly together with a piece of string.

**12.** Take the *mushrooms*, wash them, and cut off the ends of the stalks.

**13.** Arrange the *rolls of tripe and bacon* in a stewpan.

**14.** Add all the *vegetables* and the *herbs.*

**15.** Pour in a *pint of stock*, and put the stewpan on the fire.

**16.** When it just boils, remove the stewpan to the side of the fire, and let the contents simmer gently for *two hours.*

**17.** After that time, take out the *rolls of tripe* and put them on a plate.

**18.** Take a strainer, hold it over a basin, and strain the *stock.*

**19.** Put *two ounces of butter* into another stewpan, and put it on the fire to melt.

**20.** When the *butter* is melted, add to it *one ounce of flour*, and mix them smoothly together.

**21.** Now add the *stock*, and stir it over the fire until it boils and thickens.

**22.** Take *half a lemon*, and squeeze the *juice* of it into the *sauce*.

N. B.—Be careful not to let any *pips* fall in.

**23.** Stir in *one tablespoonful of Harvey sauce* and *one tablespoonful of mushroom catchup*, and season with pepper and salt.

**24.** Now place in the *rolls of tripe*, and let them warm through.

**25.** Serve the *rolls of tripe* in a circle on a hot dish, with some *purée of carrot* or *spinach* (*see* "Vegetables," Lessons Nos. 6 and 8), or with a mixture of vegetables (according to taste) in the centre, and pour the *sauce* round the edge.

# CHAPTER VII.

## *ON COOKING MEAT.*

---

### LESSON FIRST.

#### BRAISED FILLET OF VEAL.

**Ingredients.**—Three and one-half pounds of the fillet of veal. One-half a pound of the fat of bacon. A bouquet garni of parsley, thyme, and bay-leaf. One onion. Three pints of good stock. Two young carrots. Celery and turnip. Salt.

*Time required, about one hour and a half. (The stock should be made the day before.)*

To Braise a *Fillet of Veal:*

**1.** Take *three and a half pounds of the fillet of veal,* put it on a board, and cut off all the *skin* with a sharp knife.

**2.** *Lard* this *fillet* in the same way as for *fillets of beef* (*see* "Entrées," Lesson No. 3, from Note 3 to Note 7).

**3.** Place the *fillet* carefully in a clean braising-pan.

**4.** Add a *bouquet garni,* consisting of a sprig of *parsley, thyme,* and a *bay-leaf,* all tied neatly and tightly together.

**5.** Take *two young carrots,* wash them, scrape them clean with a knife, and cut them in halves.

**6.** Take an *onion* and a *quarter of a turnip*, and peel them carefully.

**7.** Add these *vegetables*, and *half a stick of celery*, to the *fillet* in the braising-pan.

**8.** Now pour in about *three pints of good stock* (the *stock* must not cover the *meat*), put the stewpan on the fire, and baste the *fillet* continually.

**9.** Take a piece of *kitchen-paper*, cut a round to the size of the braising-pan, and *butter* it.

**10.** As soon as the *stock* boils, lay this round of paper on the *fillet* in the stewpan.

N.B.—This paper is to prevent the meat from browning too quickly.

**11.** Keep the lid of the braising-pan on and place it in a hot oven, and let it cook slowly for *one hour and a quarter*.

**12.** Watch it, frequently raise the paper, and baste the *veal* with the *stock*.

**13.** Take the *veal* out of the braising-pan, and place it on a hot dish.

N.B.—Stand this dish on the hot plate, or near the fire, to keep warm until the sauce is ready.

**14.** Put the braising-pan on the fire, and let the sauce reduce to a half-glaze.

**15.** Then strain the glaze round the *meat*.

**16.** Serve it with dressed *spinach* (*see* "Vegetables," Lesson No. 8), or with dressed *carrots and turnips* (*see* "Vegetables," Lesson No. 6).

LESSON SECOND.

ROAST BULLOCK'S HEART.

**Ingredients.**—One bullock's heart.   One-quarter of a pound of suet.
Three-quarters of a pound of bread-crumbs.   A gill of milk.   Salt and
pepper.   One tablespoonful of chopped parsley.   One dessertspoonful of
chopped mixed herbs—thyme, lemon-thyme, and marjoram.   One-quarter
of a pound of dripping.   For sauce: One small onion.   Salt and pepper.
One-half ounce of flour.   One ounce of butter.   One dessertspoonful of
catchup.

*Time required, about two hours and a half.*

To Stuff a *Bullock's Heart* and Roast it:

1. Prepare the fire for roasting, as described in "Roasting," Lesson No. 1.·

2. Wash a *bullock's heart* thoroughly in *salt and water*.

3. Be careful to cleanse all the cavities of the heart, and to remove all the blood.

4. Take it out of the *salt and water* and put it into a basin of clean water, and wash it again until it is quite clean.

5. Now wipe it thoroughly on a dry cloth.

6. If the *heart* is not quite dry, it will not roast properly.

7. Put the *heart* on a board, and, with a sharp knife, cut off the *flaps* or *deaf ears* (as they are called).

N. B.—These should be put aside for gravy.

8. Take a *quarter of a pound of suet*, put it on a board, cut away all the *skin*, and chop it up as fine as possible.

9. Sprinkle a little *flour* over the *suet*, to prevent it from sticking to the board or knife.

10. Grate some *bread-crumbs* with a grater on to the board.  .

**11.** Take *two or three sprigs of parsley*, wash them in cold water, and dry them in a cloth.

**12.** Put the *parsley* on a board, and chop it up as fine as possible; when chopped, there should be about *one tablespoonful*.

**13.** Take a *sprig of thyme, lemon-thyme*, and *marjoram*, rub them through a strainer, or chop them up finely on a board; there should be about *one dessertspoonful of the mixed herbs*.

**14.** Now mix the chopped *suet* and *bread-crumbs* well · together.

**15.** Then add the *parsley* and the *herbs, one teaspoonful of salt*, and *pepper* to taste, and mix them thoroughly together.

**16.** Now mix it with *one gill of milk*.

**17.** Take the *heart* and fill all the cavities with the *stuffing*, pressing it in as firmly as possible.

N. B.—If there is any *stuffing* over, it can be put aside for the *sauce*.

**18.** Take a piece of kitchen-paper and grease it well with a piece of *butter* or *dripping*.

**19.** Place this piece of greased paper over the top of the *heart* where the cavities are, and tie it on tightly with a string.

**20.** Put the roasting-oven in front of the fire.

**21.** Put the dripping-pan, or a large dish, down on a stand within the oven, close to the fire, with the dripping-ladle or a large spoon in it.

**22.** Hang the roasting-jack up in the oven, over the dripping-pan.

N. B.—If there is no roasting-jack, you can manage with a strong piece of worsted tied to a hook in the top of the oven.

**23.** Wind up the jack with its key before you put the *meat* on.

**24.** Take the hook of the roasting-jack and pass it through the *heart*, and hang it on the jack or the worsted.

N. B.—If the *heart* is hanging to a piece of worsted, twist the worsted occasionally, to make it go round.

**25.** Put about *one ounce of clarified dripping* into the dripping-pan, and baste the *heart* occasionally.

**26.** It will take about *two hours* to roast.

**27.** Now take the *deaf ears* out of the water and put them into a saucepan, with *one pint of cold water*.

**28.** Put the saucepan on the fire to boil.

**29.** Take *one small onion*, peel it, and cut it in quarters.

**30.** When the water boils, put in the *onion*, and a little *salt and pepper* to taste.

**31.** Now move the saucepan to the side of the fire, put the lid on, and let it stew gently until *five minutes* before the *heart* is done.

**32.** Watch it, and skim it occasionally.

**33.** After that time, strain the *liquor* into a basin.

**34.** Wash out the saucepan and put in it *one ounce of butter*, and put it on the fire to melt.

**35.** When the *butter* is melted, add *one tablespoonful of flour*, and mix them smoothly together with a wooden spoon.

**36.** Now pour the liquor in by degrees, and stir smoothly until it boils and thickens.

**37.** Then stand the saucepan by the side of the fire until required for use.

**38.** When the *heart* is roasted, take it down, place it on a hot dish, and draw out the hook.

**39.** Cut the string, and take off the greased paper.

**40.** If there be any *stuffing* left over, stir it now into the sauce, and add *one dessertspoonful of mushroom catchup.*

> N. B.—If the flavoring of mushroom catchup is disliked, it may be omitted.

**41.** Pour the sauce round the *heart* on the dish, and it is ready for serving.

---

### LESSON THIRD.

#### CORNISH PASTIES.

**Ingredients.**—One-half a pound of buttock steak, or beef skirt. Half a pound of potatoes. One onion. One pound of flour. One-half a pound of dripping. Salt and pepper. One teaspoonful of baking-powder.

*Time required, about one hour.*

To make *Cornish Pasties:*

**1.** Take *half a pound of buttock steak,* or *beef skirt,* put it on a board, and cut it up into small pieces.

**2.** Take *half a pound of potatoes,* wash and peel them, put them on a board, and cut them up into small pieces.

**3.** Take *one small onion,* peel it, put it on a board, and chop it up as fine as possible.

**4.** Put *one pound of flour* into a basin, with a little *salt* and a *teaspoonful of baking-powder.*

**5.** Put in *half a pound of dripping,* and rub it well into the *flour* with your hands.

**6.** Now add enough *cold water* to mix it into a stiff *paste.*

**7.** *Flour* a board, and turn the *paste* on to it.

**8.** Take a rolling-pin, *flour* it, and roll the *paste* out into a thin sheet, about a *quarter of an inch* in thickness.

**9.** Cut the *paste* into pieces about *six or seven inches* square.

**10.** Place a little of the *meat* and *potato* in the centre of each square; sprinkle over it a little *pepper and salt,* and a very little of the *chopped onion.*

**11.** Fold the *paste* over the *meat,* joining it by pressing the edges together with your thumb and finger.

**12.** Grease a baking-tin, and put the *pasties* on it.

> N. B.—If there is no baking-tin, grease the shelf in the oven, to prevent the pasties from sticking.

**13.** Put the tin into the oven to bake for from *half an hour* to *three-quarters of an hour.*

**14.** For serving, put the pasties on a dish.

---

### LESSON FOURTH.

#### A GRILLED OR BROILED STEAK.

**Ingredients.**—One-half a pound of rump steak. Lemon, pepper, and salt. Butter and salad-oil.

*Time required, about ten minutes.*

To Grill a *Steak* (either *beef* or *rump steak* will do, but the latter is more tender):

**1.** Take a small bunch of *parsley,* wash it, dry it well in a cloth, and put it on a board.

**2.** Chop the *parsley* up very fine with a knife.

**3.** Take a *quarter of an ounce of butter* and mix it well with the *chopped parsley.*

**4.** Sprinkle over it *pepper* and *salt* (according to taste), and *six drops of lemon-juice.*

**5.** Make it all up into a small pat.

**6.** Take *half a pound of rump steak, half an inch* in thickness.

**7.** Pour about a *tablespoonful of salad-oil* on to a plate.

**8.** Dip both sides of the *steak* into the *oil*.

**9.** Take a gridiron and warm it well by the fire.

**10.** Place the *oiled steak* on the gridiron, close to the fire, to cook quickly.

> N. B.—If the meat is at all frozen, it must be warmed gradually through before putting it quite near the fire, or it will be tough.

**11.** Turn the gridiron with the *steak* occasionally; it will take from *ten to twelve minutes*, according to the brightness and heat of the fire.

**12.** When the *steak* is sufficiently cooked, place it on a hot dish; and be careful not to stick the fork into the *meat* (or the gravy will run out), but into the fat.

**13.** Take the pat of *green butter* and put it on the *steak*, spreading it all over with a knife.

---

### LESSON FIFTH.

#### LIVER AND BACON.

**Ingredients.**—Two pounds of sheep's liver. One pound of bacon. One dessertspoonful of flour. One small onion.

*Time required, about half an hour.*

To Cook *Liver and Bacon :*

**1.** Take *one pound of bacon*, put it on a board, and cut it in thin slices.

**2.** Cut the *rind* off each slice of *bacon*.

**3.** Put these slices of *bacon* into a frying-pan.

**4.** Put the frying-pan on the fire, to fry the *bacon;* it will take about *ten minutes*.

> N. B.—If the bacon is not very fat, put a small piece of dripping in the frying-pan with it.

**5.** Turn it when one side is fried.

**6.** Now take a *sheep's liver* (it will weigh about *two pounds*), put it on a board, and cut it in slices.

**7.** Put about *two tablespoonfuls of flour* on a plate.

**8.** Dip the slices of *liver* into the *flour*, and *flour* them well on both sides.

**9.** When the *bacon* is fried, take it out of the frying-pan and put it on a warm dish.

**10.** Stand the dish near the fire, to keep warm.

**11.** Put the *slices of liver* in the frying-pan, a few at a time, as they must not be on the top of each other.

> N. B.—If the flavor of onion is liked, *a small onion*, peeled and cut in slices, might be fried with the liver.

**12.** The *liver* will take about a *quarter of an hour* to fry.

**13.** Watch it occasionally, and turn it once.

**14.** To see when the *liver* is sufficiently cooked, cut a slice; the inside should be of a brownish color.

**15.** When the *liver* is all cooked, place it on the dish with the bacon.

**16.** Put a *dessertspoonful of flour* in a cup, and mix it into a smooth *paste* with nearly a *gill of water*.

**17.** Pour the *flour and water* into the frying-pan, and stir it until it boils and thickens.

**18.** Pour this *sauce* over the *liver and bacon*.

----

### LESSON SIXTH.

#### MEAT PIE (BEEF STEAK).

**Ingredients.**—One pound and a half of buttock steak. Half a pound of bullock's kidney. Seasoning. One pound of flour. One-half a pound of clarified dripping. One teaspoonful of baking-powder.

*Time required, about two hours and a quarter.*

To make *Meat Pie:*

**1.** Cut into thin slices *one pound and a half of buttock steak.*

**2.** Cut away all the skin.

**3.** Put on a plate half a pound of *bullock's kidney*, and cut it in thin slices.

**4.** Mix well together, on a plate, *one tablespoonful of flour, one teaspoonful of salt*, and a *teaspoonful of pepper*.

**5.** Dip each *slice of meat* and *kidney* into the seasoning, and roll them up into little rolls.

**6.** Arrange these rolls in a quart pie-dish, and fill it *two-thirds* full of *water*.

**7.** Put *one pound of flour* into a basin.

**8.** Add *one teaspoonful of baking-powder* and *half a salt-spoonful of salt* to the *flour*, and mix them well together.

**9.** Cut half a pound of clarified dripping in small pieces, and rub it well into the *flour* with your hands.

N. B.—Be careful that there are no lumps of dripping in the flour.

**10.** Then add, by degrees, enough *cold water* to make it into a stiff *paste*.

**11.** Take a rolling-pin and *flour* it; sprinkle *flour* on the board, and *flour* your hands, to prevent the *paste* from sticking.

**12.** Take the *paste* out of the basin and put it on a board.

**13.** Roll out the *paste* once to the shape of the pie-dish, only rather larger, and to the thickness of about *one-third of an inch*.

**14.** Wet the edge of the dish with *water*.

**15.** Take a knife, dip it in *flour*, and cut a strip of the *paste* the width of the edge of the pie-dish, and place it round the edge of the dish.

N. B.—Cut this strip of paste from round the edge of the paste, leaving the centre piece the size and shape of the top of the pie-dish.

**16.** Wet the edge of the *paste* with *water*.

**17.** Take the remaining *paste* and place it over the pie-dish, pressing it down with your thumb all round the edge.

N. B.—Be very careful not to break the paste.

**18.** Take a knife, dip it in *flour*, and trim off all the rough edges of the *paste* round the edge of the dish.

**19.** Take a knife, and with the back of the blade make little notches in the edge of the *paste*, pressing the *paste* firmly with your thumb, to keep it in its proper place.

N. B.—Ornament the top of the pie with any remaining paste, to your fancy.

**20.** Make a hole with the knife in the centre of the *pie*, to let out the steam while the *pie* is baking.

N. B.—If there be not an escape for the steam, it will sodden the inside of the crust, and so prevent it from baking properly.

**21.** Put the *pie* into the *oven*, to bake gently for *two hours*. Watch it occasionally, and turn it to prevent its burning. It should become a pale brown.

N. B.—Meat pie should be put in the hottest part of the oven first— which in most ovens is the top—to make the crust light, and then put in a cooler part, to cook the meat thoroughly.

N. B.—This pie could be made with veal or mutton, instead of *steak*.

----

LESSON SEVENTH.

MEAT PUDDING.

**Ingredients.**—Six ounces of suet. One pound of flour. One teaspoonful of baking-powder. Seasoning. One pound and a half of buttock steak. Half a pound of bullock's kidney.

*Time required, about two hours and a half.*

To make a *Meat Pudding:*

**1.** Put a large saucepan full of cold water on the fire to boil.

**2.** Put *six ounces of suet* on a board.

**3.** Cut away all the *skin* and chop up the *suet* as fine as possible, and sprinkle a little flour over it, to prevent its sticking.

**4.** Put *one pound of flour* into a basin, and add to it a *teaspoonful of baking-powder* and *half a salt-spoonful of salt*, and mix all well together.

**5.** Now add the chopped *suet*, and rub it well into the flour with your hands.

N. B.—Be careful not to have any lumps of suet.

**6.** Add, by degrees, about *half a pint* of cold water, to make it into a paste; mix it well.

**7.** Put *one teaspoonful of salt* and *one teaspoonful of pepper* on a plate, and mix them together.

**8.** Take *one pound and a half of buttock steak* on a board, and cut it in slices about *three inches long* and *two inches broad*.

N.B.—You must cut away all the skin.

**9.** Put half a pound of kidney on a board, and cut it in slices.

**10.** Dip each slice of *meat* and *kidney* into the plate of seasoning.

**11.** Take a quart basin, and grease it well inside with *dripping*.

**12.** Take a rolling-pin and *flour* it; sprinkle a very little *flour* on the board, to prevent the *paste* sticking.

N.B.—In making paste, always keep your hands well floured, to prevent its sticking to them.

**13.** Take the *paste* out of the basin and put it on the board.

**14.** Cut off about *one-third* of the *paste*, and lay it aside for the cover or top of the *pudding*.

**15.** Roll out the remainder of the *paste* to a round twice the size of the top of the basin; it should be about *one-third of an inch in thickness.*

**16.** Line the basin inside smoothly with the *paste.*

**17.** Place the slices of *meat* and *kidney* in the basin, fitting them neatly.

**18.** Pour in about *one gill and a half of water*, so as to fill the basin to within *half an inch* of the top.

**19.** Roll the remaining pieces of *paste* to a round the size of the top of the basin, and about a *quarter of an inch in thickness.*

**20.** Wet the edge of the *paste* in the basin with *cold water*, and cover over the top of the basin with the round of *paste.*

**21.** Join the *paste* together at the edge of the basin, pressing the edges together with your thumb.

**22.** Take a knife, *flour* it, and trim the edges of the *paste* neatly round.

**23.** Take a small pudding-cloth, wring it out in warm water, and *flour* it.

**24.** Put this cloth over the top of the basin, tying it on tightly with a piece of string under the rim of the basin.

**25.** Tie the four corners of the cloth together over the top of the *pudding.*

**26.** When the water in the saucepan is quite boiling, put in the *pudding*, and let it boil for *two hours.*

N. B.—The lid should be on the saucepan.

N. B.—Keep a kettle of boiling water, and fill up the saucepan as the water in it boils away.

**27.** After that time, take the *pudding* out of the saucepan, and take off the cloth.

**28.** Place a hot dish on the top of the *pudding*, turn

the basin and dish quite over, and, carefully raising the basin, leave the *pudding* in the middle of the dish, unbroken.

N. B.—This pudding might be made of beef skirt or Australian beef.

---

### LESSON EIGHTH.

#### PIG'S FRY.[1]

**Ingredients.**—One pound of pig's fry. Two and a half pounds of potatoes. One onion. Sage and seasoning.

*Time required, about an hour and a quarter.*

To cook *Pig's Fry*—"*Poor Man's Goose*" :

**1.** Take *two and a half pounds of potatoes* and put them in a basin of cold water.

**2.** Take a scrubbing-brush and wash the *potatoes* well.

**3.** Put the *potatoes* into a saucepan of cold water.

**4.** Put the saucepan on the fire to boil.

**5.** As soon as it boils, take the *potatoes* out of the water (N. B.—This is called " parboiling" *potatoes*), peel them, and cut them in slices with a sharp knife.

**6.** Take *one onion* and peel it.

**7.** Take two or three *sage-leaves* and put them on a board.

**8.** Chop up the *onion* and *sage* together on the board with a sharp knife.

**9.** Take *one pound of pig's fry* and cut it in small pieces.

**10.** Take a quart pie-dish and grease the dish with *dripping* or *fat*.

**11.** Put a layer of *sliced potatoes* in the bottom of the pie-dish.

[1] Pig's Fry is composed of the heart, liver, lights, and sweet-bread.

5

**12.** Sprinkle a little of the chopped *sage* and *onion*, *pepper* and *salt*, over the *potatoes*.

**13.** Now put in a layer of the *pig's fry*.

**14.** Sprinkle a little of the chopped *sage* and *onion*, *pepper* and *salt*, over the *pig's fry*.

**15.** Now add another layer of *sliced potatoes*, and sprinkle them with a little of the chopped *sage* and *onion*, *pepper* and *salt*.

**16.** Put in another layer of *pig's fry*, and sprinkle the remainder of the chopped *sage* and *onion*, and a little *pepper* and *salt*, on the top.

**17.** Cover these *layers* with the rest of the *sliced potatoes*.

**18.** Now fill up the pie-dish with water for gravy.

**19.** Take the *skin* usually sent with the *pig's fry* and put it over the top of the pie-dish.

**20.** If the *skin* is not sent, take a piece of whity-brown paper, and grease it with some *dripping* or *fat*, and put that over the pie-dish instead.

**21.** Put the pie-dish into a moderate oven, to bake for from *three-quarters of an hour to one hour*.

---

### LESSON NINTH.

#### BOILED PIG'S HEAD (SALTED), WITH ONION-SAUCE.

**Ingredients.**—Half a pig's head. Forty pepper-corns. Two blades of mace. Four cloves. Twelve allspice. A bunch of herbs. Two large onions.

*Time required (after salting) for boiling pig's head, about two hours; for making into brawn, two hours.*

To Boil *Pig's Head :*

**1.** Wash a *pig's head* thoroughly in plenty of tepid water.

2. Take out the *brains* and throw them away.

3. Cut out the little *veins*, and all the *splinters of bone*.

4. Wash the *head* in all parts with plenty of *salt*, thoroughly cleansing it from blood.

5. Lay the *head* in *pickle* (*see* "Pickle for Meat") for *three days*.

6. When the head is salted, put it into a saucepan, with cold water enough to cover it.

7. Put the saucepan on the fire to boil.

8. When it boils, draw the saucepan to the side of the fire, and let it simmer gently for from *one hour and a half to two hours*, according to the size and age of the pig.

> N.B.—*Boiled pig's head* is eaten with *boiled rabbit*, or with *veal*, or with *onion-sauce*.

> N.B.—If preferred, the *pig's head* can be made into *brawn* (*see* below).

### FOR ONION-SAUCE.

**Ingredients.**—Three onions. Three gills of milk. A dessertspoonful of flour. Half an ounce of butter. Pepper and salt.

For making *Onion-Sauce* :

9. Take *three or four onions*, peel them, and cut them in quarters.

10. Put them into a saucepan, with water enough to cover them.

11. Put the saucepan on the fire to boil, until the *onions* are quite tender.

12. Then strain them off, throw the water away, put the *onions* on a board, and chop them up small.

13. Throw the *onions* into a saucepan, with *three gills of milk*, put it on the fire, and let it come to the boil.

14. Put a *dessertspoonful of flour* into a basin, and mix it, with *half an ounce of butter*, into a paste with a knife.

**15.** Stir this *paste* smoothly into the boiling *milk* and *onions*, and continue to stir it until it boils.

**16.** Season the *sauce* with *pepper* and *salt* to taste, and then move the saucepan to the side of the fire, to keep warm till required for use.

**17.** Take a grater and grate some *bread-crumbs* on to a plate.

**18.** Put the plate in the stove oven, or in a tin oven, to brown the *bread-crumbs*.

**19.** When the *pig's head* is sufficiently boiled, take it out of the saucepan and put it on a hot dish.

**20.** Take out the *half tongue*, skin it, and put it back on the dish with the *head*.

**21.** Sprinkle the browned *bread-crumbs* over the *pig's head*, and pour the *onion-sauce* round it; or, if preferred, it may be served separately in a sauce-boat.

For making the *Pig's Head* into *Brawn :*

**1.** *Salt* and boil the *pig's head* in the same way as above, from Note 1 to Note 8.

**2.** When the *pig's head* is sufficiently boiled, take it out of the saucepan and put it on a board.

**3.** Cut all the *meat* off the bones, and cut it into small pieces the shape of dice; also cut up the *ear* and the *tongue* (the *tongue* should be previously skinned).

**4.** Put the *bones* back into the saucepan, with a *quart* of the *liquor* in which the *head* was boiled, *forty pepper-corns, two blades of mace, four cloves*, and *twelve allspice*.

**5.** Add also a *bunch of herbs* (viz., a *sprig of marjo-ram, thyme,* and *two bay-leaves*), tied tightly together.

**6.** Peel *two onions*, cut them in quarters, and put them in the saucepan.

**7.** Put the saucepan on the fire and let it come to a

boil; then remove the lid, and let the *liquor* reduce for about *half an hour*.

**8.** Then strain the *liquor* into a basin.

**9.** Pour *one pint and a half of the strained liquor* back into the saucepan, and put it on the fire.

**10.** Now put the pieces of *meat* into the *liquor*, season it with pepper (and salt, if necessary) to taste, and let it come to boiling.

**11.** Rinse a basin or tin mould in cold water.

**12.** Then pour the *meat* and the *liquor* together into the wet basin or tin, and stand it aside to get cold and set.

**13.** For serving, turn the *brawn* out of the basin on to a dish.

---

### LESSON TENTH.

#### PORK PIE.

**Ingredients.**—One-quarter of a pound of lard. One pound of pork (either loin or leg). Seasoning. One pound of flour. One egg.

*Time required, two hours and a half.*

To make a *Pork Pie:*

**1.** Put a *quarter of a pound of lard* and a *quarter of a pint of cold water* into a large saucepan.

**2.** Put the saucepan on the fire to boil.

N. B.—Watch it, as, if it boils over, it will catch fire.

**3.** Take one pound of *lean pork* (cut either from the loin or leg), put it on a board, and cut it in pieces about *one inch square*.

**4.** Put *one pound of flour* into a basin.

**5.** When the *lard* and *water* are quite boiling, pour them into the middle of the *flour*, and mix them well with a spoon.

**6.** When the *paste* is cool enough, knead it well with your hands.

N. B.—More water must not be added, as the paste is required to be rather stiff.

**7.** Take the *paste* out of the basin and put it on a floured board.

**8.** Cut off a *quarter of the paste*, and mould the remainder into the shape of a *basin*, pressing it inside with one hand and supporting it outside with the other.

**9.** Shape it as evenly as possible, and it should be about *one-third of an inch* in thickness all round.

**10.** Take a knife, flour it, and cut the top of the shape level all round.

**11.** Dip the pieces of *pork* into cold water, then season them well with *pepper* and *salt*.

**12.** Put these *pieces* inside the mould of *paste*, as close together as possible.

N. B.—The pie can be flavored, if liked, with chopped sage—about a teaspoonful—sprinkled well among the pieces of pork.

**13.** Take the remainder of the *paste* and roll it out with a floured rolling-pin, and cut it to the size of the top of the mould, and to about the thickness of *one-third of an inch.*

**14.** Take an *egg* and break it into two cups, separating the *yolk* from the *white.*

**15.** Take a paste-brush, dip it into the *white of egg,* and *egg* the edge of the mould of *paste.*

**16.** Take the piece of *paste* and put it over the top of the *pie,* pressing the edges together with your thumb.

**17.** Cut little leaves out of the remaining paste, dip them in the *white of egg,* and stick them on the top of the pie.

**18.** Wet the *pie* all over with the *yolk of egg.*

**19.** Put the *pie* in a moderate oven, to bake for *two hours.*

---

LESSON ELEVENTH.

S A U S A G E - R O L L S .

**Ingredients.**—One-half pound of cooked (or uncooked) meat. One pound of flour. One-half pound dripping. One teaspoonful of baking-powder. Seasoning. One-half a shallot. One small onion. Four sage-leaves. One egg.

*Time required, half an hour.*

To make *Sausage-Rolls :*

**1.** Put *half a pound of meat* (cooked or uncooked) on a board, take away all the fat, and mince it up as fine as possible.

**2.** Put the *mince-meat* in a basin and season it well with pepper and salt.

**3.** Put four sage-leaves on a board and chop them up as fine as possible with a knife.

**4.** Peel *half a shallot* and *one small onion,* and chop them up on a board.

**5.** Mix the chopped sage, shallot, and onion well into the mince-meat with a spoon.

**6.** Put *one pound of flour* into a basin.

**7.** Add to it *one teaspoonful of baking-powder,* a *quarter of a salt-spoonful of salt,* and *half a pound of clarified dripping.*

**8.** Rub the *dripping* well into the *flour* with your hands.

N. B.—Mix it thoroughly, and be careful not to leave any *lumps.*

**9.** Add enough *water* to the *flour* to make it into a stiff *paste.*

**10.** Flour the paste-board.

**11.** Turn the *paste* out on the board.

N. B.—Divide the *paste* in two, so as not to handle it too much.

**12.** Take a rolling-pin, flour it, and roll out *each portion* into a thin sheet, about *one-eighth of an inch* in thickness.

**13.** Cut the *paste* into pieces about *six inches* square.

**14.** Collect all the scraps of *paste* (so that none is wasted), fold them together, and roll them out and cut them into squares.

N. B.—There should be about *one dozen squares* of paste.   ·

**15.** Put about a *tablespoonful* of the *mince-meat* and *herbs* into the centre of each square of *paste*.

**16.** Fold the *paste* round the *meat*, joining it smoothly round the centre, and pressing the *ends* of the *paste* together with your finger and thumb.

**17.** Take a baking-tin, grease it well, and place the *sausage-rolls* on it.

**18.** Break *one egg* on to a plate, and beat it slightly with a knife.

**19.** Take a paste-brush, dip it in the *egg*, and paint over the tops of the *rolls*.

**20.** Place the tin in a hot oven, to bake for *fifteen minutes*, if the *meat* is already *cooked;* but if *raw meat* is used, then *half an hour* is required.

N. B.—Look at them once or twice, and turn them if necessary, so that they shall be equally baked.

**21.** For serving, take the *rolls* off the tin and place them on a hot dish.

## LESSON TWELFTH.

### SEA PIE.

**Ingredients.**—Two pounds of buttock steak. Two onions. One small carrot. One-half a turnip. Pepper and salt. Three-quarters of a pound of flour. One-quarter of a pound of suet. One teaspoonful of baking-powder.

*Time required, two hours.*

To make *Sea Pie :*

1. Cut *two pounds* of *steak* into thin slices on a board, with a sharp knife.

2. Peel *two onions*, and slice them as thin as possible.

3. Take a *small carrot* and *half a turnip*, wash them, scrape the carrot clean with a knife, peel the turnip, and cut them in thin slices.

4. Season the *slices of meat* with *pepper* and *salt* to taste.

5. Put the *slices of meat* in layers in a two-quart saucepan, sprinkling a little of the *sliced vegetables* on each layer of the *meat*.

6. Pour in enough *cold water* just to cover the *meat*.

7. Put the saucepan on the fire, just bring it to the boil, and then move it to the side of the fire to simmer.

N. B.—During this time make the crust.

8. Take a *quarter of a pound of suet*, put it on a board, cut away all the *skin*, and chop it up as fine as possible.

9. Sprinkle a little *flour* over the *suet*, to prevent it sticking to the board or knife.

10. Put *three-quarters of a pound of flour* into a basin, and mix into it *half a salt-spoonful of salt* and *one tea-spoonful of baking-powder*.

**11.** Now put in the chopped *suet*, and rub it well into the *flour* with your hands.

**12.** Add enough *cold water* to mix it into a stiff *paste*.

**13.** Flour a board and turn the *paste* out on it.

**14.** Take a rolling-pin, flour it, and roll out the *paste* to the size of the saucepan.

**15.** This quantity of *paste* will roll out to the size of a *two-quart saucepan*, so that, if a smaller saucepan is used, less *paste* will be required.

**16.** Put this *paste* over the *meat* in the saucepan, and let it simmer gently for *one hour and a half*.

N.B.—The lid should be on the saucepan.

**17.** Watch it, and be careful to pass a knife round the sides of the saucepan, or the *paste* will stick.

N.B.—Sailors add *sliced potatoes* to the *pie* when they can get them.

**18.** For serving, carefully remove the *crust*, turn the *meat*, *vegetables*, and *gravy* on to a hot dish, and place the *crust* over it.

---

## LESSON THIRTEENTH.

### SHEEP'S HEAD.

**Ingredients.**—One sheep's head. Salt. Four pepper-corns. Two turnips. One carrot. One onion. One-half a small head of celery. One sprig of thyme. Two sprigs of parsley. Toasted crusts of bread. Half an ounce of flour. One ounce of clarified dripping, or half an ounce of butter.

*Time required (after the sheep's head has been soaked for two hours), one hour and a half.*

To cook *Sheep's Head :*

**1.** Put in a basin of warm water a *sheep's head* (which has been chopped half-way through by a butcher), with a *dessertspoonful of salt*.

**2.** Wash the head thoroughly, remove the brains (which should be put aside), and all the *splinters* of the *bones*.

**3.** Wash all the *blood* and *matter* from the passages of the *nose*, *throat*, and *ears*, and clean round the gums.

N. B.—If this is not well done, the sheep's head will be spoiled.

**4.** Now put the *sheep's head* in a basin of *salt* and water, to soak for *two hours*.

**5.** After the head has been soaked, take it out of the water and cut out the tongue with a knife.

**6.** Tie the head together with a piece of string, to keep it in shape.

**7.** Put the head and tongue in a large saucepan.

**8.** Pour in sufficient *lukewarm water* to cover the *head*.

**9.** Add a good *salt-spoonful of salt* and *four pepper-corns*.

N. B.—If liked, one ounce of pearl barley or rice, previously washed, may now be added.

**10.** Put the saucepan on the fire and let it boil very gently for *one hour*.

**11.** Watch it, and skim it occasionally with a spoon, removing as much of the *fat* as possible.

**12.** Take *two turnips*, wash them in cold water, peel them, and cut them in quarters with a sharp knife.

**13.** Take a *carrot*, scrape it clean with a knife, and cut it in pieces.

**14.** Take a *good-sized onion*, peel it, and cut it in quarters.

**15.** Take *half a small head of celery* and *two sprigs of parsley*, and wash them in cold water.

**16.** When the *sheep's head* has boiled for *an hour*, add all these *vegetables*.

**17.** Add also *one sprig of thyme.*

**18.** Now move the saucepan to the side of the fire, and let it simmer gently for *one hour and a half.*

N. B.—The lid should be on the saucepan.

**19.** *Half an hour* before the *sheep's head* is finished, wash the *brains* well in cold water (removing all the skin).

**20.** Tie the *brains* up in a piece of muslin and put them in the saucepan with the *head*, to boil for *ten minutes.*

**21.** Put *one ounce of clarified dripping*, or *half an ounce of butter*, into a small saucepan.

**22.** Put the saucepan on the fire, to melt the *dripping*, and then add *half an ounce of flour*, and mix them well together with a spoon.

**23.** Take *one gill of broth* from the saucepan in which the *head* is boiling, and add it by degrees to the *sauce*, stirring it as smoothly as possible until it boils and thickens.

**24.** Now move the saucepan to the side of the fire.

**25.** When the *brains* have boiled for *ten minutes*, take them out of the saucepan, take them out of the muslin, and chop them up in small pieces with a knife.

**26.** Add the *brains* to the *sauce.*

**27.** When the *sheep's head* is sufficiently cooked, take it out of the saucepan, cut away the string, and place it on a warm dish.

**28.** Take the *tongue*, skin it carefully, and place it on the same dish.

**29.** Take out the *turnips*, put them in a basin, and mash them with a fork.

**30.** Take out the *carrot*, and arrange it alternately with the *mashed turnips* round the *sheep's head.*

**31.** Take the *brain-sauce* and pour it over the *sheep's head.*

**32.** Pour the *broth* carefully into a basin, without the *bread* or *vegetables*.

> N. B.—Bread or vegetables should never be kept in broth, as they would turn it sour.

**33.** Put the basin of *broth* away until required for use.

> N. B.—All the fat should be removed from the broth before it is used.
> N. B.—When the broth is required for use, a few toasted crusts of bread might be added, and a little chopped parsley.
> N. B.—The fat from the broth should be melted down into dripping.

If the *Sheep's Head* be preferred browned:

**1.** Proceed as above (*see* from Note 1 to Note 17).

**2.** Then move the saucepan to the side of the fire, and let it simmer gently for *one hour*.

> N. B.—The lid should be on the saucepan.

**3.** Take a piece of *stale bread*, and grate a *tablespoonful of bread-crumbs* with a grater.

**4.** Mix with these *crumbs* a *teaspoonful of parsley* and a *teaspoonful of mixed herbs*, chopped fine.

**5.** When the *head* has simmered for *one hour*, take it out of the saucepan.

**6.** Cut the string round it, and lay it on a dish.

**7.** Sprinkle the bread-crumbs and herbs over the head, and put a few tiny pieces of dripping on it.

**8.** Put the dish in the oven, or in front of the fire, for *ten* or *fifteen minutes*. It will then be ready for serving.

**9.** Take the *brains* and wash them well in cold water (removing all skin).

**10.** Tie them up in a piece of muslin and put them in the saucepan of *broth* (in which the sheep's head was boiled), to boil for *ten minutes*.

> N. B.—For serving, the tongue should be skinned, as above, and served separately with the brain-sauce (*see* above, from Note 21 to Note 27).

**11.** Proceed with the broth the same as above, from Note 32.

LESSON FOURTEENTH.

S T E W E D   S T E A K .

**Ingredients.**—One pound of rump steak.  One carrot.  One turnip.  Two sticks of celery.  One onion.  One ounce of butter.  One tablespoonful of flour.  Pepper and salt.

*Time required, about one hour.*

To Stew a *Steak* (either beef or rump—the latter is more tender):

1. Put *one pound of rump steak, one and a half inch* in thickness, on a board.

2. Cut off all the *skin* and *fat* from the *steak*.

3. Wash one carrot, one turnip, and a few celery-leaves, in cold water.

4. Scrape the carrot clean with a sharp knife.

5. Cut the turnip in half (as not all will be required), and peel off the outside skin.

6. Peel the carrot and turnip into thin ribbons with a sharp knife, leaving just the centre of each vegetable.

7. Peel one onion and put it on a board.

8. Shred the *onion* and *celery*.

9. Put *one ounce of butter* in a stewpan, and lay the steak in it to brown.

10. Put the *onion, celery,* and the remains of the *carrot* and *turnip*, after peeling, into the stewpan with the steak.

11. Put the stewpan on the fire.

12. Look occasionally at the *steak*, and when it is sufficiently browned on one side, turn it carefully over, to brown the other.

13. When the *steak* is sufficiently browned on both sides, then put in the vegetables.

**14.** Take a basin and put in it a *tablespoonful of flour*, *half a teaspoonful of salt*, *half a salt-spoonful of pepper*, and mix them together with a wooden spoon, and *one pint of water* or *stock*.

**15.** Stir them all well together into a smooth *sauce*.

**16.** Pour this *sauce* into the stewpan with the *steak* and vegetables, and stir all together until it boils and thickens.

**17.** Let it gently simmer *one hour*.

**18.** Take the fat which you have cut off the *steak*, and cut it into small pieces.

**19.** Put the pieces of fat on a tin dish.

**20.** Put the fat in the oven to cook till brown.

N. B.—It is better for stewed steak to cook the fat separately, as it keeps the gravy of the steak free from grease.

**21.** Take the thin peelings from the *carrot* and *turnip*, and put them on a board and shred them finely with a sharp knife.

**22.** Put these *shredded vegetables* into a small saucepan, with about a *gill of cold water*.

**23.** Put the saucepan on the fire, and let it boil until the *vegetables* are quite tender when tried with a fork.

**24.** When the *steak* is sufficiently stewed, put it on a hot dish.

**25.** Take a strainer and strain the gravy, in which the *steak* has·been stewed, over the *steak*.

**26.** The *stewed vegetables* must be thrown away, as all the goodness is out of them.

**27.** Take the tin dish out of the oven, and place the pieces of fat about on the *steak*.

**28.** Take the boiled *shredded vegetables* and garnish the *steak* with them.

N. B.—Any other vegetables can be used for garnishing—i. e., peas, French beans, asparagus, etc.

## TOAD-IN-THE-HOLE.

**Ingredients.**—Six ounces of flour.  One egg.  One pint of milk.  One and
a half pound of meat (beef or mutton).  Seasoning.

*Time required, about one hour and three-quarters.*

To make *Toad-in-the-Hole :*

**1.** Put *six ounces of flour* into a basin, with *half a
salt-spoonful of salt.*

**2.** Break *one egg* into the *flour*, and stir in smoothly,
and by degrees, *one pint of milk.*

N. B.—Be careful that it is not lumpy.

**3.** Beat it up as much as possible, as it will make the
*batter* lighter.

**4.** Take *one pound of meat*, put it on a board, and cut
it in neat pieces.

N. B.—*Buttock steak, beef skirt,* or any pieces of *mutton,* might be used ;
    for instance, the *short bones* from the *neck of mutton.   Sausages* or
    *cold meat* might very well be used.

**5.** Take a pie-dish, or a tin, and grease it inside with
*clarified dripping.*

**6.** Season the pieces of *meat* with *pepper* and *salt*, and
place them in the greased dish.

**7.** Pour the *batter* over the *meat*, and put the dish in
the oven to bake for *one hour*.

**8.** After that time it is ready for serving.

# CHAPTER VIII.

## *COOKING POULTRY.*

### TRUSSING A FOWL FOR ROASTING.

**Ingredients.**—One fowl. One ounce of butter. One large roll. One onion. Half a pint of milk. Five pepper-corns. Salt. One tablespoonful of cream.

*Time required, about three-quarters of an hour.*

To prepare a *Fowl* and Truss it for Roasting:

**1.** Take a suitable *fowl* that has been already plucked, and put it on a board.

**2.** Turn the *fowl* on its breast, and make an incision of *an inch* long down the neck, *three inches* below the head.

**3.** Pass your thumb round this incision, and loosen the skin.

**4.** Take a sharp knife and put it under the *skin*, and cut off the neck as low down as possible.

**5.** Be careful, in cutting off the neck, to leave a piece of *skin* to fold over on to the back of the neck and cover the opening.

**6.** Take out the crop, which lies in the front of the neck.

**7.** Then, with your finger, loosen the *liver* and the other parts at the breast-end.

**8.** Now turn the *fowl* round, and make an incision at the vent, about *one inch and a half* wide.

**9.** Put your hand through this incision into the body, and draw out all the interiors carefully, so as not to mess the *fowl*.

**10.** Be very careful not to break the gall-bag, or the *liver* will be spoiled.

> N. B.—Take the *liver*, *heart*, and *gizzard*, and put them in a basin of water, with about half a teaspoonful of salt; the other interiors should be thrown away.

> N. B.—Look through the fowl from one end to the other, and see that it is perfectly cleared out.

**11.** Take a damp cloth and wipe out the inside of the *fowl*, to clean it thoroughly.

> N. B.—If the fowl is not quite fresh, use a little vinegar and water on the cloth in cleaning it, and then take a clean cloth and wipe it quite dry.

**12.** Take a sharp knife and cut off the claws from the legs of the *fowl*.

**13.** Take a basin of boiling water, and hold the ends of the legs of the *fowl* in the water for a minute or two.

**14.** Then take off the outside *skin* as far as to the first joint.

**15.** Take a twist of paper, or a taper, and light it.

**16.** Take the *fowl* up by its legs, and hold the lighted paper under it, to singe off the little hairs.

**17.** Then hold the *fowl* up by its wings and singe the other end.

> N. B.—Be careful, in singeing, not to blacken or mark the fowl in any way.

**18.** Turn the *fowl* on its breast, and draw tightly the breast-skin over the incision on to the back of the neck.

**19.** Cross the ends of the wings over the back of the neck.

**20.** Now turn the *fowl* on its back, with the neck toward you.

**21.** Take a trussing-needle and thread it with fine twine.

**22.** Hold the legs up and press the thighs well into the sides of the *fowl*, forcing the breast up, to give the *fowl* a good shape.

**23.** Take the threaded trussing-needle and pass it through the bottom of one thigh, through the body, and out on the other side through the other thigh.

> N. B.—If liked, a part of the *gizzard* and *liver*, when cleaned (*see* note at the end of "Trussing a Fowl for Boiling"), can be put into the *wings* of the *fowl*.

**24.** Now turn the fowl on its breast, and take the threaded trussing-needle again and pass it through the middle of the pinion or wing, through the little bone called the sidesman or step-mother's wing, catching up the skin which folds over the incision, and out through the other little bone and wing.

**25.** Pull this twine very tightly, and tie it as firmly as possible at the side of the fowl.

**26.** Turn the fowl over on its back, keeping the neck still toward you.

**27.** Put your finger in the incision (made for drawing the *fowl*), and lift up the end of the breast-bone.

**28.** Take the threaded trussing-needle and pass it through the skin over the bottom of the breast-bone, over the end of one leg, back through the body close to the back-bone, and tie it firmly over the other leg at the side.

> N. B.—If there is no gravy ready for serving with the roast fowl, prepare it now (*see* note at the end).

**29.** Now put the tin oven, with the jack and dripping-pan, before the fire.

**30.** Make up the fire in the same manner as described in "Roasting."

N. B.—You do not require such a large fire as for roasting meat.

**31.** Take the trussed fowl, and pass the hook of the jack through the back of the fowl, and hang it up on the jack.

N. B.—If the fire is very fierce, you should take a piece of whity-brown paper, butter it, and tie it over the fowl, so as to prevent it from burning.

**32.** Put one ounce of butter in the dripping-pan to melt.

**33.** Use this melted butter to baste the fowl; as the fowl is not very fat, there will not be much dripping from it.

**34.** The fowl will take from half an hour to three-quarters of an hour to roast, according to its size.

**35.** Baste the fowl frequently.

**36.** When the fowl is quite done, take it off the jack and put it on a hot dish.

**37.** Take a knife and cut the twine, and draw it all out of the fowl, and take off the paper before serving.

For making *Bread-Sauce* :

**1.** Take a *French penny-roll* and cut it in half.

**2.** Pull out all the inside *crumb* and put it on a plate.

**3.** Pull this *crumb* apart into small pieces.

N. B.—If a French roll cannot be procured, bread-crumbs can be used instead—about one ounce and a half.

**4.** Take a small *onion* and peel it with an onion-knife.

**5.** Take a small stewpan and put in it the peeled *onion*.

**6.** Pour in *half a pint of milk*.

**7.** Now put in the *crumb* of the *roll*.

**8.** Add *five pepper-corns*, and salt to taste.

**9.** Stand the stewpan aside, with the lid on, for a *quarter of an hour*, to soak the *crumb*.

**10.** After that time, put the stewpan on the fire, and stir the *sauce* smoothly with a wooden spoon, until it boils.

**11.** Now add a *tablespoonful of cream*, and stir the *sauce* until it just boils again.

**12.** Before serving the *sauce*, take out the *onion*, and then pour it into a sauce-tureen.

> N.B.—The *neck, gizzard, liver*, and *claws* of the fowl, when properly prepared (*see* note at the end of " Trussing a Fowl for Boiling "), can be used for soup or gravy, to be served with the *roast fowl*. For making the gravy, put the *giblets* into a saucepan, with enough water to cover them (about *half a pint*); also add *half an onion* (peeled), *six pepper-corns*, and *salt* to taste. Put the saucepan on the fire, and, when it comes to the boil, move it to the side, to simmer while the *fowl* is roasting.

> N.B.—For serving, strain the gravy into a basin, and color it, if necessary, by stirring in a quarter of a teaspoonful of "*Liebig's Extract*," or ten or twelve drops of *caramel* (*see* note at the end of " Australian Meat," Lesson No. 2, " Brown Purée "); then pour it in a sauce-tureen, or round the *fowl*.

---

## LESSON SECOND.
### TRUSSING A FOWL FOR BOILING.

**Ingredients.**—One fowl. One and a quarter ounce of butter. Stock or water. One carrot. One small onion. A bouquet of herbs. Two eggs. One ounce of flour. One-half a pint of milk. A gill of cream.

*Time required, about one hour and a quarter.*

To prepare a *Fowl* and Truss it for Boiling:

**1.** Take a *fowl* that has been already plucked and put it on a board.

**2.** Prepare it and clean it in the same way as described in " Trussing a Fowl for Roasting," from Note 1 to Note 12.

**3.** Take a sharp knife and cut off the claws and the ends of the legs of the *fowl*, to the first joint.

**4.** Take a twist of paper, or taper, and light it.

**5.** Take the *fowl* up by its legs, and hold the lighted paper under it, to singe off the little hairs.

**6.** Then hold the *fowl* up by its wings and singe the other end.

N. B.—Be careful, in singeing, not to blacken or mark the fowl in any way.

**7.** Turn the *fowl* on its back, with the tail toward you.

**8.** Put your hands through the incision (made for drawing the *fowl*), and pass two fingers round the inside of the leg, so as to loosen the outside skin.

**9.** Draw this outside skin right off the legs, and press the legs well into the sides of the *fowl*, forcing the breast up, so as to give the *fowl* a good shape.

**10.** Pull this outside skin, and turn it neatly inside the *fowl*, over the joints of the legs.

**11.** Turn the *fowl* on its breast, and draw tightly the breast-skin over the incision on to the back of the neck.

**12.** Cross the ends of the wings over the back of the neck.

**13.** Now turn the *fowl* on its back, with the neck toward you.

**14.** Take a trussing-needle and thread it with fine twine.

**15.** Take the threaded trussing-needle and pass it through the bottom of one thigh, through the body, and out on the other side through the other thigh.

**16.** Now turn the *fowl* on its breast, and take the threaded trussing-needle again and pass it through the middle of the pinion or wing, through the little bone called the sidesman or step-mother's wing, catching up the skin which folds over the incision, and out through the other little bone and wing.

**17.** Pull this twine very tightly, and tie it as firmly as possible at the side of the *fowl*.

**18.** Turn the *fowl* over on its back, keeping the neck still toward you.

**19.** Put your finger in the incision (made for drawing the *fowl*), and lift up the end of the breast-bone.

**20.** Take the threaded trussing-needle and pass it through the skin over the bottom of the breast-bone, over one leg, back through the body close to the back-bone, and tie it firmly over the other leg at the side.

**21.** Take a piece of kitchen-paper and butter it well.

**22.** Take this piece of buttered paper and wrap it well round the *fowl*.

**23.** Take a large saucepan half full of hot *second white stock* or *water*, and put it on the fire.

> N. B.—The reason why second white stock should be used is, that the goodness which comes from the fowl after boiling adds to the goodness of this stock, which can afterward be used for soup.
> N. B.—If hot water is used, the goodness which comes from the fowl after boiling is only wasted, as it is not of sufficient strength to make the large quantity of water of any use.

**24.** When the water is quite boiling, place the *fowl* in the saucepan, with its breast downward.

**25.** Put into the saucepan one carrot which has been scraped, a small onion which has been peeled, and a bouquet of herbs, for flavoring.

**26.** The *fowl* will take from *three-quarters of an hour to one hour* to boil, according to its size.

To make the *Egg-Sauce* to be served with the *Boiled Fowl*:

**1.** Take a small saucepan full of hot water, and put it on the fire to boil.

2. When the water is quite boiling, put in two eggs to boil for ten minutes.

3. Take a stewpan and put in it *one ounce of butter* and *one ounce of flour*.

4. Mix them well together with a wooden spoon.

5. Pour in *half a pint of milk*.

6. Put the stewpan on the fire, and stir the mixture with a wooden spoon until it boils and thickens.

7. Then remove the stewpan to the side of the fire until required for use.

8. When the eggs are sufficiently boiled, take them carefully out of the saucepan with a spoon.

9. Knock the eggs against the edge of a basin, to break off all the shell.

10. Take a small basin of cold water.

11. Cut the eggs in half and take out the yolks.

12. Put the whites into cold water, to prevent their turning yellow.

13. Take the whites of the eggs out of the water and cut them to the shape of small dice.

14. Add the pieces of white of egg to the sauce in the stewpan.

15. Now add one gill of cream to the sauce.

16. Move the stewpan to the centre of the fire, and stir well till it boils again.

N. B.—Be careful, in stirring, not to break the pieces of egg.

17. When the *fowl* is sufficiently boiled, take it out of the stewpan; take off the buttered paper, and place the *fowl* on a hot dish.

18. With a knife cut the twine, and draw it all out of the *fowl*.

19. Take the stewpan off the fire, and pour the *sauce* over the *fowl*.

**20.** Take a wire sieve, with the hard-boiled *yolks* of the *eggs*, place it over the *fowl*, and rub the *yolks* through on to the breast.

N. B.—The neck, gizzard, liver, heart, and claws of the fowl—namely, the *giblets*—should be put aside, and, when properly prepared, can be used for soup (*see* "Soups," Lesson Sixth), or should be put in the *stock-pot*.

N. B.—To clean and prepare the *giblets* for use:

A.—Take the *gizzard*, cut it very carefully with a knife down the centre, where there is a sort of seam (be sure only to cut the first or outer skin), and draw off the outer skin without breaking the inside, which should be thrown away.

B.—Take the *outer skin* of the *gizzard*, the *heart*, and *liver*, wash them well in water, and dry them in a cloth.

C.—Take the *neck*, cut off the *head*, which is of no use, draw the skin off the *neck*, and wash the latter well in water, so as to remove the blood and any impurities.

D.—Put the *claws* and ends of *legs* in a basin of boiling water for some minutes; then take a knife, cut off the *nails*, and draw off the *outer skin*, which can be pulled off like a glove.

6

# CHAPTER IX.

## STOCK AND SOUPS.

### LESSON FIRST.

#### STOCK.

**Ingredients.**—Four pounds of shin of beef, or two pounds of knuckle of veal, and two pounds of beef. Four young carrots, or two old ones. One turnip. One onion. One leek. Half a head of celery. Salt.

*Time required, about five hours.    It should be made the day before it is required for use.*

To make *Stock* for *Soup:*

1. Take *four pounds of shin of beef* and put it on a board.

2. Cut off all the *meat* from the bone with a sharp knife.

3. Cut off all the *fat* from the *meat.*   (Put it aside for other purposes.)

4. Take a chopper and break the bone in half.

5. Take out all the marrow and put it aside for other uses.

> N.B.—If the fat and marrow were to go into the stock, it would make it greasy.[1]

6. Take a stock-pot, or a large stewpan, and put the *meat* and *bone* into it.

[1] Which is no great matter, as appears from 21.

**7.** Pour in *five pints of cold water.*

> N. B.—One pint of water is allowed for each pound of meat, and one pint over.[1]

**8.** Put in *half a teaspoonful of salt.* This will assist the scum to rise.

**9.** Put the stock-pot on the fire with the lid on, and let it come to the boil quickly.

**10.** Take *four young carrots,* scrape them clean with a knife, and cut them in pieces.

**11.** Take *one turnip* and *one onion,* peel them, and cut them in quarters.

**12.** Take a *leek* and *half a head of celery,* and wash them well in cold water.

**13.** Take a spoon and remove the scum from the *stock* as it rises.

**14.** Now put in all the *vegetables,* and let it simmer gently for *five hours.*

**15.** Watch and skim it occasionally, and add a little *cold water,* to make the scum rise.

**16.** Take a clean cloth and put it over a good-sized basin.

**17.** Put a hair-sieve on the top of the cloth over the basin.

**18.** When the *stock* has been simmering for *five hours,* take the stock-pot off the fire.

**19.** Pour the contents into the sieve which contains the *meat, bone,* and *vegetables;* and the cloth very effectually strains the *stock.*

> N. B.—The meat and bone can be used again, with the addition of fresh vegetables and water, and you thus make what is called second stock.[2]

[1] One pint of water extra is added to every two quarts, on account of evaporation.

[2] Second stock cannot be used for clear soup unless it is first clarified, as shown in Lesson Third.

**20.** Take the basin (into which the *stock* has been strained) and put it in a cool place till the next day, when it will be a stiff jelly.

**21.** When this stock-jelly is required for use, take off the hardened fat from the top with a spoon.

**22.** Take a clean cloth and dip it in hot water, and wipe over the top of the jelly, to remove every particle of fat.

**23.** Now take a clean dry cloth, and wipe the top of the jelly dry.

> N.B.—This is brown stock; but for some soups and purées, as well as for many other purposes, white stock is required. This is made in the same way, only with veal instead of beef. It can also be made of veal and beef mixed, or rabbit and beef; but veal alone is considered best.

---

LESSON SECOND.

VEGETABLE STOCK.

**Ingredients.**—One cabbage. Three large or six small onions. Two carrots. One turnip. Two ounces of butter. Three cloves. Thirty pepper-corns. A bunch of herbs (thyme, marjoram, and a bay-leaf). Salt.

*Time required, about two hours and a quarter.*

To make *Vegetable Stock:*

**1.** Take *one cabbage,* wash it well in cold water, and cut it in quarters.

**2.** Take *two carrots,* wash them, scrape them clean, and cut them in quarters.

**3.** Take *one turnip,* peel it, and cut it in quarters.

**4.** Take *three large* or *six small onions* and wash them clean. (The skins are to be left on.)

**5.** Put all these *vegetables* into a saucepan, with *two ounces of butter.*

**6.** Add a *bunch of herbs* (namely, a *sprig of thyme, marjoram,* and a *bay-leaf*), tied tightly together, *three cloves,* and *thirty pepper-corns.*

**7.** Put the saucepan on the fire, and let the *vegetables* and *herbs* sweat in the butter for *ten minutes.* Stir them, to prevent burning.

**8.** Now pour in *three quarts of cold water,* and add *salt* according to taste.

**9.** When the water boils, move the saucepan to the side of the fire, and let it simmer gently for *two hours.* Watch it, and skim it occasionally.

**10.** After that time, strain the *stock* into a basin, and it is ready for use. It is now reduced to two quarts and one-half a pint.

N. B.—This stock can be used for thick vegetable soups.

---

## LESSON THIRD.

### CLEAR SOUP.

**Ingredients.**—Two quarts of stock. Three-quarters of a pound of gravy-beef. Two carrots. Two turnips. One and one-half a leek. One cabbage-lettuce. One tablespoonful of young peas. Salt. One lump of sugar.

*Time required (the stock should be made the day before), about one hour and a half.*

To make *Clear Soup:*

**1.** Take two quarts of stock[1] (*see* Lesson First on "Stock"), and be careful to remove from it all fat.

---

[1] This lesson only applies to second stock, or stock that, for any reason, has become turbid. Stock carefully made by the directions in Lesson First on "Stock" is already clear, if a little care is taken to separate the sediment at the bottom of the jelly. It is only second stock, or stock made from odds and ends of meat and bones, cooked and uncooked, that requires to be clarified.

**2.** Put the *stock* into a stewpan.

**3.** Take three-quarters of a pound of gravy-beef (from the shin of beef), put it on a board, and cut off all the fat and skin with a sharp knife.

**4.** Chop the beef up very fine.

> N.B.—The proportion of beef for clarifying stock is one pound to every five pounds of meat with which the stock is made.

**5.** Put the chopped *gravy-beef* into the stewpan.

**6.** Take *one carrot, one turnip,* and *one leek,* and wash them well in cold water.

**7.** Take the *vegetables* out of the water and put them on a board.

**8.** Take a sharp knife and scrape the *carrot* quite clean, and slice it up.

**9.** Take the *turnip,* peel it, and cut it in small pieces.

**10.** Take the *leek* and cut off part of the long green leaves and the little straggling roots, and chop up the remainder fine.

**11.** Put all these vegetables into the stewpan, and stir them with an iron spoon until they are well mixed with the *beef* and *stock.*

**12.** Put the stewpan on the fire, and stir the contents till boiling begins.

**13.** Now take a large spoon and carefully skim the surface.

**14.** Stand the stewpan by the side of the fire, and let it simmer gently for *twenty minutes.*

**15.** Take a clean soup-cloth and fix it on the soup-stand.[1]

**16.** Take a large basin and place it below the cloth.

---

[1] A soup-stand is easily improvised by turning bottom upward a seat which has no back, and tying the four corners of your napkin to the ends of its four legs.

**17.** Take the stewpan off the fire and pour the contents into the cloth, and let it all pass into the basin.

N. B.—The chopped gravy-beef acts as a filter to the soup.

**18.** After the *soup* has all passed through, remove the basin and put a clean one in its place.

**19.** Take a soup-ladle and pour a little of the *soup* at a time over the *meat* in the cloth, and let it pass through very slowly.

N. B.—Be careful not to disturb the deposit of chopped beef which settles at the bottom of the cloth.

N. B.—If *savory custard* is preferred in the soup instead of *shredded vegetables, see* No. 31.

**20.** Take a small *carrot, turnip, half a leek, cabbage-lettuce,* and a *tablespoonful of young peas,* and wash them in cold water.

**21.** Put the vegetables on a board, scrape the *carrot* clean, peel the *turnip* with a sharp knife, and cut off all the outside leaves of the *lettuce,* and the long green leaves of the *leek.*

**22.** Shred the *carrot, turnip, leek,* and *cabbage-lettuce* very finely in equal lengths.

**23.** Put the shredded *carrot, turnip,* and *leek* into a small saucepan of cold water, with *half a salt-spoonful of salt.*

**24.** Put the saucepan on the fire, and let it just come to the boil.

N. B.—This is to blanch the vegetables.

**25.** Take the saucepan off the fire, and strain the water from the vegetables.

**26.** Take a stewpan and put in the blanched vegetables and *cabbage-lettuce* and *peas;* add a lump of sugar and *half a pint* of the *clear soup.*

27. Put the stewpan on the fire, to boil fast, and reduce the *soup* to a glaze over the vegetables.

28. Take the basin of strained *soup*, and pour the *soup* on the vegetables in the stewpan, and let it just boil.

29. Then remove the stewpan to the side of the fire, and let it boil gently for half an hour.

30. For serving, pour the soup into a hot soup-tureen.

### FOR SAVORY CUSTARD.

**Ingredients.**—Two eggs.  Butter.

31. Take the yolks of *two eggs* and the white of *one*, and put them in a small basin.

32. Add *one gill* of the *clear soup* and a *quarter of a salt-spoonful of salt.*

33. Whisk up the *eggs* and the *stock* well together.

34. Take a small gallipot[1] and butter it inside.

35. Pour the mixture into the gallipot.

36. Take a piece of whity-brown paper and butter it.

37. Put this buttered paper over the top of the gallipot, and tie it on with a piece of string.

38. Take a saucepan of hot water and put it on the fire.

39. When the water is quite boiling, stand the little gallipot in it.

> N.B.—The water must not quite reach the paper with which the gal-
> lipot is covered.

40. Draw this saucepan to the side of the fire, and let it simmer for a *quarter of an hour.*

> N.B.—It must not boil, or the custard will be spoiled.

41. Take the gallipot out of the saucepan, take off the

---

[1] Any earthen cup or bowl that will stand fire will do equally well.

buttered paper, and turn the *custard* out on to a plate to cool.

**42.** Cut the *custard* into small pieces the shape of diamonds.

**43.** Just before serving, pour the soup into the hot tureen, and add the *savory custard* to the *soup*.

---

LESSON FOURTH.

### TAPIOCA CREAM.

**Ingredients.**—One pint of white stock. One ounce of tapioca. Yolks of two eggs. Two tablespoonfuls of cream or good milk. Pepper and salt.

*Time required (the stock should be made the day before), about a quarter of an hour.*

To make *Tapioca Cream :*

**1.** Take *one pint of white stock* (*see* Lesson on " Stock ") and pour it in a stewpan.

**2.** Put the stewpan on the fire to boil.

**3.** Take *one ounce of prepared tapioca.*

**4.** When the white stock boils, stir in gradually the *tapioca.*

**5.** Move the saucepan to the side of the fire, and let it all simmer until the *tapioca* is quite clear.

**6.** Now prepare the *liaison.*

**7.** Put the *yolks of two eggs* in a basin, and add to them *two tablespoonfuls of cream* or *good milk.*

**8.** Just stir it with a wooden spoon, and then pour the mixture through a strainer into another basin.

**9.** Now take the stewpan with the *white stock* off the fire, and stand it on a piece of paper, or wooden trivet, on the table.

**10.** When the stock is cooled a little, add, by degrees,

two or three tablespoonfuls of it to the *liaison,* stirring well all the time.

N. B.—Be careful that the eggs do not curdle.

**11.** Now add this mixture to the remainder of the stock in the stewpan, and stir well.

**12.** Add pepper and salt to the soup, according to taste.

**13.** Place the stewpan of soup on the fire, to warm before serving.

N. B.—It must not boil.  For serving, pour it into a hot soup-tureen.

---

### LESSON FIFTH.

#### BONNE FEMME SOUP.

**Ingredients.**—Two lettuces.  Two leaves of sorrel.  Four sprigs of tarragon.  Four sprigs of chervil.  One-half a cucumber.  Half an ounce of butter.  Salt.  One salt-spoonful of sugar.  One and one-half pint of white stock.  The yolks of three eggs.  One gill of cream or milk.  The crust of a French roll.

*Time required (the stock should be made the day before), about half an hour.*

To make *Bonne Femme Soup :*

**1.** Take *two lettuces, two leaves of sorrel, four sprigs of tarragon, four sprigs of chervil,* and wash them well in cold water.

**2.** Take these *vegetables* and *herbs* out of the water, put them upon a board, and shred them finely.

**3.** Take a *cucumber* and cut it in half.

**4.** Peel half the *cucumber* and cut it up in thin slices, and then shred it with a sharp knife.

**5.** Put half an ounce of butter in a stewpan, and put it on the fire to melt.

**6.** Place all the shredded *vegetables* and *herbs* in the stewpan, to sweat for *five minutes.*

**7.** Sprinkle over them half a salt-spoonful of salt and a salt-spoonful of castor sugar.[1]

**8.** Watch it occasionally, as the *vegetables* must not burn, or in any way discolor.

**9.** Take *a pint and a half of white stock* (*see* Lesson on "Stock") and put it in another saucepan.

**10.** Put the saucepan on the fire to boil.

**11.** Now make a *liaison*.

**12.** Take the yolks of *three eggs*, put them in a basin, and beat them well.

**13.** Stir in *one gill* of cream or milk.

**14.** When the *stock* is quite boiling, pour it into the stewpan with the *vegetables*, and let all boil gently for *ten minutes*, until the *vegetables* are quite tender.

**15.** After that time, take the stewpan off the fire and stand it on a piece of paper on the table.

**16.** Take a *French roll* and cut off all the *crust*.

**17.** Put the crust on a tin, and put it in the oven to dry for a minute or two.

**18.** When the *stock* has cooled a little, stir in the *liaison*, straining it through a hair-sieve into the stewpan.

**19.** Stand the stewpan by the side of the fire, to keep warm until required for use.

N. B.—Do not let it boil, as, now the *liaison* is added, it would curdle.

**20.** Take the tin out of the oven and turn the dried *crust* on to a board.

**21.** Cut this *crust* into small pieces, and into any fancy shape, according to taste.

**22.** Place these pieces of crust in a hot soup-tureen, and pour the soup over them.

[1] Ordinary pulverized sugar.

## PURÉE OF POTATOES.

**Ingredients.**—One pound of potatoes. One small onion. Two leaves of celery. One ounce of butter. One and one-half pint of white stock. Salt. One gill of cream. Fried bread.

*Time required (the stock should be made the day before), about three-quarters of an hour.*

To make a *Purée of Potatoes :*

**1.** Take *one pound of potatoes*, put them in a basin of cold water, and scrub them clean with a scrubbing-brush.

**2.** Take a sharp knife and peel the *potatoes*, and cut them in thin slices.

**3.** Take a *small onion*, wash it well in cold water, and peel it.

**4.** Take *two leaves of celery* and wash them.

**5.** Take a stewpan and put in it *one ounce of butter.*

**6.** Now add the sliced *potatoes*, the *onion*, and the *celery.*

**7.** Put the stewpan on the fire and let the *vegetables* sweat for *five minutes ;* take care that they do not discolor.

**8.** Pour into the stewpan *one pint of white stock*, and stir frequently with a wooden spoon, to prevent it from burning.

**9.** Let it boil gently till the *vegetables* are quite cooked.

**10.** Put *half a pint of white stock* into a stewpan, and put it on the fire to heat.

**11.** Now place a tammy-sieve over a basin, and pass the contents of the stewpan through the sieve with a wooden spoon, adding, by degrees, the *half pint of hot white stock*, which will enable it to pass through more easily.

**12.** Take the stewpan and wash it out.

**13.** Pour the *purée* back into the stewpan.

**14.** Add *salt* according to taste, and *one gill of cream*, and stir smoothly with a wooden spoon until it boils.

**15.** For serving, pour it into a hot soup-tureen.

N. B.—Fried bread, cut in the shape of dice, should be served with the purée (*see* "Vegetables," Lesson Eighth, from Note 13 to 17).

---

LESSON SEVENTH.

SPRING VEGETABLE SOUP.

**Ingredients.**—Two pounds of the shin of beef. Two pounds of the knuckle of veal. Salt. Two young carrots. One young turnip. One leek. Half a head of celery. One cauliflower. One gill of peas. One-quarter of a salt-spoonful of carbonate of soda.

*Time required for making, about five hours.*

To make two quarts of *Spring Vegetable Soup:*

**1.** Take *two pounds of shin of beef* and *two pounds of knuckle of veal,* and put them on a board.

**2.** Cut off all the meat from the bone with a sharp knife.

**3.** Cut off all the fat from the meat. (Put the fat aside for other purposes.)

**4.** Take a chopper and break the *bones* in halves.[1]

**5.** Take out all the *marrow* inside the *bones,* and put it aside for other uses.

N. B.—If the fat and marrow were to go into the soup, they would make it greasy.

**6.** Take a stock-pot, or a large stewpan, and put the *meat* and *bones* into it.

**7.** Pour in *five pints of cold water.*

[1] The butcher will always do this for a customer.

**8.** Put in a *teaspoonful of salt.* This will assist the scum to rise.

**9.** Put the stock-pot on the fire, with the lid on, and let it come to the boil quickly.

**10.** Take a spoon and remove all the *scum* as it rises.

**11.** Now draw the stock-pot rather to the side of the fire, and let it simmer gently for *five hours.*

**12.** Take *two young carrots,* scrape them clean with a knife, and cut them in *slices.*

**13.** Take *one young turnip,* peel it, and cut it in *slices.*

**14.** Take *half a head of celery* and *one leek,* wash them well in cold water, and cut them in *squares* with a knife.

**15.** Take *one cauliflower,* wash it in cold water, and put it in a basin of cold water, with a *dessertspoonful of salt,* for two or three minutes.

**16.** Then take the cauliflower out of the water and squeeze it dry in a cloth.

**17.** Take a knife and cut off all the green leaves and the stalks from the *cauliflower,* and pull the flower into sprigs.

**18.** Watch and skim the *soup* occasionally, and you should add a little cold water, to make the *scum* rise.

**19.** One hour before serving the soup, add the vegetables.

**20.** You first put in the sliced *carrots* and the cut-up *celery* and *leek.* (These vegetables take the longest to boil.)

**21.** In half an hour add the sliced *turnips,* and, fifteen minutes after that, the cut-up flower of the *cauliflower.*

**22.** Take a saucepan full of hot water, and put it on the fire to boil.

**23.** When the water is quite boiling, put in *one gill of shelled peas,* a *teaspoonful of salt,* and a *quarter of a* *salt-spoonful of carbonate of soda*, and let it boil from *fif-teen* to *twenty minutes*, according to the age of the peas.

N. B.—The cover should be off the saucepan.

**24.** After that time try the *peas*, and, if they are quite soft, take them out of the saucepan and drain them in a colander.

**25.** For serving, put the boiled peas into a hot soup-tureen, and ladle the soup, and the other vegetables from the stock-pot, out into the tureen.

---

### LESSON EIGHTH.

#### GIBLET SOUP.

**Ingredients.**—Two sets of giblets. One-quarter of a head of celery. One carrot. One turnip. Two small onions. Two cloves. One blade of mace. A bouquet garni of parsley, thyme, lemon-thyme, basil, marjoram, and bay-leaf. Two quarts of second white stock. One and a half ounce of clarified butter. One ounce of flour. Half a pint of Madeira. Thirty drops of lemon-juice. A few grains of Cayenne pepper. Salt.

*Time required (the stock should be made the day before), about three hours and a half.*

To make *Giblet Soup :*

**1.** Take *two sets of goose* or *four of duck giblets*, scald and skin the *claws, ends of legs*, etc., and wash them clean in cold water (*see* note for " Cleaning Giblets," at the end of Lesson on " Trussing a Fowl for Boiling ").

**2.** You should put them into boiling water, to blanch them, for *five minutes*.

**3.** Then lay them in a basin of cold water, and wash and scrape them clean.

**4.** Take them out of the water and drain them.

**5.** Take a knife and cut the *giblets* in pieces, to about *one and a half inch* in length.

**6.** Put the pieces of *giblet* into a stewpan.

**7.** Take a *quarter of a head of celery* and wash it well in cold water.

**8.** Take *one carrot*, wash it in cold water, and scrape it clean with a knife.

**9.** Take *one turnip* and *two small onions*, wash them in cold water, and peel them.

**10.** Add these *vegetables* to the *giblets* in the stewpan.

**11.** Also put in *two cloves, one blade of mace*, and a *bouquet garni*, consisting of *parsley, one sprig of thyme, lemon-thyme, basil, marjoram*, and *one bay-leaf*, all tied tightly together.

**12.** Pour in two quarts of *second white stock*.

**13.** Put the stewpan on the fire, and let it boil gently for *two hours ;* skim it occasionally.

**14.** After that time, take out the best pieces of the *giblets* and trim them neatly.

**15.** Put these pieces aside until required for use.

**16.** Leave the stewpan on the fire, to boil for *half an hour*.

**17.** Put *an ounce and a half of clarified butter* and *one ounce of flour* into a stewpan.

**18.** Put the stewpan on the fire, and let the *flour* and *butter* fry for a few minutes, stirring it well with a wooden spoon.

**19.** Now add the *stock*, and stir it well until it boils.

**20.** Now remove the stewpan to the side of the fire, and let it boil gently for *twenty minutes*. (The cover of the saucepan should be only half on.)

**21.** After that time, take a spoon and carefully skim off all the *butter* that will have risen to the top of the *soup*.

**22.** Now strain the soup into a basin ; add to it *half a pint* of Madeira, thirty drops of lemon-juice, a few grains of Cayenne pepper, and salt according to taste.

**23.** For serving, pour the *soup* into a hot soup-tureen, and add to it the pieces of *giblet* that were put aside.

N. B.—If disliked, the wine may be omitted.

----

### MOCK-TURTLE SOUP.

**Ingredients.**—Half a calf's head. Three ounces of butter. Half a table-spoonful of salt. One-quarter of a pound of lean ham. One shallot. One clove of garlic. Six mushrooms. One carrot. Half a head of celery. One leek. One onion. Half a turnip. Bouquet garni (sprig of thyme, marjoram, parsley, and a bay-leaf). One blade of mace. Six cloves. Three ounces of flour. Two wineglasses of sherry. The juice of half a lemon. One dozen force-meat balls.

*Time required, about six hours.*

N. B.—If the soup is required to be made in one day, the stock should be made early in the morning, so as to give it time to get cold, that the fat may be removed.

To make *Mock-Turtle Soup:*

**1.** Take *half a calf's head* and wash it well in water, to remove all blood and impurities.

**2.** Cut all the *flesh* from the *bones*, and tie it up in a very clean cloth or napkin.

**3.** Put it in a large stewpan, with the *bones*, and *four quarts of cold water* and *half a tablespoonful of salt.*

**4.** Put the stewpan on the fire and let it come to the boil.

**5.** As soon as it boils, skim it well with a spoon, and move the stewpan to the side of the fire, to stew gently for *three hours.*

N. B.—Watch it, and skim it occasionally.

**6.** After that time, take out the *calf's head*, and pour the *stock* through a strainer into a basin.

**7.** Set it aside to get cold; then remove every particle of *fat* from the top of the *stock.*

**8.** Now make some *force-meat* (*see* "Beef Olives," "Entrées," Lesson Eighth, from Note 4 to Note 12), and make it up into little balls—about *one dozen.*

**9.** Take *six mushrooms* (cut off the ends of the stalks), *one onion,* and *half a turnip,* wash, peel, and cut them up in slices.

**10.** Take *one carrot,* wash, scrape clean, and cut in slices.

**11.** Take *half a head of celery* and *one leek,* wash them, and cut them up in slices. (Throw away the long green leaves.)

**12.** Put a quarter of a pound of lean ham on a board and cut it up in slices.

**13.** Put *one ounce of butter* in a stewpan, and put it on the fire to melt.

**14.** Add the ham and all the sliced *vegetables* to the *butter* in the stewpan.

**15.** Also add *one shallot* (peeled), *one clove of garlic, one blade of mace, six cloves,* and a *bouquet garni* (a *sprig of thyme, marjoram, parsley,* and a *bay-leaf,* tied tightly together).

**16.** Let all these *vegetables, herbs,* etc., fry in the *butter* for *ten minutes.* Stir them occasionally.

**17.** Then add *three ounces of flour,* and stir well.

**18.** Now add the *stock,* and stir it till it boils; then move the stewpan to the side of the fire, and let it simmer about *ten minutes.*

**19.** Take a spoon and remove every particle of scum.

**20.** Now strain the soup into another stewpan.

**21.** Take the *calf's head* out of the cloth and cut it up in small, neat pieces.

**22.** Add the pieces of *calf's head* to the *soup*, also *two wineglasses of sherry*, the dozen *force-meat balls*, and squeeze in, through a strainer, the *juice of half a lemon*.

**23.** Let the *soup* just come to the boil, and then pour it in a hot soup-tureen for serving.

---

### LESSON TENTH.

#### POT-AU-FEU, OR SOUP.

**Ingredients.**—Four pounds of beef, or four pounds of the meat of the ox-cheek. Sago or tapioca for soup. Half an ounce of salt. Two turnips. Two carrots. Two leeks. One parsnip. One small head of celery. Two or three sprigs of parsley. One cabbage. One bay-leaf, thyme, and marjoram, and one onion stuck with three cloves.

*Time required, about four hours.*

To make *Pot-au-feu :*

**1.** Put *six quarts of water* in a large pot.

**2.** Take *four pounds of the sticking piece of beef*, or *four pounds* of the meat off the *ox-cheek*, without any bone, tie it up firmly into a shape with a piece of string, and put it into the pot.

**3.** Put the pot on the fire to boil.

**4.** When the water is quite boiling, put in *half an ounce of salt*, and then move the pot to the side of the fire to simmer.

**5.** Take *two carrots, two leeks, two turnips, one parsnip, one small head of celery*, and wash them well in cold water.

**6.** Scrape the *carrots* and the *parsnip*, and cut them in quarters with a knife.

**7.** Take the *leeks* and cut off the long *green leaves*, as only the white part is required.

**8.** Take the *head of celery* and cut off the *green tops* of the *leaves*.

**9.** Tie the *leeks*, the *celery*, and the *parsnip* and *carrot* together with a piece of string.

**10.** Take a *cabbage*, cut it in two, and wash it thoroughly in cold water, and tie it firmly together with a piece of string.

**11.** Skim the *pot-au-feu* occasionally with a spoon.

**12.** When it has boiled very gently for *one hour*, add to it all the *vegetables* except the *cabbage*.

**13.** Take *one bay-leaf*, a *sprig of parsley*, a *sprig of thyme*, a *sprig of marjoram*, and tie them together with a piece of string.

**14.** Put these *herbs* into the pot.

**15.** Take *one onion*, peel it, and stick *three cloves* in it.

**16.** Put the *onion* into the pot.

**17.** When the *vegetables* have been *two hours* in the pot, put in the *cabbage*.

**18.** When the contents of the pot have simmered gently for *four hours*, take out the *meat* and put it on a hot dish.

**19.** Garnish the *meat* with the *carrots*, *turnips*, and *parsnips*, and pour over it about half a pint of the *liquor* for gravy.

**20.** Take out the *cabbage* and serve it in a hot vegetable-dish.

**21.** Strain the *liquor* through a colander, or cloth, into a basin, and put it by to cool.

**22.** Do not remove the fat until the liquor is required for use; it keeps the air from it.

To make a Soup of the *liquor*:

**23.** Put *two quarts* of the *liquor* in a saucepan, and put it on the fire to boil.

**24.** Take two ounces of crushed tapioca, or small sago; and when the liquor boils, sprinkle in the tapioca or sago, and let it boil for fifteen minutes, stirring occasionally.

**25.** Then pour it into the soup-tureen, and it is ready for use.

N. B.—If liked, Beef à-la-mode, or rissoles (*see* "Cooked Meat," Lesson Sixth), can be made from the meat of the Pot-au-feu.

For *Beef à-la-mode:*

**1.** Put two ounces of dripping into a saucepan, and put it on the fire to melt.

**2.** Stir in one tablespoonful of flour.

**3.** Take one pound and a half of the meat and cut it in neat pieces.

**4.** Put these pieces of meat into the saucepan.

**5.** When it comes to the boil, turn over the slices of meat and pour in half a pint of cold water.

**6.** Wash and scrape clean one carrot, and cut it in slices.

**7.** Put the carrot into the saucepan; add a bunch of herbs (namely, a sprig of marjoram and thyme and a bay-leaf), tied tightly together.

**8.** Let it just come to a boil, and then move the saucepan to the side of the fire, and let it simmer gently for three hours.

**9.** Watch it, and stir it occasionally.

**10.** For serving, turn the meat on to a hot dish, and place the carrot on the top of the meat.

### LESSON ELEVENTH.

#### DR. KITCHENER'S BROTH.

**Ingredients.**—Four ounces of Scotch barley.  Four ounces of sliced onion.
Four ounces of dripping.  Three ounces of bacon.  Four ounces of oatmeal.  Pepper and salt.  Five quarts of liquor.

*Time required, about two hours.*

To make *"Dr. Kitchener's Broth"* :

1. Take *four ounces of Scotch barley*, wash it well,
and let it soak in a basin of cold water for *two hours*.

2. Put *five quarts of liquor* into a saucepan, and put
it on the fire to boil.

3. Take *two or three onions*, peel them, and cut them
in slices.  (There should be about *four ounces*.)

4. Drain off the *barley* and put it and the *onions* into
the *liquor*, and let it boil gently for *one hour*.

5. Put *three ounces of bacon* into another saucepan,
with *two ounces of clarified dripping*.

6. Put the saucepan on the fire to fry the *bacon* brown.

7. Then add, by degrees, *four ounces of oatmeal*, stirring it well until it is a paste.

8. Now stir in, by degrees, the *broth*, and season it
with *pepper* and *salt* according to taste.

9. Move the saucepan to the side of the fire, and let it
simmer gently for at least *half an hour*.

10. For serving, pour the *broth* into a hot soup-tureen
or basin.

## LESSON TWELFTH.

### CROWDIE.

**Ingredients.**—Two gallons of liquor from meat. Half a pint of oatmeal. Two onions. Salt and pepper.

*Time required, half an hour.*

### To make " *Crowdie*," or *Scotch Broth :*

1. Take two gallons of any meat-liquor, either salt or fresh, remove all the fat from it, and put it into a saucepan.

2. Put the saucepan on the fire to boil.

3. Take half a pint of oatmeal, put it into a basin, and mix it into a smooth paste with about a gill of the liquor.

N. B.—Half a pint of oatmeal is enough to thicken two gallons of liquor.

4. Peel two onions, put them on a board, and chop them up as fine as possible.

5. Stir the chopped onions into the paste, and add salt and pepper to taste.

N. B.—If salt liquor is used, salt should not be added.

6. When the liquor in the saucepan is quite boiling, stir in the paste smoothly.

7. Let it boil for twenty minutes, stirring it occasionally ; it must not get lumpy.

8. For serving, pour it into the soup-tureen or basin.

## LESSON THIRTEENTH.

### MILK SOUP.

**Ingredients.**—Four potatoes. Two leeks or onions. Two ounces of butter. One-quarter of an ounce of salt. Pepper. One pint of milk. Three tablespoonfuls of tapioca.

*Time required, about two hours and a half.*

To make *Milk Soup :*

**1.** Put *two quarts of water* into a large saucepan, and put it on the fire to boil.

**2.** Take *four large potatoes*, wash and scrub them clean in cold water, peel them, and cut them in quarters.

**3.** Take *two leeks*, cut off the *green tops* of the *leaves*, wash them well in cold water, and cut them up.

> N.B.—*Onions* can be used instead of *leeks*, only they would give a stronger flavor.

**4.** When the water is quite boiling, put in the *potatoes* and *leeks*.

**5.** Put in *two ounces of butter, a quarter of an ounce of salt*, and *pepper* to taste.

**6.** Let it boil till done to a mash.

**7.** Then strain off the *soup* through the colander.

**8.** Rub the *vegetables* through the colander with a wooden spoon.

**9.** Return the *pulp* and the *soup* to the saucepan, add *one pint of milk* to it, and put it on the fire to boil.

**10.** When it boils, sprinkle in, by degrees, *three table-spoonfuls of crushed tapioca*, stirring it well the whole time.

**11.** Let it boil gently *fifteen minutes.*

**12.** For serving, pour the *soup* in a hot tureen.

## LESSON FOURTEENTH.

### CABBAGE SOUP.

**Ingredients.**—One cabbage.  Two ounces of butter.  Three-quarters of a pint of milk.  Pepper and salt.  A slice of bread.

*Time required, about one hour and a quarter.*

To make *Cabbage Soup :*

1. Put three pints of water into a saucepan, and put it on the fire to boil.

2. Take a good-sized cabbage, wash it well in cold water, and trim off the outside dead leaves.

3. Cut the cabbage up as you would cut a lettuce up for a salad, but not into small pieces.

4. When the water in the saucepan is quite boiling, put in the cabbage.

5. Add two ounces of butter, and pepper and salt for seasoning, and let it boil one hour.

6. Then pour in three-quarters of a pint of milk, and let it boil up.

7. Stick a slice of bread on a toasting-fork, and toast it slightly on both sides in front of the fire.

8. Cut the toasted bread in pieces the size of dice, and put them into a hot soup-tureen or basin.

9. Pour the cabbage soup on to the bread in the soup-tureen, and it is ready for serving.

7

LESSON FIFTEENTH.

PEA SOUP.

**Ingredients.**—One quart of split peas.  Two onions.  One turnip.  One carrot.  One head of celery.  Teaspoonful of salt.  Half a teaspoonful of pepper.  Cooked or uncooked bones.

*Time required (after the peas have been soaked all night), about two hours and a half.*

To make *Pea Soup :*

**1.** Put a *quart of split peas* into a basin, with cold water to cover them, and let them soak for *twelve hours.*

N. B.—This should be done over night.

**2.** Put *two quarts* of cold water and the *split peas* into a saucepan, and put it on the fire to boil.

N. B.—If there is any liquor from boiled meat, it would of course be better than water for the soup.

**3.** Take *two onions* and *one turnip*, wash them in cold water, peel them, and cut them in halves.

**4.** Take *one carrot*, wash it, and scrape it clean with a knife.

**5.** Take *one head of celery*, cut off the ends of the root, and wash it well in cold water.

**6.** When the water in the saucepan is boiling, put in all the *vegetables.*

**7.** Add any *cooked or uncooked bones* that are at hand, and season it with *one teaspoonful of salt* and *half a tea-spoonful of ground pepper.*

N. B.—If some liquor (in which meat or pork has been boiled) is used, the addition of bones will not then be necessary.

**8.** Let it all boil slowly for *two hours*, and you must watch it, and skim it occasionally.

**9.** After that time, take the *bones* out of the saucepan.

**10.** Place a colander or wire sieve over a basin.

**11.** Pour the contents of the saucepan into the colander, and rub them through into the basin with a wooden spoon.

**12.** The *pea soup* is then ready for serving.

**13.** *Powdered* (*dried*) *mint* and *toasted bread,* cut to the shape of dice, should be handed with the *soup,* either put in, or served separately on plates.

---

### LESSON SIXTEENTH.

### GERMAN PEA SOUP.

**Ingredients.**—Quarter of a stick of German pea-soup sausage.  Three pints of water.

*Time required, about a quarter of an hour.*

To make *Pea Soup* from the German *pea-soup sausage :*

**1.** Put *three pints* of warm water into a saucepan, and put it on the fire to boil.

**2.** Take a *quarter of a stick of German pea-soup sausage* and scrape it into a basin.

**3.** Add to it a very little warm water, let it soak, and then mix it into a smooth paste.

N. B.—Be very careful that there are no lumps in the *paste.*

**4.** When the water in the saucepan is quite boiling, stir the *paste* in smoothly.

**5.** It is now ready for use, and should be poured into a hot soup-tureen.

N. B.—If the soup is preferred thinner, more water might be added.

N. B.—A *dessertspoonful of chopped mint* might be added to the *soup,* if the flavor is liked.

LESSON SEVENTEENTH.

MACARONI SOUP.

**Ingredients.**—Bones. One tablespoonful of salt and pepper-corns. One good-sized turnip and four leeks. Two carrots. Four onions. Two cloves, and a blade of mace. A bunch of herbs (marjoram, thyme, lemon-thyme, and parsley). One-quarter of a pound of macaroni.

*Time required, about two hours and a half.*

To make *Soup* from *Bones:*

1. Cut off from the bones all the meat that can be used.

N. B.—Cooked or uncooked bones can be used.

2. Break up the *bones* in pieces and put them into a saucepan, with *cold water* enough to cover them, and one quart more.

3. Put the saucepan on the fire to boil.

4. When it just boils, put in a tablespoonful of salt, to help the scum rise.

5. Peel one good-sized turnip and cut it in quarters.

N. B.—When turnips are used only for flavoring, they can be peeled thinner than if for eating.

6. Take *two carrots*, wash them, scrape them, and cut them in quarters; take *four leeks*, wash them, and shred them up finely.

N. B.—As soon as these vegetables are prepared, they should be thrown into cold water, to keep them fresh.

7. Take *four onions*, peel them, and stick *two cloves* into them.

N. B.—The outer skins of the onions can be put into a saucepan by the side of the fire, to brown; when browned, they are used for coloring gravies or soups.

8. Skim the *soup* well, and then put in the *vegetables;* also add a blade of *mace* and a *teaspoonful of pepper-corns.*

**9.** Move the saucepan to the side of the fire, and let it simmer gently for *two hours and a half*.

**10.** Raise the lid slightly to let out the steam.

N. B.—The soup can be thickened with macaroni, vermicelli, barley, or rice.

**11.** If the *soup* is thickened with *macaroni*, take a *quarter of a pound of macaroni* and wash it well in two or three waters.

**12.** Put the *macaroni* into a saucepan with plenty of cold water, and sprinkle a little *salt* over it.

**13.** Put the saucepan on the fire, and let it boil until the *macaroni* is quite tender; it will take about *half an hour*.

**14.** Try the *macaroni* with your fingers, to see that it is quite soft and tender.

**15.** When it is sufficiently boiled, strain the water off and pour some cold water on it, and wash the *macaroni* again.

**16.** Put it on a board and cut it into small pieces, about *a quarter of an inch* in length; it is then ready to be put into the *soup*.

N. B.—If barley is used instead of macaroni, it will take a much longer time to boil; but if vermicelli is used, it takes a very short time to boil.

**17.** When the *soup* is ready for use, put the *macaroni* into a soup-tureen, and strain the hot *soup* over it.

N. B.—It is better to boil macaroni separately, as the first water is not clean.

# CHAPTER X.

## *FISH.*

---

### BOILED TURBOT AND LOBSTER-SAUCE.

**Ingredients.**—Lobster. Two ounces of butter. One tablespoonful of cream. Half an ounce of flour.

*Time required, about half an hour.*

To Boil *Turbot* and make *Lobster-Sauce :*

**1.** Put the *turbot* in a basin of cold water and wash it well.

**2.** Get a fish-kettle and fill it with cold water ; add to it as much *salt* as will make the water taste salt, and put it on the fire to boil.

**3.** Take the turbot out of the basin.

**4.** Put it on the drainer of the fish-kettle, and put it in the kettle of boiling water, so that it will be covered with water.

**5.** Let it boil for *twenty* or *thirty minutes.*

**6.** Watch it, and skim the water if necessary.

N. B.—While the *turbot* is boiling, make the *lobster-sauce* (*see* below).

**7.** When the fish is sufficiently boiled, the flesh will divide from the bones.

**8.** Now take the drainer out of the fish-kettle, stand it across the kettle a *minute* to drain, and slip the fish carefully on to a hot dish for serving.

While the turbot is boiling, make the *Lobster-Sauce:*

**1.** Take a small lobster—it should be a hen-lobster, if possible.

**2.** Put the lobster on a board.

**3.** Take a chopper and break the shell of the lobster, by hitting it with the blade of the chopper, not with the edge; first, because it would cut the lobster in pieces, and second, because it would spoil the edge of the chopper.

**4.** Break all the shell off the claws and back with your fingers, and take out all the flesh.

**5.** Cut this flesh up with a sharp knife to the size of small dice.

**6.** If the lobster is a hen-lobster, you will find a bit of coral in the neck, and a strip of it down the back.

**7.** Take all this coral out of the lobster and wash it carefully in cold water in a small basin.

**8.** Take the coral out of the basin and put it in a mortar, with one ounce of butter.

**9.** Pound the coral and the butter well with the pestle.

**10.** Take it out of the mortar, and scrape the mortar out quite clean with a palette-knife, for none must be lost.

**11.** If you have not a palette-knife, you can manage as well with a piece of uncooked potato cut into the shape of a knife-blade with a thick back; with this you can scrape all out of the mortar.

**12.** Take a hair-sieve and put it over a plate.

**13.** Rub the pounded mixture through the sieve with the back of a wooden spoon.

**14.** Turn up the sieve when all the mixture has passed

through, and you will find some sticking on the under part.

**15.** Scrape all this carefully off with the spoon.

**16.** Make it all into a little pat.

**17.** Take a stewpan and put in it one ounce of butter and half an ounce of flour.

**18.** Mix them well together with a wooden spoon.

**19.** Add one gill and a half of cold water.

**20.** Put the stewpan on the fire.

**21.** Stir the mixture smooth with a wooden spoon until it boils and thickens. Add a large tablespoonful of cream, and stir well till it boils again.

**22.** Then take the stewpan off the fire and stand it on a piece of paper on the table.

**23.** Add to the mixture in the stewpan the pat of coral butter, by degrees, to color it.

N.B.—If there is no coral, the sauce might be colored with half a teaspoonful of *essence of anchovy.*

**24.** Stir it quite smoothly with a wooden spoon; it must not be lumpy.

**25.** Now add pepper and salt, and a few grains of Cayenne pepper, according to taste.

**26.** Take the chopped lobster and mix it into the sauce, and add a little lemon-juice.

**27.** Pour the sauce into a sauce-boat, and serve it with the turbot.

## LESSON SECOND.

**Ingredients.**—Haddock. Two pounds of potatoes. Three ounces of butter. One egg.

### For Sauce.

**Ingredients.**—Two ounces of butter. Half an ounce of flour. Half a gill of cream. Two eggs, and salt.

*Time required, about one hour and a half.*

To make a *Fish Pudding* of a *Haddock :*

**1.** Take a fish-kettle of warm water and put in it a little salt, and put it on the fire to boil.

**2.** Take a haddock and put it into a basin of cold water, and wash it well.

**3.** Take the haddock out of the basin and put it into the fish-kettle of boiling water, laying it carefully on the drainer, so that it will be covered with water.

**4.** Let it simmer for *fifteen minutes.*

**5.** Take *six potatoes*, put them into a basin of cold water, and scrub them well with a scrubbing-brush.

N. B.—Any cold potatoes can, of course, be used, instead of boiling fresh ones.

**6.** Take the potatoes out of the basin and dry them with a cloth.

**7.** Take a sharp knife and peel the potatoes.

**8.** Take a saucepan of cold[1] water and lay the potatoes in it.

**9.** Put the saucepan on the fire to boil. It must not boil less than *twenty minutes*, or more than *forty-five*, according to the size of the potatoes.

**10.** When you think the potatoes are sufficiently done,

[1] *See* Lessons First, Second, Third, and Fourth, on the cooking of potatoes, in the chapter on "Vegetables."

take a steel fork and try them, to see if they are tender all through.

11. When they are quite boiled, drain off all the water from the saucepan, and sprinkle the potatoes with a little salt.

12. Put the lid of the saucepan on, and stand the saucepan by the side of the fire, to steam the potatoes until they have become quite mealy and dry.

13. Shake the saucepan every now and then, to prevent the potatoes from sticking to the bottom.

14. When the haddock is sufficiently boiled, take it carefully out of the fish-kettle.

15. Take a sharp knife and cut off the head and tail of the fish.

16. Skin the fish from the head to the tail.

17. Cut up the fish, and take out all the bones.

18. Cut the fish up into small pieces the size of dice, and put them in a large basin.

19. When the potatoes are steamed, take them out of the saucepan with a spoon.

20. Have a wire sieve ready standing over a large plate.

21. Rub the potatoes quickly through the sieve with a wooden spoon.

22. Add the sifted potatoes to the haddock, and mix them well together with a wooden spoon.

23. Add salt and pepper, and a few grains of Cayenne pepper, to taste.

24. Put in two ounces of butter.

25. Take one egg and beat it slightly in a basin.

26. Pour the egg into the above mixture, and mix all together to a thick paste.

27. Take a large-sized flat tin and butter it well with your fingers.

**28.** Put the mixture on to this tin, and shape it as well as you can like a haddock.

> N. B.—If preferred, the mixture can be formed into cutlets, or croquette shapes, or as fish-cakes, and egged and bread-crumbed and fried in dripping, as for *lobster cutlets* (*see* " Fish," Lesson Seventh, Note 34 to Note 40).

**29.** Put some little bits of butter all about on the shape.

**30.** Put the tin into a quick oven for a *quarter of an hour*. It should become a pale-brown color.

Now make the *Sauce :*

**1.** Take a stewpan and put in it *two ounces* of butter and *one ounce and a half* of flour.

**2.** Mix them well together with a wooden spoon.

**3.** Add *half a teaspoonful* of salt.

**4.** Pour in *half a pint* of cold water.

**5.** Put the stewpan on the fire, and stir all smooth with a wooden spoon until it boils.

**6.** Now add *two tablespoonfuls* of cream, and let it boil, stirring all the time.

**7.** Stand the stewpan by the side of the fire. The mixture must not boil again, but only keep warm.

**8.** Take a saucepan of warm water and put it on the fire to boil.

**9.** When the water boils, put in *two* eggs, to boil for *ten minutes*.

**10.** Put the eggs into cold water for a minute, and then shell them.

**11.** Cut the eggs with a sharp knife into little square pieces.

**12.** Take the stewpan of sauce off the fire and stand it on a piece of paper on the table.

**13.** Add the cut-up eggs to the sauce, and stir them lightly in, not to break the pieces of egg.

**14.** For serving, move the *fish pudding* carefully on to a hot dish, and pour the *egg-sauce* round.

LESSON THIRD.

W H I T E B A I T.[1]

To Fry *Whitebait:*

**1.** Wash the whitebait in *iced water*, pick them over carefully, and dry them well in a cloth.

**2.** Take a sheet of paper and put on it a good *teacupful of flour*.

**3.** Take the whitebait and sprinkle them in the flour. They must not touch each other, and you must finger them as little as possible.

**4.** Take up the paper and shake the whitebait in the flour, so that they will be well covered with it.

**5.** Turn the whitebait from the paper of flour into a frying-basket, and sift all the loose flour back on to the paper.

**6.** Take a saucepan and put in it *one pound and a half* of lard or clarified dripping.

**7.** Put the saucepan on the fire, to heat the fat. When the fat smokes, it will then be hot enough.

> N. B.—The fat requires to be much hotter for frying whitebait than for anything else.

> N. B.—If possible, the fat should be tested by a frimometer, and the heat should rise to 400° Fahr.

**8.** Then turn the whitebait, a few at a time, into the frying-basket, and put it into the fat for *one minute*. The whitebait should be quite crisp.

**9.** Put a piece of whity-brown paper on a plate, stand the plate near the fire, and turn the fried whitebait on to

[1] We have no whitebait, but this lesson applies to smelts equally well.

the paper, to drain off the grease. Serve them on a napkin on a hot dish. *Lemon* cut, and thin slices of *brown bread* and *butter*, should be served with them.

---

## SOLE[1] AU GRATIN.

**Ingredients.**—One sole. Parsley, and a quarter of a shallot. Four mushrooms. A teaspoonful of lemon-juice. Salt and pepper. Two tablespoonfuls of glaze. Half an ounce of butter. Crumbs.

*Time required, about one hour.*

To Cook *Sole au Gratin :*

1. Take a small sole and cut off, with a sharp knife, the outside fins.

2. Cut through the skin only, across the head and the tail, on both sides of the fish.

3. Take the skin off from the tail to the head.

4. Wash the sole in cold water and dry it with a cloth, and nick it with a knife on both sides.

5. You can cook the sole in fillets if required, or whole. (N. B.—If in fillets, then fillet the sole the same as for the fried fillets in Lesson Sixth.) You are now going to cook the sole whole.

6. Take a small bunch of parsley and dry it well in a cloth.

7. Chop the parsley up fine on a board.

8. Chop a *quarter* of a shallot up fine, and mix it with the parsley.

9. The chopped parsley and shallot should fill a tablespoon.

---

[1] All the directions here given for cooking sole, apply perfectly to the dressing and cooking of the American flounder.

**10.** Take *four* small mushrooms, cut off the roots, and then wash the mushrooms well in a basin of cold water.

**11.** Take them out of the water, dry them in a cloth, and peel them.

**12.** Chop them up fine.

**13.** Take a dish and spread a little butter on it with your fingers.

**14.** Sprinkle *half* the chopped parsley, shallot, and mushroom over the bottom of the buttered dish.

**15.** Pour *half a teaspoonful* of lemon-juice over the chopped parsley, shallot, and mushroom in the dish; also sprinkle *half a salt-spoonful* of salt and a *quarter of a salt-spoonful* of pepper.

**16.** Lay the *sole* carefully in the dish, and sprinkle over it the *remainder* of the chopped parsley, shallot, and mushroom.

**17.** Sprinkle over the *sole* a little pepper and salt, and squeeze over it *half a teaspoonful* of lemon-juice.

**18.** Take *half an ounce* of butter and cut it in small pieces, and put them over the *sole*.

**19.** Pour over it *two tablespoonfuls* of half glaze.

> N.B.—*Glaze* can be bought, or it can be made by reducing some strong stock over the fire.

**20.** Take a wire sieve and put it over a piece of paper.

**21.** Take some *crumb of bread* and rub it through the sieve.

**22.** Take these bread-crumbs and put them on a flat tin. Put this tin into the oven, to dry and slightly brown the bread-crumbs.

**23.** When the crumbs are done, sift them over the sole.

**24.** Now put the dish into a brisk oven for *ten minutes*.

Take a fork and prick in the thick part of the sole, to see if the fish is tender.

25. Carefully move the sole with a slice on to a clean dish, and pour the sauce round.

---

LESSON FIFTH.

FILLETS OF SOLES À LA MAÎTRE D'HÔTEL.

**Ingredients.**—Sole. Lemon-juice. Half an ounce of butter. Three-quarters of an ounce of flour. Half a gill of cream.

*Time required, about half an hour.*

To Cook *Fillets of Soles à la Maître d'Hôtel :*

1. Take one sole and fillet it the same way as the *fried fillets* in Lesson Sixth.

2. Take the *bones* and *fins* of the sole and put them into a stewpan, with *half a pint* of water, and put it on the fire to boil.

3. Take a flat tin pan and butter it with your fingers.

4. Fold the fillets loosely over and lay them in the buttered tin.

5. Sprinkle a little salt and squeeze a little lemon-juice over them, and cover them with a piece of buttered paper.

6. Put the tin with the fillets into a sharp oven for *six minutes.*

Now make the *Sauce :*

1. Take a small bunch of *parsley*, wash it, dry it, and chop it fine with a knife on a board.

2. Take a stewpan and put in it *one ounce* of butter and *three-quarters* of an ounce of flour.

3. Mix them smoothly together with a wooden spoon.

**4.** Take the saucepan of *fish-stock* and pour it by degrees through a strainer into the stewpan of butter and flour, stirring well.

**5.** Put the stewpan on the fire, and stir the mixture smooth with a wooden spoon. Now add *two tablespoonfuls* of cream, and stir it well until it boils.

**6.** Take the stewpan off the fire and stand it on a piece of paper on the table.

**7.** Add the chopped parsley to the mixture.

**8.** Add *half a teaspoonful* of lemon-juice, salt and pepper to taste, and stir the sauce well.

**9.** Now take the fillets out of the oven and arrange them on a hot dish for serving; add the liquor from the fillets of soles, out of the tin, to the sauce.

**10.** Pour the *sauce* over the *fillets of soles*.

> N.B.—If there is no cream, the sauce can be made with milk; the bones of the fish should therefore be boiled in half a pint of milk, instead of water.

---

### LESSON SIXTH.

#### FRIED SOLES.

**Ingredients.**—Sole. One egg. Crumbs.

*Time required, about half an hour.*

To Fry *Filleted Soles :*

**1.** Take *one* sole, wash it well, and lay it on a board.

**2.** Take a sharp knife and cut off all the outside *fins*, the *head*, and the *tail*.

**3.** Take the *skin* off the sole, from the tail to the head.

**4.** Cut down the centre of the fish.

**5.** Slide the knife along carefully between the flesh and the bones, holding the flesh in one hand and drawing it gently away as the knife cuts it away from the bone.

**6.** Do both sides of the fish alike, and it will make *four fillets*.

**7.** Put each fillet separately on a plate, and rub it over with flour.

**8.** Take a wire sieve and stand it over a piece of paper.

**9.** Take some crumb of bread and rub it through the sieve.

**10.** Take *one* egg and beat it on a plate with a knife.

**11.** Lay the fillets in the egg, and egg them well all over with a brush.

**12.** Then put them in the bread-crumbs and cover them well. Be careful to finger them as little as possible.

**13.** Take a saucepan and put in it *one pound and a half* of lard or clarified dripping.

Now make the *Butter-Sauce* with *Anchovy* (*see* next page).

**14.** Put the saucepan on the fire, to heat the fat. Test the heat of it by throwing in a piece of *bread*, and if it makes a fizzing noise, it is ready.

N. B.—The heat is tested best by a frimometer; it should rise to 345°.

**15.** Take a frying-basket and place in it the fillets.

**16.** They should be slightly bent, or folded over, to prevent their being flat when fried.

**17.** When the fat is quite hot, put in the frying-basket with the fillets for *three minutes*.

**18.** Put a piece of whity-brown paper on a plate.

**19.** When the fillets are done, they should be a pale brown. Turn them out on to the paper on the plate, to drain off the grease.

**20.** Serve them in a hot dish on a napkin, garnished with a little fried *parsley*. (Refer to " Fish," Lesson Seventh, Note 41.)

### ANCHOVY-SAUCE.

**Ingredients.**—One ounce of butter.   Half an ounce of flour.   Anchovy-sauce.

1. Take a stewpan and put in it *one ounce* of butter and *half an ounce* of flour.

2. Mix them well with a wooden spoon.

3. Add *one gill and a half* of cold water.

4. Put the stewpan on the fire, and stir well with a wooden spoon until the mixture is quite smooth and boils.

5. Take the stewpan off the fire and stand it on a piece of paper on the table.

6. Now add *one tablespoonful* of anchovy-sauce, and stir it well into the butter-sauce.

7. For serving, pour it into a sauce-boat.

---

### LESSON SEVENTH.

### LOBSTER CUTLETS.

**Ingredients.**—One lobster.   One and one-half ounce of butter.   Half a gill of cream.   Seasoning and flavoring.   One ounce of flour.   One egg.   Bread.   Parsley.

*Time required, about three hours.*

To make *Lobster Cutlets :*

1. Take a small lobster—it should be a hen-lobster, if possible.

2. Put the lobster on a board.

3. Take a chopper and break the shell of the lobster, by hitting it with the blade of the chopper, not with the edge ; first, because it would cut the lobster in pieces, and second, because it would spoil the edge of the chopper.

4. Break all the shell off the claws and back with your fingers, and take out all the flesh.

5. Cut this flesh up in pieces with a sharp knife, to the size of small dice.

6. If the lobster is a hen-lobster, you will find a bit of coral in the neck, and a strip of it down the back.

7. Take all this coral out of the lobster, and wash it carefully in cold water in a small basin.

8. Take the coral out of the basin and put it in a mortar, with one ounce of butter.

9. Pound the coral and the butter well with the pestle.

10. Take it out of the mortar, and scrape it out quite clean with a palette-knife or slice of raw *potato*, for none must be lost.

11. Take a hair-sieve and put it over a plate.

12. Pass the pounded mixture through the sieve with a wooden spoon.

13. Turn up the sieve when all the mixture has passed through, and you will find some sticking inside.

14. Scrape all this carefully off with the spoon.

15. Make it all into a little *pat*.

16. Take a stewpan and put in it *one ounce* of flour and *half an ounce* of butter. Mix them well together with a wooden spoon.

17. Add *one gill* of cold water. Put the stewpan on the fire, and stir the mixture with a wooden spoon till it boils and thickens.

18. Add *one tablespoonful* of cream, and stir smooth until it boils.

19. Take the stewpan off the fire and stand it on a piece of paper on the table.

20. Now stir in, by degrees, the pat of coral-butter. Be sure the *sauce* is quite smooth, and not lumpy.

21. Add salt and pepper, and a few grains of Cayenne

pepper, according to taste, and about *six drops* of lemon-juice, and mix well.

**22.** Add the chopped lobster, and stir lightly—not to break up the lobster, but only to mix it with the *sauce*.

**23.** Take a clean plate and pour the mixture from the stewpan on to it, smoothing it with a knife.

**24.** Take a piece of paper and cut it round to the size of the plate.  Butter it with a knife.

**25.** Put the buttered paper over the mixture which is in the plate, to prevent the dust from getting in.

**26.** Take the plate and stand it on ice (if possible), or put it in a cold place to cool.

**27.** Take a wire sieve and put it over a piece of paper.

**28.** Take a piece of the crumb of bread and rub it through the wire sieve.

**29.** Take *one* egg and beat it slightly with a knife on a plate.

**30.** Take a saucepan and put in it *one pound and a half* of lard or clarified dripping.

**31.** Put the saucepan on the fire, to heat the fat.  It must not burn.

**32.** Take the plate of lobster mixture, which should by this time be cold and rather stiff.

**33.** Shape the mixture into cutlets.  This quantity will make *seven*.

**34.** Dip the cutlets into the egg, and egg them well all over with a brush.

**35.** Take them carefully out of the egg, and cover them well with the bread-crumbs.

N.B.—If the cutlets are not well covered with egg and bread-crumbs, they will burst in the frying.

**36.** Take a frying-basket and lay in it the lobster cutlets, a few at a time, so as not to touch each other.

**37.** When the fat is quite hot, test it by throwing into it a piece of bread. If it makes a sharp, fizzing noise, it is ready.

**38.** Put the frying-basket into the fat for *three minutes*, or perhaps less. The cutlets should become a pale brown.

**39.** Get a plate, with a piece of whity - brown paper on it, ready to receive the cutlets when they come out of the boiling fat. This is to strain all the grease from them.

**40.** Take the small claws of the lobster and stick them into the end of each cutlet, to represent the bone.

**41.** Take a few sprigs of parsley and put them into the frying-basket.

**42.** Just toss the basket with the parsley into the boiling fat for a second.

**43.** Arrange the cutlets on a napkin on a hot dish, and garnish them with the fried parsley.

---

### LESSON EIGHTH.

#### BOILED CODFISH AND OYSTER-SAUCE.

**Ingredients.**—One dozen oysters. Half an ounce of butter. One-quarter of an ounce of flour. One tablespoonful of cream. Lemon-juice and Cayenne pepper.

*Time required, about twenty minutes.*

To Cook *Codfish* and make *Oyster-Sauce :*

**1.** Take a slice of cod weighing *one pound*.

**2.** Put it in a basin of cold water and wash it well.

**3.** Take a small fish-kettle of boiling water and add to it as much salt as will make the water taste salt.

**4.** Put the fish-kettle on the fire.

**5.** Take the cod out of the basin and place it on the drainer in the fish-kettle, and let it boil for *fifteen minutes*.

N. B.—It must not boil fast.

**6.** When the slice of cod is sufficiently cooked, the flesh will leave the bones.

N. B.—The bone is usually left in, or the fish would break to pieces.

**7.** Serve the slice of cod on a folded napkin on a hot dish, with oyster-sauce.

### FOR OYSTER-SAUCE.

**1.** Take *one dozen* oysters and the liquor that is with them, and put them into a small saucepan.

**2.** Put the saucepan on the fire and bring them to the boil; this is to blanch the oysters.

**3.** Take the saucepan off the fire as soon as it boils.

**4.** Take a basin and pour into it the oyster-liquor through a strainer.

**5.** Take the oysters out of the saucepan and lay them on a plate.

**6.** Take off the beards and all the hard parts of the oysters, leaving only the soft part.

**7.** Take a stewpan and put in *half an ounce* of butter and a *quarter of an ounce* of flour.

**8.** Mix the flour and the butter well together with a wooden spoon.

**9.** Now add to the contents of the stewpan the oyster-liquor which is in the basin.

**10.** Put the stewpan on the fire, and stir the mixture well with a wooden spoon until it boils and thickens.

**11.** Now add *one tablespoonful* of cream, and stir again until it boils.

**12.** Take the stewpan off the fire and stand it on a piece of paper on the table.

**13.** Add six drops of lemon-juice and a few grains of Cayenne pepper, according to taste.

**14.** Take the trimmed oysters and cut them into small pieces.

**15.** Add the pieces of oyster to the mixture in the stew-pan, and mix all together with a wooden spoon.

---

LESSON NINTH.

BROILED SALMON AND TARTARE-SAUCE.

**Ingredients.**—Two eggs. Salt and pepper. A tablespoonful of French vinegar. Parsley. Gherkins or capers. One gill of oil.

*Time required, about fifteen minutes.*

To Cook *Salmon :*

**1.** Take a thick slice of salmon weighing *one pound*.

**2.** Cut it into two thin slices, as it will cook better than in a thick piece.

**3.** Put the salmon in a basin of cold water and wash it well.

**4.** Take it out of the basin and dry it well with a cloth.

**5.** Take a plate and pour on it about a *gill* of salad-oil.

**6.** Dip the slices of salmon into the oil on both sides; the *oil* will prevent the fish from drying while cooking.

**7.** Season the slices on both sides with pepper and salt.

**8.** Take a gridiron and heat it on both sides by the fire ; this is to prevent the fish sticking.

**9.** When the gridiron is hot, place on the slices of salmon, and let them grill for a *quarter of an hour*.

**10.** Turn the gridiron occasionally, so as to cook the fish on both sides, which should become of a pale-brown color.

**11.** When the fish is quite done, remove the bone in the centre of each slice. Serve the salmon on a napkin on a hot dish.

## FOR TARTARE-SAUCE.

**1.** Take *two* eggs, and put the yolks into one basin, and the whites (which will not be wanted) into another basin.

**2.** Take a wooden spoon and just stir the yolks enough to break them.

**3.** Add to them a *salt-spoonful* of salt and *half a salt-spoonful* of pepper, and a *tablespoonful* of French vinegar.

**4.** Take a bottle of salad-oil, and, putting your thumb half over the top, pour in, drop by drop, the oil, stirring well with a whisk the whole time; a *gill* of oil will be sufficient.

**5.** If the sauce is not sharp enough to taste, add a little more vinegar, stirring it in smooth.

**6.** Now stir in a *teaspoonful* of ready-made mustard, or tarragon-vinegar if it is liked.

**7.** Take a small bunch of parsley and put it in a small saucepan of boiling water, with a little salt and soda, for two or three seconds.

N. B.—Soda is to keep the parsley green.

N. B.—This is called " blanching " or " parboiling " parsley.

**8.** Take the parsley out and dry it thoroughly by squeezing it in a cloth. Put it on a board and chop it up fine. There should be a teaspoonful.

**9.** Take a few gherkins or capers and chop them up fine on a board. There should be enough to fill a table-spoon.

**10.** Take these chopped gherkins or capers, and the chopped parsley, and put them all into the sauce, and mix them in with a spoon.

**11.** Serve the sauce in a sauce-tureen.

## LESSON TENTH.

### BAKED MACKEREL OR HERRING.

**Ingredients.**—Two mackerel or herrings. One dessertspoonful of chopped herbs and onions. One dessertspoonful of chopped parsley. One dessertspoonful of bread-crumbs. Pepper and salt. Two ounces of dripping.

*Time required, about forty minutes.*

To Bake *Mackerel* or *Herrings* with *herbs* and *bread-crumbs :*

1. Wash the mackerel or herrings in cold water, dry them in a cloth, and put them upon a board.

2. Take a sharp knife, cut off the *heads* of the fish, carefully split open each fish, and take out the *back-bone.*

3. Lay one fish open flat on a tin (*skin downward*).

4. Take a *sprig of parsley*, wash it in water, and dry it in a cloth.

5. Put the parsley on a board, take away the *stalks*, and chop it up as fine as possible. There should be about a *dessertspoonful.*

6. Take half an onion, peel it, put it on a board with a sprig of *thyme* and *marjoram*, and chop it up fine. There should be about a *dessertspoonful.*

7. Take a grater, stand it on a board, and grate a few *bread-crumbs.* There should be about a *dessertspoonful.*

8. Mix the onions, herbs, and bread-crumbs together.

9. Sprinkle *pepper* and *salt* to taste over the fish in the tin.

10. Then sprinkle over the fish the mixture of *herbs* and *bread-crumbs.*

11. Take the other fish and lay it over the one in the tin (*skin upward*).

8

**12.** Put two ounces of *clarified dripping* in a saucepan, and put it on the fire to melt.

**13.** Pour the *melted dripping* over the fish in the tin.

**14.** Cover the tin with a dish, and stand it on the hot plate or in the oven, to bake for *half an hour.*

**15.** Watch it, and baste it occasionally with the dripping.

**16.** For serving, turn the fish carefully out of the tin on to a *hot dish.*

LESSON ELEVENTH.

BAKED STUFFED HADDOCK.

**Ingredients.** — One haddock. Bread-crumbs. One dessertspoonful of chopped parsley. One teaspoonful of chopped herbs. Pepper and salt. Two ounces of suet. One egg. Two ounces of dripping.

*Time required, about three-quarters of an hour.*

To Stuff a *Haddock* and Bake it :

**1.** Take a *haddock,* wash it, clean it carefully in cold water, and dry it in a cloth.

**2.** Stand a grater on a piece of paper, and grate some *bread-crumbs.*

**3.** Take a *sprig of parsley,* wash it in cold water, and dry it in a cloth.

**4.** Put the *parsley* on a board and chop it up fine. There should be about a dessertspoonful.

**5.** Take a small *sprig of thyme* and *marjoram,* remove the stalks, and chop the herbs up fine on a board. There should be about a teaspoonful.

N. B.—The *stalks* will do for flavoring, but they cannot be eaten, as they are bitter.

**6.** Mix all the *herbs* together with two tablespoonfuls of the *bread-crumbs.*

N. B.—The remainder of the bread-crumbs will be required to roll the fish in.

**7.** Add *pepper* and *salt* to taste, and mix the stuffing together with *two ounces of suet.*

**8.** Stuff the belly of the fish with the stuffing, and sew it up.

**9.** Break an *egg* into a plate, and brush the fish over with it; then roll it in the *bread-crumbs*, covering it well all over.

**10.** Grease a dish or tin with a piece of dripping.

**11.** Lay the *fish* on the dish or tin, and put it into the oven, to bake for from *half* to *three-quarters of an hour,* basting it frequently with dripping.

---

LESSON TWELFTH.

FISH BAKED IN VINEGAR.

**Ingredients.**—Six herrings. Thirty pepper-corns. One blade of mace. One shallot. One bay-leaf. One gill of vinegar. Salt.

*Time required, about six hours.*

To Bake *Fish* (such as *herrings* or *mackerel*) in *Vinegar :*

**1.** Wash the fish and clean them thoroughly in cold water.

**2.** Put the fish on a board and cut them into thick pieces.

**3.** Lay these pieces close together in a stone jar, with *thirty pepper-corns* and *half a teaspoonful of salt.*

**4.** Add *one blade of mace* and a *bay-leaf.*

**5.** Take *one shallot,* peel it, and add it, or part of it (according to taste), to the *fish.*

**6.** Pour in *one gill of vinegar,* and tie a piece of brown paper tightly over the top of the jar with a piece of string.

**7.** Put the jar into a very slow oven, to bake for *six hours ;* or it may stand in a baker's oven all night.

N. B.—The *fish* is to be eaten cold.

---

## LESSON THIRTEENTH.

### FRIED PLAICE.

**Ingredients.**—One plaice. One egg. Bread-crumbs. Dripping for frying. *Time required, about half an hour.*

To Fry *Plaice* in *Egg* and *Bread-crumbs,* or *Batter :*

**1.** Put about *half a pound of clarified dripping* into a saucepan, and put it on the fire to heat.

**2.** Take the *plaice,* wash it in cold water, and dry it in a cloth.

**3.** Put the *plaice* on a board, and, with a sharp knife, carefully remove the skin from the back side of the fish, and cut off the head and the tail.

**4.** Hold a grater over a piece of paper, and grate some *bread-crumbs.*

**5.** Cut up the *fish* into slices or fillets.

**6.** Break an *egg* on to a plate, and beat it lightly with a knife.

**7.** Dip the slices of fish into the egg, and egg them well all over.

**8.** Then roll them in the *bread-crumbs,* covering them well.

N. B.—Shake off the loose *crumbs.*

**9.** When the *dripping* is quite hot and smoking, carefully put in the *fish,* fingering it as little as possible, so as not to take off any of the egg or bread-crumbs.

N. B.—Do not put too many pieces at a time into the dripping, as they must not touch each other.

**10.** Put a piece of whity-brown paper on to a plate, and as the fish is fried, take it out of the dripping carefully with a slice, and lay it on the paper, to drain off the grease.

> N. B.—Soles, or any fish, can be fried in the same way.

> N. B.—For frying fish in batter, dip each piece of fish in the batter, made as for meat fritters (*see* "Cooked Meat," Lesson Second), and fry it in the same way as above.

---

### LESSON FOURTEENTH.

### BOILED FISH.

**Ingredients** (for Sauce).—One dessertspoonful of corn-flour or arrow-root. One teaspoonful of vinegar or lemon-juice.

*Time required for boiling fish, about twenty minutes to three-quarters of an hour, according to the size of the fish.*

To Boil *Fish* and make the *Sauce*:

**1.** Put a saucepan or fish-kettle of water on the fire to boil.

**2.** Take the *fish* and clean it thoroughly in cold water.

**3.** When the water is quite boiling, put in the *fish* on a strainer or a plate. There should be enough water just to cover the fish.

**4.** Also put in some *salt*—enough to make the water taste salt.

**5.** Put the lid on the saucepan and move it to the side of the fire, to simmer gently for from twenty minutes to three-quarters of an hour (according to the size of the fish).

**6.** You must watch it, and skim it occasionally.

**7.** When you find that the skin of the *fish* is cracking, you may know that it is sufficiently boiled.

While the *fish* is boiling, make the *Sauce :*

**8.** Put a *dessertspoonful of corn-flour* or *arrow-root* into a small saucepan, and mix it into a smooth paste with cold water.

**9.** Now add to it *half a pint* of the water in which the *fish* was boiled.

**10.** Put the saucepan on the fire, and stir it until it boils and thickens.

**11.** Then take the saucepan off the fire and stand it on a piece of paper on the table.

**12.** Flavor the *sauce* with a *teaspoonful of vinegar* or *lemon-juice*, and season it with *pepper* and *salt* according to taste.

> N.B.—If liked, the *sauce* can be colored with *half a teaspoonful of caramel* (burnt sugar). (*See* note at end of "Brown Purée," "Australian Meat," Lesson Second.)

**13.** For serving, take the fish carefully out of the saucepan and place it on a hot dish. Pour the sauce into a sauce-boat or a basin, or round the fish.

# CHAPTER XI.

## *VEGETABLES.*

---

### LESSON FIRST.

#### BOILED AND STEAMED POTATOES.

*Time required for boiling: Old potatoes, about half an hour; new potatoes, about twenty minutes; steamed potatoes, half an hour.*

To Boil *Old Potatoes:*

**1.** Wash *two pounds of potatoes* well in cold water, and scrub them clean with a scrubbing-brush.

> N. B.—If the *potatoes* are diseased, take a sharp knife, peel them, and carefully cut out the eyes and any black specks about the *potato;* but it is much better to boil them in their skins.

**2.** Put them in a saucepan with cold water enough to cover them, and sprinkle over them a *teaspoonful of salt.*

**3.** Put the saucepan on the fire, to boil the potatoes for from twenty minutes to half an hour.

**4.** Take a fork and put it into the potatoes, to try if the centre is quite tender.

**5.** When they are sufficiently boiled, drain off all the water, and place a clean cloth over the potatoes in the saucepan.

**6.** Stand the saucepan by the side of the fire, with the lid on, to steam the potatoes.

7. When the potatoes have become quite dry, take them carefully out of the saucepan, peel them without breaking them, and place them in a hot vegetable-dish for serving.

To Boil *New Potatoes :*

1. Wash two pounds of potatoes in cold water.
2. Take a knife and scrape them.
3. Take a saucepan of warm water and put it on the fire to boil.
4. When the water is quite boiling, put in the new potatoes, and sprinkle over them a teaspoonful of salt.
5. Let them boil for a quarter of an hour; you should take a fork and put it into the potatoes, to feel if the centre is quite tender.
6. Then drain off all the water, and place a clean cloth in the saucepan over the potatoes, and stand the saucepan by the side of the fire, with the lid on.
7. When they have become quite dry, take them out of the saucepan and arrange them on a hot vegetable-dish for serving.

To Steam *Potatoes :*

N.B.—Old potatoes only can be steamed.

1. Wash the potatoes well in cold water, and scrub them clean with a scrubbing-brush.

N.B.—It is best to steam the potatoes in their skins, but they can be peeled if preferred.

2. Take a potato-steamer, fill the saucepan with hot water, and put it on the fire to boil.
3. When the water is quite boiling, put the potatoes in the steamer, and sprinkle them over with salt.

**4.** Place the steamer on the saucepan of boiling water, and cover it down tight, to keep the steam in.

**5.** Let the potatoes steam for *half an hour*.

**6.** Take a fork and put it into the potatoes, to feel if the centre is quite tender.

**7.** When they are sufficiently steamed, take them carefully out of the steamer and arrange them on a hot vegetable-dish for serving.

---

LESSON SECOND.

MASHED, SAUTÉ, AND BAKED POTATOES.

**Ingredients** (for Mashed Potatoes).—Two pounds of old potatoes. One ounce of butter. One gill of milk. Pepper and salt.

**Ingredients** (for Sauté Potatoes).—New Potatoes. Two ounces of butter. Salt.

*Time required for mashed potatoes, forty minutes ; for sauté potatoes, half an hour ; for baked potatoes, three-quarters of an hour.*

For a dish of *Mashed Potatoes :*

**1.** Take *two pounds* of old potatoes, wash them, and steam them, as for steaming potatoes (*see* "Vegetables," Lesson First).

**2.** Take a stewpan and put in it *one ounce of butter*, *one gill of milk*, and *pepper* and *salt* to taste.

**3.** Put the stewpan on the fire to boil.

**4.** Place a wire sieve over a plate.

**5.** Take the steamed potatoes one at a time out of the steamer, put them on the sieve, and pass them through on to the plate as quickly as possible, rubbing them with a wooden spoon.

**6.** Take the sifted potato and stir it into the boiling milk in the stewpan.

7. Now beat it all lightly together, and then turn it into a hot vegetable-dish for serving.

For *Sauté Potatoes :*

1. Take some *new potatoes*, as small as possible, wash them in cold water, and scrape them clean.

> N.B.—If the potatoes are large, they should be cut in halves, or even in quarters, and trimmed.

2. Put them in a saucepan with cold water.

3. Put the saucepan on the fire, and only just bring them to the boil.

4. Then drain off the water, and wipe the potatoes dry in a clean cloth.

5. Take a thick stewpan and put in it *two ounces of butter* and the potatoes.

6. Put the stewpan on a quick fire for about *twenty minutes*, to brown the potatoes. Watch them, and when they have begun to brown, toss them occasionally in the stewpan, so as to brown them on all sides alike.

7. Then strain off the butter, sprinkle them over with salt, and serve them on a hot vegetable-dish.

For *Baked Potatoes :*

1. Take the potatoes, wash and scrub them well with a scrubbing-brush, in a basin of cold water.

2. Take them out of the water and dry them with a cloth.

3. Put them in a brisk oven to bake. They will take from half to three-quarters of an hour to bake, according to the heat of the oven and the size of the potatoes.

4. Take a steel fork, or skewer, and stick it into the potatoes, to see if they are done. They must be soft inside.

5. Take a table-napkin, fold it, and place it on a hot dish.

6. When the potatoes are done, take them out of the oven and arrange them on the napkin for serving.

---

### LESSON THIRD.

#### FRIED POTATOES.

**Ingredients.**—One pound of potatoes. Salt. The use of one and one-half pound of clarified fat or lard, for frying.

*Time required, about eight minutes.*

For *Potato Chips :*

1. Wash the potatoes well in cold water, and scrub them clean with a scrubbing-brush.

2. Take a sharp knife, peel them, and carefully cut out the eyes and any black specks about them.

3. Now peel the potatoes very thinly in ribbons, and twist them into fancy shapes.

4. Take a saucepan and put in it *one pound and a half of clarified fat or lard.*

5. Put the saucepan on the fire, to heat the fat. Test the heat of it with a piece of bread (*see* Lesson on "Frying").

6. Take a frying-basket and put in it the ribbons of potato.

7. When the *fat* is quite hot, put in the frying-basket with the potatoes for about six minutes.

8. Place a piece of whity-brown paper on a plate.

9. When the chips are done, they should be quite crisp and of a pale-brown color. Turn them out on to the paper, to drain off the grease, and sprinkle over them a little salt.

10. Serve them on a hot dish.

For Fried *Slices of Potato :*

**1.** Take the potatoes, wash them clean, and peel them with a sharp knife.

**2.** Put the potatoes on a board, and cut them in slices about *one-eighth of an inch* in thickness.

**3.** Take a saucepan and put in it *one and a half pound of clarified dripping* or *lard.*

**4.** Take a frying-basket and place in it the sliced potatoes.

**5.** Put the saucepan on the fire, to warm the *fat.*

**6.** When the *fat* is warm, but not very hot, place in it the frying-basket with the slices of potatoes, and let them boil in the fat until they are quite tender.

> N. B.—You should take out a piece of potato and press it between the thumb and finger, to feel that it is quite tender.

**7.** Now take out the frying-basket with the potatoes and place it on a plate.

**8.** Leave the fat on the fire to heat.

**9.** When the *fat* is quite hot, place in the frying-basket with the *potatoes* for about *two minutes.*

**10.** Put a piece of whity-brown paper on a plate.

**11.** When the potatoes are fried, they should be a pale-brown color. Turn them out on to the paper, to drain off the grease.

**12.** Sprinkle a little salt over them.

**13.** For serving, arrange them on a hot dish.

## LESSON FOURTH.

### POTATO CROQUETTES.

**Ingredients** (for eighteen croquettes).—Two pounds of potatoes. One ounce of butter. One tablespoonful of milk. Three eggs. A small bunch of parsley. Bread-crumbs. Pepper and salt.

*Time required, about one hour.*

To make *Potato Croquettes:*

**1.** Take *two pounds of potatoes*, wash, scrub, and boil or steam them (*see* " Vegetables," Lesson First).

> N. B.—Any remains of *cold potatoes* could be used up in this way, instead of boiling fresh ones.

**2.** Place a wire sieve over a plate.

**3.** Take the *potatoes* one at a time, place them on the sieve, and rub them through with a wooden spoon as quickly as possible on to the plate.

> N. B.—The *potatoes* can be passed through the sieve much quicker while they are hot.

**4.** Put *one ounce of butter* and a *tablespoonful of milk* into a stewpan, and put it on the fire.

**5.** When the milk and butter are hot, stir in smoothly the sifted potato.

**6.** Take the stewpan off the fire and stand it on a piece of paper on the table.

**7.** Break *two eggs*, put the *whites* in a cup (as they are not required for present use), and stir the *yolks*, one at a time, into the *potato* in the stewpan.

**8.** Take two or three sprigs of parsley, wash them in cold water, dry them in a cloth, and chop them up finely on a board. There should be about a teaspoonful.

**9.** Sprinkle the *parsley* into the stewpan, and season the potato according to taste with *pepper* and *salt*.

**10.** Turn the potato mixture on to a plate, and stand it aside till cold.

**11.** Put *one pound of clarified dripping* into a deep stewpan, and put it on the fire to heat; be careful that it does not burn.

**12.** Take some crumb of bread and rub it through a wire sieve on to a piece of paper.

**13.** When the potato mixture is cold, form it into croquettes or balls, according to taste.

**14.** Break an *egg* on to a plate, and beat it up slightly with a knife.

**15.** Dip the croquettes into the egg, and egg them well all over with a paste-brush.

**16.** Now roll them in the bread-crumbs, covering them well all over.

N. B.—Be careful to cover them smoothly, and not too thickly.

**17.** Take a frying-basket and arrange the croquettes in it; but you must finger them as little as possible, and not allow them to touch each other.

**18.** When the *fat* on the fire is quite hot and smoking (test the heat by throwing in a piece of *bread*, which should fry brown directly), put in the frying-basket for *two minutes* or so, to fry the *croquettes* a pale-yellow.

**19.** Put a piece of whity-brown paper on a plate, and as the croquettes are fried, turn them on to the paper, to drain off the grease.

**20.** Put three or four small sprigs of parsley (washed and dried) into the frying-basket, and just toss the basket into the boiling fat for a second or so.

**21.** For serving, arrange the croquettes tastily on a hot dish, with the fried parsley in the centre.

## LESSON FIFTH.

### BRUSSELS SPROUTS.

**Ingredients.**—Brussels sprouts. Salt. One-quarter of a salt-spoonful of carbonate of soda. One ounce of butter. Pepper.

*Time required, about half an hour.*

To Dress *Brussels Sprouts :*

**1.** Take the Brussels sprouts, wash them well in two or three waters, and trim them.

**2.** Take a saucepan with plenty of warm water in it.

**3.** Put the saucepan on the fire to boil.

**4.** When the water is quite boiling, add a tablespoonful of salt and a quarter of a salt-spoonful of carbonate of soda.

**5.** Put in the sprouts, and let them boil quickly for from ten to twenty minutes, according to their age.

N. B.—Young sprouts take the shortest time to boil.

**6.** Keep the lid off the saucepan the whole time.

**7.** After that time, pour the sprouts into a colander to drain.

**8.** When the sprouts are quite dry, put them in a sauté-pan with *one ounce* of butter.

**9.** Sprinkle over them a little *pepper* and *salt,* and toss them over the fire for a few minutes ; but they must not fry.

**10.** For serving, arrange them tastily on a hot vegetable-dish.

## LESSON SIXTH.

### CARROTS AND TURNIPS.

**Ingredients.**—Carrots or turnips. Two tablespoonfuls of salt. Half a pint of good stock. Dessertspoonful of castor-sugar. Half an ounce of butter.

*Time required, about three-quarters of an hour.*

For *Carrots :*

**1.** Take a saucepan of water and put it on the fire to boil.

**2.** When the water is quite boiling, add a *tablespoonful of salt.*

**3.** Take the carrots, and if they are quite young, put them into the saucepan of boiling water, to boil for *twenty minutes.*

**4.** Take a fork and stick it in the carrots, to feel that they are quite tender all through.

**5.** You should let them boil for from half an hour to three-quarters of an hour.

**6.** After that time, take them out of the saucepan and rub them clean with a cloth.

> N. B.—If the carrots are old, you should wash, scrape them clean with a knife, and cut them to the shape of young carrots, or cut them out with a round cutter, before boiling.

**7.** Take a stewpan and put the boiled carrots in it.

**8.** Pour in some good stock—enough to cover them.

**9.** Put in a piece of *butter* the size of a nut, and sprinkle a little white castor-sugar over them.

**10.** Put the stewpan on the fire to boil, and reduce to a glaze over the carrots.

**11.** Then take them out of the stewpan, and they are ready for use.

For *Turnips :*

**1.** Take the turnips and wash them well in cold water.

**2.** Take them out of the water, put them on a board, peel them with a sharp knife, and cut them in quarters, or cut them out with a round cutter.

**3.** Take a saucepan of water and put it on the fire to boil.

**4.** When the water is quite boiling, add a tablespoonful of salt.

**5.** Now put in the cut-up turnips, and let them boil for from *ten* to *fifteen* minutes.

**6.** When they are sufficiently boiled, take them out of the saucepan and put them into a stewpan with some good *stock*—enough to cover them.

**7.** Add to them a piece of *butter*, and sprinkle over them about a *teaspoonful of castor-sugar.*

**8.** Put the stewpan on the fire to boil, and reduce to a glaze over the turnips.

**9.** Then take them out of the stewpan, and they are ready for serving.

> N.B.—Turnips and carrots as prepared above may be served with braised veal (*see* "Braised Fillet of Veal"), or separately as a vegetable.

---

### LESSON SEVENTH.

#### BOILED CAULIFLOWER, AND CAULIFLOWER AU GRATIN.

**Ingredients.**—Cauliflower. Salt. Half an ounce of butter. One ounce of flour. Tablespoonful of cream. Two ounces of Parmesan cheese. Cayenne pepper.

*Time required, about one hour.*

To Dress a *Cauliflower :*

**1.** Take a cauliflower and wash it well in two or three

waters, and take a knife and cut off the end of the stalk and any withered outside leaves.

**2.** Put it in a basin of cold water with a *dessertspoonful of salt*, and let it stand for *two* or *three* minutes.

**3.** Take a large saucepan full of water and put it on the fire to boil.

**4.** When the water is quite boiling, put in a tablespoonful of salt.

**5.** Take the cauliflower out of the salt and water and place it in a saucepan, with the flower downward, and let it boil till it is quite tender—from *fifteen* to *twenty* minutes.

**6.** Take it out with a slice, and feel the centre with your finger, to see that it is quite tender.

**7.** When done, take it out of the saucepan and put it on a sieve.

**8.** For serving, place it on a hot vegetable-dish.

If *Cauliflower au Gratin* be required:

**1.** Take the cauliflower and wash it, and boil it in the same way as described above, from Note 1 to Note 6.

**2.** When the cauliflower is sufficiently boiled, take it out of the saucepan with a slice and put it on a plate.

**3.** Take a knife and cut off all the outside green leaves.

**4.** Take a cloth and squeeze all the water out of the cauliflower.

**5.** Put half an ounce of butter and one ounce of flour into a stewpan, and mix them well together with a wooden spoon.

**6.** Pour in one gill of *cold water*.

**7.** Put the stewpan on the fire, and stir smoothly until it boils and thickens.

**8.** Now add *one tablespoonful of cream,* a little *salt*, and a few grains of *Cayenne pepper*, according to taste.

**9.** Stand the stewpan by the side of the fire, until the sauce is required for use.

**10.** Take two ounces of Parmesan cheese and grate it with a grater on to a piece of paper.

**11.** Now take the stewpan off the fire and stand it on a piece of paper on the table.

**12.** Stir rather more than half the grated cheese into the *sauce*.

**13.** Place the cauliflower on a tin dish.

**14.** Pour the sauce all over the *cauliflower*.

**15.** Take the remainder of the grated *cheese* and sprinkle it over the cauliflower, and brown the top of it with a hot salamander.

**16.** The cauliflower should become a pale-brown, and be served hot.

---

### LESSON EIGHTH.

#### SPINACH.

**Ingredients.**—Two pounds of spinach. Salt. Three ounces of butter. Half a gill of cream. Pepper. A slice of bread.

*Time required, about half an hour.*

To Dress *Spinach :*

**1.** Take *two pounds of spinach* and place it on a board.

**2.** Pick off all the stalks from the leaves.

**3.** Put the leaves in plenty of cold water, and wash them two or three times.

**4.** Turn the spinach on to a colander to drain.

**5.** Take a large saucepan and put the spinach into it; sprinkle a *salt-spoonful of salt* over it, and put it on the fire to boil. The drops of water on the leaves and their own juice are sufficient, without adding any water.

**6.** Let it boil quickly for *ten minutes*, with the cover off.

**7.** Then pour the spinach into the colander to drain.

**8.** Now press all the water out of the spinach, squeezing it quite dry.

**9.** Put it on a board and chop it up as finely as possible.

N. B.—If preferred, the spinach might be rubbed through a wire sieve, instead of being chopped up.

**10.** Take a stewpan and put in it one ounce of butter.

**11.** Put the *spinach* into the stewpan, and add about *half a salt-spoonful of pepper* and a *salt-spoonful of salt*, or more, according to taste, and *half a gill of cream*, and mix all together with a wooden spoon.

**12.** Put the stewpan on the fire, and stir until it is quite hot.

**13.** Cut a slice of crumb of bread about a quarter of an inch in thickness, put it on a board, and cut it up into triangular pieces.

**14.** Take a frying-pan and put into it *two ounces of butter* or *clarified dripping*.

**15.** Put the frying-pan on the fire, to heat the fat.

**16.** When the fat is quite hot, throw in the pieces of bread, and let them fry a pale-brown.

**17.** Take the pieces of fried bread and arrange them round a hot vegetable-dish, to form a wall.

**18.** Serve the dressed spinach in the centre.

## LESSON NINTH.

### PEAS.

**Ingredients.**—Half a peck of peas. Salt. Quarter of a salt-spoonful of carbonate of soda. Half an ounce of butter. Castor-sugar.

*Time required, about half an hour.*

To Dress *Peas :*

**1.** Take the *peas* and shell them.

**2.** Take a saucepan full of warm water and put it on the fire to boil.

**3.** When the water is quite boiling, put in the shelled peas, a *teaspoonful of salt,* and a *quarter of a salt-spoonful of carbonate of soda.*

N.B.—The soda will keep the peas a good color.

**4.** Let them boil for from *fifteen* to *twenty minutes,* according to the age of the peas. (The cover should be off the saucepan.)

**5.** After that time, feel the peas, that they are quite soft ; then take them out of the saucepan, and drain off all the water in a colander.

**6.** Now turn the peas into a sauté-pan, with *half an ounce of butter.*

**7.** Sprinkle *half a teaspoonful of salt* and a *teaspoonful of castor-sugar* over the peas, and toss them over the fire for a few minutes ; but they must not fry.

**8.** For serving, arrange them on a hot vegetable-dish.

LESSON TENTH.

HARICOT BEANS.

**Ingredients.**—One pint of beans.  One ounce of butter.  A sprig of parsley.  Pepper and salt.  Quarter of an ounce of clarified dripping.

*Time required (after the beans are soaked), about two hours and ten minutes.*

To Boil *Haricot Beans*, and serve them with *parsley* and *butter :*

1. Soak *one pint of haricot beans* in cold water all night.

2. Put them into a saucepan with three pints of cold water and a quarter of an ounce of clarified dripping.

3. Put the saucepan on the fire, and when it boils, move it rather to the side of the fire, and let it boil very gently for *two hours.*

4. After that time, turn the beans on to a colander, drain off the water, and put the beans back into a dry saucepan, with *one ounce of butter.*

5. Take a *sprig of parsley*, wash it, and dry it in a cloth, put it on a board, and chop it up as finely as possible.

6. Sprinkle the parsley over the beans, and season them with *pepper* and *salt.*

7. Put the saucepan on the fire, and stir the contents carefully for about *five minutes.*

8. For serving, turn the beans on to a hot dish.

TURNIPS.

**Ingredients.**—Four large turnips.   One ounce of butter.   Pepper and salt.

*Time required, about three-quarters of an hour.*

To Boil *Turnips* and Mash them:

**1.** Put *two quarts of warm water* and a *tablespoonful of salt* into a saucepan, and put it on the fire to boil.

**2.** Take some turnips, wash them in cold water, and peel them thickly with a sharp knife.

**3.** If the turnips are very large, cut them in quarters.

**4.** When the water in the saucepan is quite boiling, put in the turnips, and let them boil gently until they are quite tender.

**5.** Feel them with a fork, to see if they are tender all through.

**6.** Then turn them into a colander and drain them very dry.

**7.** For serving, put them on to a hot dish.

If *Mashed Turnips* are required:

**8.** Boil them as above.

**9.** Squeeze them as dry as possible in the colander, pressing them with a plate.

**10.** When the turnips are quite free from *water*, hold the colander over a saucepan and rub them through with a wooden spoon.

**11.** Put *one ounce of butter* into the saucepan with the *turnips,* and *pepper* and *salt* to taste.

**12.** Put the saucepan on the fire, and stir the contents

until the butter is well mixed with the turnips and they are thoroughly warmed through.

**13.** For serving, turn them on to a hot dish.

---

LESSON TWELFTH.
CARROTS.

To Boil *Carrots:*

**1.** Put *two quarts of warm water* into a saucepan, with *one good tablespoonful of salt* and a small piece of *soda* the size of a chestnut, and put it on the fire to boil.

**2.** Take the carrots and cut off the green tops, and wash them well in cold water.

**3.** Scrape the carrots clean with a sharp knife, and carefully remove any black specks.

**4.** If the carrots are very large, cut them in halves and quarters.

**5.** When the water in the saucepan is quite boiling, put in the carrots and let them boil until they are tender.

> N. B.—*Young carrots* need not be cut up, nor do they take so long to boil as *old ones.*

**6.** For serving, turn the carrots into a colander to drain, and then put them on a hot dish.

---

LESSON THIRTEENTH.
RICE.

To Boil *Rice:*

**1.** Take a large stewpan and pour in it *four quarts of water*.

**2.** Put the stewpan on the fire to boil the *water*.

**3.** Take *half a pound of rice*, put it in a basin of cold water, and wash it well.

**4.** Drain off the water and rub the *rice* with your hands.

**5.** Be careful to pick out all the yellow grains and bits of black.

**6.** Wash the rice in this manner four times.

**7.** Just before putting the rice on to boil, you must pour some fresh cold water over it.

**8.** When the water in the stewpan is quite boiling, throw the rice into it, stirring it round with a spoon.

**9.** Add one-quarter of a teaspoonful of salt, which will make the scum rise.

**10.** Take a spoon and skim it occasionally.

**11.** The *rice* should boil fast from *fifteen* to *twenty minutes*.

> N. B.—To test if the rice is sufficiently boiled, take out a grain or two, and press it between the thumb and finger, and if quite done, it will mash.

**12.** Now pour the rice out of the saucepan into a colander, to drain off the water.

**13.** Take the colander which contains the rice and hold it under the tap.

**14.** Turn the tap and let the cold water run on to the *rice* for *one* or *two seconds*. This is to separate the grains of rice.

**15.** Take a clean dry stewpan and put it at the side of the fire.

**16.** When the water is quite drained from the rice, turn it from the colander into the dry stewpan at the side of the fire.

**17.** Put the lid half on the stewpan.

**18.** Watch it, and stir it occasionally, to prevent the grains from sticking to the bottom of the stewpan.

**19.** When the rice is quite dry, take it out carefully with a wooden spoon, and place it lightly on to a hot dish.

9

LESSON FOURTEENTH.

MACARONI.

**Ingredients.**—One-half a pound of macaroni. Salt. One quart of skimmed milk. Two ounces of cheese. One ounce of butter. Pepper and Cayenne pepper.

*Time required, about one hour and three-quarters.*

### To Cook *Macaroni* :

**1.** Take *half a pound of macaroni*, wash it, and put it in a saucepan of *cold water*, with *one tablespoonful of salt*.

**2.** Put the saucepan on the fire, bring it to the boil, and let it boil gently for *half an hour*.

**3.** After that time, pour the water out of the saucepan.

**4.** Put *one quart of skimmed milk* into the saucepan.

**5.** Put the saucepan on the fire, just bring it to the boil, and then move it to the side of the fire, and let it simmer gently for *one hour*.

**6.** When the macaroni is sufficiently cooked and quite tender, turn it out on a hot dish, and it can be eaten with sugar or treacle.

N. B.—If liked, *macaroni* and *cheese* can be made of it.

**7.** For *macaroni* and *cheese*, take *two ounces of cheese* and grate it with a grater on to a piece of paper.

**8.** Take a dish, or a tin, and grease it well inside with a piece of dripping or butter.

**9.** When the macaroni is sufficiently cooked (as above), turn it out of the saucepan on to the greased dish.

**10.** Sprinkle over it *pepper* and *salt*, and two or three grains of *Cayenne pepper*, according to taste; or, about *half a teaspoonful of mustard* might be mixed with it.

**11.** Stir part of the grated cheese into the macaroni, and sprinkle the remainder over the top.

**12.** Take *one ounce of butter*, cut it in small pieces, and put these pieces of butter about on the top of the macaroni.

**13.** Put the dish in the oven (the heat should rise to 240°), or in a Dutch oven before the fire, for *ten minutes ;* it should become a pale-brown.

**14.** It will then be ready for serving.

---

LESSON FIFTEENTH.

STEWED MACARONI.

**Ingredients.**—Half a pound of macaroni. Salt and pepper. One pint of stock.

*Time required, about forty minutes.*

To Stew *Macaroni :*

**1.** Take *half a pound of macaroni*, wash it, and put it in a saucepan, with plenty of *cold water* and a *dessert-spoonful of salt.*

**2.** Put the saucepan on the fire, bring it to the boil, and let it boil gently for *ten minutes.*

**3.** After that time, put the macaroni into a colander, take it to the tap, and turn some cold water on it.

**4.** Now let the macaroni drain in the colander.

**5.** Then turn it on a board and cut it up in pieces.

**6.** Put one pint of stock into a saucepan.

**7.** Put the macaroni into the stock, and season it with *pepper* and *salt* according to taste.

**8.** Put the saucepan on the fire, just bring it to the boil, and then move the saucepan to the side of the fire, and let it simmer gently for *twenty minutes.*

N. B.—The lid should be on the saucepan.

**9.** For serving, turn the macaroni out on a hot dish.

# CHAPTER XII.

## SAUCES.

LESSON FIRST.

### WHITE SAUCE.

**Ingredients.**—One pint of white stock. Two ounces of butter. One and one-half ounce of flour. Six mushrooms. Half a pint of cream.

*Time required (if the stock is made), about half an hour.*

To make *White Sauce:*

1. Put *two ounces of butter* into a stewpan.

2. Put the stewpan on the fire, and when the butter is melted, stir in *one ounce and a half of flour* with a wooden spoon.

3. Add one pint of white stock, and stir it until it boils (*see* Lesson on "Stock").

4. Take half a dozen mushrooms, wash them, and peel them.

5. Add them to the sauce.

6. Let it come to the boil again; then move the stewpan to the side of the fire, with the lid half on, to simmer for *twenty minutes*, to throw up the butter.

7. As the butter rises, skim it off with an iron spoon.

**8.** Strain the sauce through a tammy-cloth into another saucepan.

**9.** Put this saucepan on the fire, and stir till it boils; then add half a pint of cream.

**10.** Pour it into a basin and stir while it cools. It is then ready for use.

---

LESSON SECOND.

BROWN SAUCE.

**Ingredients.**—One pint of brown stock.  One and one-half ounce of flour.  Salt and pepper.  Two ounces of butter.  Four mushrooms.

*Time required, about fifteen minutes.*

To make *Brown Sauce :*

**1.** Put *two ounces of butter* into a stewpan, and put it on the fire to melt.

**2.** Take *four mushrooms*, if large, or six small, wash them well in cold water, cut off the ends of the stalks, and peel them.

**3.** When the butter in the stewpan is melted, stir in *two ounces of flour*, and mix them into a smooth paste with a wooden spoon.

**4.** Now add one pint of brown stock and the mushrooms, and stir the sauce smoothly over the fire until it boils and thickens.

> N. B.—The *mushrooms* might be omitted if liked, and the *sauce* flavored according to the dish with which it is to be served.

**5.** Then move the stewpan to the side of the fire, and let it simmer gently for ten minutes.

**6.** Watch it carefully, and skim off all the *butter* as it rises to the top of the *sauce*.

**7.** Season the *sauce* with *pepper* and *salt* according to taste.

N. B.—If the *sauce* is not brown enough in color, a *teaspoonful of caramel (burnt sugar)* might be stirred into it.

**8.** Now strain the sauce through a tammy-sieve into a basin, and it is then ready for use.

---

LESSON THIRD.

MAYONNAISE SAUCE.

**Ingredients.**—Two eggs. Salt and pepper. One teaspoonful of French vinegar. One teaspoonful of mustard. One teaspoonful of tarragon vinegar. One gill of salad-oil.

*Time required, about ten minutes.*

To make *Mayonnaise Sauce:*

**1.** Take *two eggs*, and put the *yolks* in one basin and the whites (which will not be wanted) into another basin.

**2.** Take a wooden spoon and just stir the yolks enough to break them.

**3.** Add to them a *salt-spoonful of salt* and *half a salt-spoonful of pepper*, and a *tablespoonful of French vinegar*.

**4.** Take a bottle of *salad-oil*, and, putting your thumb half over the top, pour in, drop by drop, the oil, stirring well with a whisk the whole time. A gill of the oil will be enough.

N. B.—Add a *teaspoonful* of ready-made mustard, or tarragon vinegar if liked, stirring it in smoothly.

**5.** The sauce is now ready for use.

---

LESSON FOURTH.

SAUCE PIQUANTE.

**Ingredients.**—One shallot. Half a carrot. Three mushrooms. One ounce of butter. One ounce of flour. Half a pint of good brown stock. One sprig of thyme. One bay-leaf. Salt and Cayenne pepper. Two table-spoonfuls of vinegar.

*Time required, about twenty-five minutes.*

To make *Sauce Piquante,* or *Sharp Sauce :*

**1.** Take a shallot and three mushrooms, and peel them, scrape half a carrot, and then chop them up very finely on a board.

**2.** Put the shallot, carrot, and mushrooms into a stew-pan with *one ounce of butter.*

**3.** Put the stewpan on the fire and fry them brown.

**4.** Then stir in *one ounce of flour* and *half a pint of good brown stock* (*see* Lesson on "Stock").

**5.** Also add *one sprig of thyme,* a *bay-leaf,* and *one tablespoonful of Harvey sauce,* and stir the sauce well until it boils.

**6.** Then remove the stewpan to the side of the fire, and let it simmer for *twenty minutes.*

**7.** Season the sauce with *salt* according to taste, a few grains of Cayenne pepper, and two tablespoonfuls of vinegar.

**8.** Strain the sauce, and it is then ready for use.

## LESSON FIFTH.

### DUTCH SAUCE.

**Ingredients.**—Half a pint of melted butter.   Five yolks of eggs.   Salt and Cayenne pepper.   Two teaspoonfuls of lemon-juice.

*Time required, about ten minutes.*

To make *Dutch Sauce:*

1. Take half a pint of melted butter and put it into a stewpan.

2. Add the yolks of five eggs.

3. Stand the stewpan in a saucepan of hot water over the fire, and stir well with a wooden spoon.

4. Season it with salt and a few grains of Cayenne pepper.

5. Stir continually until it thickens; and you must not let the sauce boil, or it will curdle.

6. Just before the sauce is finished, stir in two teaspoonfuls of lemon-juice.

# CHAPTER XIII.

## *PASTRY.*

---

### PUFF-PASTE.

**Ingredients.**—Quarter of a pound of flour.   Quarter of a pound of fresh butter.   Yolk of one egg.   Salt.   A few drops of lemon-juice.

*Time required, one hour and a quarter.*

To make *Puff-Paste :*

**1.** Take a *quarter of a pound of flour* and put it in a heap on a clean board, and make a well in the centre of the flour.

**2.** Put half of the yolk of an egg in the well.

**3.** Add six drops of lemon-juice.

**4.** Lay a quarter of a pound of butter in a clean cloth.

**5.** Fold the cloth over the butter and squeeze it, to get all the water out of the butter.

**6.** Mix all these ingredients together with your hands, adding water to make the paste of the same consistence as the squeezed butter.

**7.** Take a rolling-pin and flour it, and also sprinkle a little flour on the board, to prevent the paste from sticking.

**8.** Roll out the paste rather thin, to about a quarter of an inch in thickness.

**9.** Place the pat of squeezed butter on one-half of the paste, and fold the other half over the butter so as to cover it entirely, pressing the edges together with your thumb.

**10.** Let it stand on a plate in a cool place for a quarter of an hour.

> N. B.—It is not necessary to do this in cold weather; it might be rolled at once.

**11.** Bring the paste back and place it on the board; roll it out with the rolling-pin, and fold it over in three.

**12.** Turn it round, with the rough edges toward you.

**13.** Roll it again and fold it in three.

**14.** Put it aside again for a quarter of an hour.

**15.** Bring it back on the board and roll it with a rolling-pin, and fold in three twice, as before.

**16.** Put it aside again for a quarter of an hour.

**17.** Bring it back to the board and roll it and fold it in three as before.

**18.** Put it aside for another quarter of an hour.

**19.** Bring it back to the board and roll it out ready either to cover an apple-tart, to make tartlets, or patty-cases.

**20.** If the paste is used for an apple-tart, put it over the apples in the same way as the short crust over the fruit-tart (*see* " Pastry," Lesson Second).

**21.** If the paste is used for tartlets, it should be one-eighth of an inch thick.

**22.** Take the *tartlet-tins* and wet them with the *paste-brush*.

**23.** Cut the paste out with a cutter a size larger than the tins. The cutter must be floured, or the paste will stick to it.

**24.** Fix the paste into the tins, and put a *dummy*, to prevent the paste rising straight.

**25.** Put the tins on a baking-sheet.

**26.** Put the baking-sheet in a hot oven for *six minutes;* the *heat* of the *oven* should rise to 300° Fahr., according to the thermometer fixed in the oven.

**27.** When the *tartlets* are baked sufficiently, take them out of the oven.

**28.** Take out the dummies, and turn the paste out of the tin.

**29.** Fill in the tartlets with jam.

If *Patty-Cases* are required:

**1.** Take the *puff-paste* (it should be half an inch thick) and stamp it out with a round cutter, the usual size of an oyster patty.

**2.** Take these cut rounds and place them on a baking-sheet.

**3.** Take a round cutter, three sizes smaller, and dip it in hot water, and stamp the cut rounds of paste in the centre, but not right through.

**4.** Put the baking-sheet in a *hot* oven for *six minutes.*

N. B.—The *heat* of the *oven* should be the same as for *tartlets.*

**5.** When the *patties* are sufficiently baked, take the baking-sheet out of the oven.

**6.** The cut centre of each patty-case will have risen so that we can take it off.

**7.** Take a small knife, and with the point cut out all moist paste from the centre of the patty-case.

**8.** Now the cases are ready to be filled in with either prepared oysters, minced veal, chicken, or pheasant, etc., according to taste.

## LESSON SECOND.

### SHORT CRUST.

**Ingredients.**—Six ounces of flour. Four ounces of butter. One ounce of powdered sugar. Yolk of one egg. Salt. A teaspoonful of lemon-juice.

*Time required for making, about a quarter of an hour.*

To make *Short Crust :*

**1.** Take *six ounces of flour* and *four ounces of butter.*

**2.** Put these on a clean board and mix them well together, rubbing them lightly with your hands until there are no lumps of butter left, and the flour and butter resemble sifted bread-crumbs.

**3.** Take a large tablespoonful of powdered sugar.

**4.** Mix the sugar well into the buttered flour.

**5.** Heap it on the board, making a well in the centre.

**6.** Take the *yolk of one egg* and place it in the well.

**7.** Sprinkle a quarter of a salt-spoonful of salt over the egg.

**8.** Add a teaspoonful of lemon-juice.

**9.** Add a large tablespoonful of cold water.

**10.** Slowly and lightly mix all these ingredients with your fingers until they are formed into a stiff paste.

**11.** Keep your hands and the board well floured, that the *paste* may not stick.

**12.** Fold the paste over, and knead it lightly with your knuckles.

**13.** Take a rolling-pin and *flour* it, and roll out the paste to the size and thickness required.

**14.** If the paste is for a fruit-tart, roll it out to the shape of the pie-dish, only a little larger, and to the thickness of about a *quarter of an inch.*

15. Arrange the fruit in the pie-dish, heaped up in the centre.

16. Sprinkle a tablespoonful of moist sugar over the fruit, or more or less, according to the fruit used.

17. Take a paste-brush, and wet the edge of the dish with water or a little white of egg.

18. Cut a strip of the paste the width of the edge of the pie-dish, and place it round the edge of the dish.

19. Take the paste-brush again, and wet the edge of the paste with water or white of egg.

20. Take the remaining paste and lay it over the pie-dish, pressing it down with your thumb all round the edge.

21. Be very careful not to break the paste.

22. Take a knife and trim off all the rough edges of the paste round the edge of the dish.

23. Take a knife and with the back of the blade make little notches in the edge of the paste, pressing the paste firmly with your thumb, to keep it in its proper place.

24. Take a skewer and make a little hole through the *paste* on either side of the tart, to let out the steam.

25. Take the paste-brush and wet the tart all over with water.

26. Sprinkle some powdered sugar over it; this is to glaze it.

27. Now put the tart into a hot oven (the *heat* of the *oven* should rise to 240° Fahr.) for *half an hour* or *three-quarters of an hour*, according to the size of the tart. Watch it occasionally, and turn it, to prevent its burning. It should become a pale-brown.

LESSON THIRD.

### GENOESE PASTRY.

**Ingredients.**—Six ounces of flour.  Six ounces of butter.  Eight ounces of powdered sugar.  Seven eggs.

*Time required, about one hour.*

To make *Genoese Pastry :*

**1.** Take a small stewpan and put in it *six ounces of butter.*

**2.** Put the stewpan on the fire, to melt the butter. Be careful that it does not burn or boil.

**3.** Take a round tin two inches deep, and fit into it a sheet of paper, cut round so that it will allow one inch of paper to be above the edge of the tin.

**4.** Butter the paper with a paste-brush dipped in the melted butter.

**5.** Stand a wire sieve over a plate, and rub through it *six ounces of flour.*

**6.** Take a large basin and break into it *seven eggs.*

**7.** Add *half a pound of powdered sugar.*

**8.** Take a large saucepan of boiling water and put it on the fire.

**9.** Stand the basin with the eggs and sugar in the saucepan of boiling water, and whip the eggs and sugar for twenty minutes ; they must not get very hot.

**10.** Take the basin out of the saucepan and stand it on the table.

**11.** Now add the butter, and then sprinkle in the sifted flour, stirring lightly with a wooden spoon all the time.

**12.** Pour this mixture into the prepared tin.

**13.** Put the tin into a quick oven, to bake for half an hour.  The mixture should become a pale-brown.

N. B.—When the paste is sufficiently baked, no mark should remain on it if pressed with the finger.

**14.** When it is quite baked, take the tin out of the oven and turn the cake upside down on a hair-sieve, to cool.

**15.** When it is cold, cut it into little shapes with a cutter. Sandwiches of jam can be made with it if required.

---

LESSON FOURTH.

ROUGH PUFF-PASTE.

**Ingredients.**—Eight ounces of flour. Six ounces of butter. The yolk of one egg. Salt. One-half a teaspoonful of lemon-juice.

*Time required, about a quarter of an hour.*

To make *Rough Puff-Paste:*

**1.** Take *eight ounces of flour* and *six ounces of butter*, and put them on a clean board.

**2.** Take a knife and chop up the butter in the flour.

**3.** Heap it on the board, making a well in the centre.

**4.** Take the yolk of one egg and place it in the well.

**5.** Sprinkle a *quarter of a salt-spoonful of salt* over the egg, and squeeze *half a teaspoonful of lemon-juice.*

**6.** Add a *large tablespoonful of cold water*, and beat it up slightly with a knife.

**7.** Now slowly, and lightly, mix it all with your fingers, adding more water if necessary, until it is formed into a stiff paste.

**8.** Keep your hands and the board well floured, that the paste may not stick.

**9.** Take a rolling-pin, flour it, and roll out the paste, and fold it over in half.

**10.** Turn it round with the rough edges toward you.

**11.** Roll it again, and fold it in half.

**12.** Roll out the paste and fold it twice more, as before.

> N.B.—The paste is now ready to be used for a meat-pie, apple-tart, tartlets, etc. The *heat* of the *oven* should rise to 280°, but it must be reduced down to 220° after the first *quarter of an hour.*

---

## LESSON FIFTH.

### SUET-CRUST FOR BEEF-STEAK PUDDING.

**Ingredients.**—Half a pound of flour. Five ounces of beef-suet. Two pounds of rump or beef steak. Pepper and salt. One dozen oysters. One gill of stock.

*Time required, about three hours and a half.*

To make *Suet-Crust,* to be used for either a *Beef-steak Pudding* or *Roly-Poly,* etc.:

**1.** Take *five ounces of beef-suet* and put it on a board.

**2.** Take a knife and cut away all the skin, and chop up the *suet* as fine as possible.

**3.** Put *half a pound of flour* into a basin, and add to it the *chopped suet* and *a teaspoonful of salt.*

**4.** Rub the suet well into the flour with your hands.

**5.** Then add, by degrees, enough cold water to make it into a smooth paste. You should mix it well.

**6.** Take the paste out of the basin, and put it on a board.

**7.** Take a rolling-pin and flour it. Sprinkle flour on the board, to prevent the paste from sticking.

**8.** Roll out the paste once, to the thickness of rather more than one-eighth of an inch.

> N.B.—Now the paste is ready for use; and if it is required for beef-steak pudding—

9. Take a quart pudding-basin and butter it well inside.

10. Line the basin smoothly inside with paste.

11. Take a knife, flour it, and cut away the paste that is above the edge of the basin.

12. Fold this paste together, and roll it out to a round the size of the top of the basin, one-eighth of an inch in thickness.

13. Take *two pounds of rump or beef steak*, put it on a board, and cut it into thin slices.

14. Flour the slices well (using about *a tablespoonful of flour*), and season them with plenty of *pepper* and *salt*.

15. Take *one dozen oysters* and the liquor that is with them, and put them into a saucepan.

16. Put the saucepan on the fire, and just bring them to the boil.

N. B.—This is to blanch the oysters.

17. Take the saucepan off the fire, and strain the *oyster-liquor* into a basin.

18. Take the oysters and lay them on a plate.

19. Cut off the beards and all the hard parts of the oysters, leaving only the soft part.

20. Roll up the slices of beef-steak, and fill the basin with the meat and the oysters.

N. B.—If oysters be disliked, kidneys might be used instead, or the pudding might be flavored with shallot, parsley, and mushrooms, according to taste.

21. Now pour into the basin the liquor from the oysters, and *one gill of stock* (*see* Lesson on "Stock").

22. Wet the paste round the edge of the basin with *cold water*, and cover over the top of the basin with the round of paste.

**23.** Join the paste together at the edge of the basin, pressing down with your thumb.

**24.** Flour a pudding-cloth and lay it over the top of the basin, tying it on tightly with a piece of twine.

**25.** Put a large saucepan of warm water on the fire to boil.

**26.** When it is quite boiling, put in the pudding and let it boil for three hours.

**27.** For serving, take off the cloth and turn the pudding out of the basin on to a hot dish.

---

### LESSON SIXTH.

#### SHORT CRUST FOR APPLE TURNOVERS AND APPLE DUMPLINGS.

**Ingredients.**—Three-quarters of a pound of flour. One-quarter of a pound of clarified dripping or butter. Half a teaspoonful of baking-powder. Three apples. Three teaspoonfuls of moist sugar.

To make *Apple Turnovers :*

**1.** Peel, quarter, and core three apples, and cut them into thin slices.

> N. B.—One apple is required for each turnover.

> N. B.—To make fruit-pie or apple dumplings, *see* below.

**2.** Put *three-quarters of a pound* of *flour* into a basin, and mix into it half a teaspoonful of baking-powder.

**3.** Rub well into the flour, with your hands, a quarter of a pound of clarified dripping or butter.

**4.** Add enough *cold water* to moisten, and mix into a stiff paste.

**5.** Flour a board and turn the paste on to it.

**6.** Flour a rolling-pin, and roll out the paste to about a quarter of an inch in thickness.

**7.** Cut the paste into rounds; each round should be about the size of a small plate.

**8.** Lay the apple on one-half of the round of paste, and sprinkle over it one teaspoonful of moist sugar.

**9.** Wet the edges of the paste, fold the paste over the apple, pressing the edges together with your thumb.

> N. B.—Be careful to join the paste together on all sides, or the juice of the apple will run out while it is cooling.

**10.** Grease a tin with a little dripping, and place the turnovers on it.

**11.** Put the tin into the oven (the heat of it should rise to 220°) to bake for *a quarter of an hour*.

**12.** For serving, place the turnovers on a hot dish.

For *Baked Apple Dumplings :*

**1.** Divide the paste into three portions.

**2.** Take three apples, peel them, and cut out the core from the centre.

> N. B.—Do not cut the apples in pieces.

**3.** Fill the centre of the *apples* with *moist sugar*.

**4.** Press each *apple* into the centre of each *portion of paste*, and gradually work the *paste* over the *apple*, until the *apple* is entirely covered in.

> N. B.—You must be very careful to join the paste together as neatly as possible, so as not to show the join; and there must be no cracks in the paste.

**5.** Grease a tin as described above, place the dumplings

on it, and put it in the oven (the heat should rise to 220°) to bake for *a quarter of an hour*.

6. For serving, take the dumplings off the tin, and put them on a hot dish.

1. If the *paste* is for a *Fruit-Pie*, roll it out to the shape of the pie-dish, only a little larger, and to the thickness of about *a quarter of an inch*.

2. Arrange the fruit in the pie-dish, heaped up in the centre.

3. Sprinkle a tablespoonful of moist sugar over the fruit, or more or less, according to the *fruit* used.

4. Take a paste-brush and wet the edge of the dish with water, or a little white of egg.

5. Cut a strip of the paste the width of the edge of the pie-dish, and place it round the edge of the dish.

6. Take the paste-brush again and wet the edge of the paste with water or white of egg.

7. Take the remaining paste and lay it over the pie-dish, pressing it down with your thumb all round the edge.

8. Be very careful not to break the paste.

9. Take a knife and trim off all the rough edges of the paste round the edge of the dish.

10. Take a knife, and with the back of the blade make little notches in the edge of the paste, pressing the paste firmly with your thumb to keep it in its proper place.

11. Take a *skewer* and make a little *hole* through the *paste* on either side of the *tart*, to let out the steam.

12. Take the paste-brush and wet the tart all over with water.

13. Sprinkle some pounded loaf-sugar over the tart, to glaze it.

14. Now put it into the oven (the heat should rise to

240°) for half or three-quarters of an hour, according to the size of the tart. Look at it occasionally, and turn it to prevent its burning. It should become a pale-brown.

N. B.—If better crust is wanted for apple turnovers, *see* "Pastry," Lesson Second.

---

## LESSON SEVENTH.

### FLAKY CRUST FOR PIES AND TARTS.

**Ingredients.**—One pound of flour. Half a pound of butter. Two eggs. One teaspoonful of baking-powder.

*Time required to make the pastry, about a quarter of an hour.*

To make *Flaky Crust* for *Pies* or *Tarts :*

1. Put *one pound of flour* into a basin, and mix into it a *teaspoonful of baking-powder.*

2. Break *two eggs*, put the *whites* on a plate (the yolks put aside in a cup), and whip them to a stiff froth with a knife.

3. Add the whipped whites of the eggs to the flour, and mix it into a stiff paste with water (about one gill).

4. *Flour* a board and turn the paste out on it.

5. Take a rolling-pin, flour it, and roll out the paste to a thin sheet.

6. Divide the *half pound of butter* into *three portions.*

7. Take one portion of the butter and spread it all over the paste with a knife.

8. Sprinkle a little flour over the butter, and fold the *paste* into three.

9. Flour the rolling-pin and roll out the paste, and spread another portion of the butter over it.

10. Fold the paste as before, roll it out, and add the remainder of the butter.

**11.** Then fold the paste again, and roll it out to the size and thickness required either for a fruit-pie or an open tart.

N. B.—This crust should be baked in a quick oven (the heat should rise to 240°).

N. B.—The top of a fruit-pie should be brushed over with *water*, and then sprinkled with pounded white sugar.

N. B.—For an open tart, take a tin (the size required) and grease it with clarified dripping or butter. Roll out the *paste* to a thin sheet about a quarter of an inch in thickness, and rather larger than the size of the tin. Place the paste in the greased tin, pressing it into the shape of the tin with your thumb. Place a dummy, or a piece of crust of bread, in the centre of the paste, to prevent the paste from rising while baking. Put the tin in the oven to bake for twenty minutes. The jam should be put into the tart after it is baked.

# CHAPTER XIV.

## PUDDINGS.

LESSON FIRST.

### CABINET PUDDING.

**Ingredients.**—One dozen cherries or raisins, and two or three pieces of angelica. One dozen finger-biscuits and half a dozen ratafias. One ounce of loaf-sugar and fifteen drops of essence of vanilla. Four eggs. One pint of milk.

*Time required, about one hour.*

To make a *Cabinet Pudding :*

**1.** Take a *pint-and-a-half mould* and *butter* it inside with your fingers.

**2.** Take a *dozen raisins* or *dried cherries*, and two or three pieces of *angelica,* and ornament the bottom of the mould with them.

**3.** Take *one dozen* stale sponge *finger-biscuits* [1] and break them in pieces.

**4.** Partly fill the mould with pieces of cake and half a dozen *ratafias.* [2]

**5.** Take *four yolks* and *two whites of eggs* and put them in a basin.

---

[1] To be had at the baker's.
[2] For sale at all large grocery-houses.

**6.** Add to the eggs one ounce of white sugar, and whip them together lightly.

**7.** Stir in, by degrees, one pint of milk.

**8.** Flavor it by adding fifteen drops of essence of vanilla.

**9.** Pour this mixture over the cakes in the mould.

**10.** Place a piece of *buttered paper* over the top of the mould.

**11.** Take a saucepan half full of boiling water, and stand it on the side of the fire.

**12.** Stand the mould in the saucepan, to steam for from three-quarters of an hour to an hour.

> N. B.—The water should only reach half-way up the mould, or it would boil over and spoil the *pudding*.

**13.** For serving, turn the pudding carefully out of the mould on to a hot dish.

> N. B.—For a *cold* "Cabinet Pudding," *see* "Puddings," Lesson Twenty-seventh.

---

LESSON SECOND.

LEMON PUDDING.

**Ingredients.**—Three lemons. Six ounces of sugar. Six eggs. One gill of cream. One gill of milk. Three ounces of cake-crumbs. One inch of cinnamon-stick.

*Time required, about one hour.*

To make a *Lemon Pudding:*

**1.** Take *three lemons,* wipe them clean in a cloth, and grate the rind of them on *six lumps of sugar.*

**2.** Take an inch of the stick of cinnamon and put it in a mortar.

**3.** Pound the cinnamon well in the mortar with the sugar.

**4.** Put this into a basin.

**5.** Take three ounces of cake-crumbs and add to the above in the basin, and mix all well together.

**6.** Take the three lemons, cut them in halves, and squeeze the juice of them into the basin through a strainer.

**7.** Add the *yolks of six eggs*, and beat them in with the above. (Two of the whites of eggs put on a plate, the others put aside.)

**8.** Stir in well and smoothly *one gill of cream* and *one gill of milk* with a wooden spoon.

**9.** Whip the whites of the two eggs to a stiff froth with a knife, and add them at the last moment to the above mixture, stirring it lightly.

**10.** Take a pie-dish and line the edge of it with puff-paste (*see* "Pastry," Lesson First).

**11.** Pour the mixture into the pie-dish.

**12.** Put the pie-dish in the oven (the heat of it should rise to 220°), to bake till the mixture is set and of a light-brown color. It is then ready for serving.

<hr>

LESSON THIRD.

APPLE CHARLOTTE.

**Ingredients.**—Two pounds of apples. Half a pound of loaf-sugar. The rind of one lemon. Bread and clarified butter.

*Time required, about two hours and a half.*

To make an *Apple Charlotte:*

**1.** Take *two pounds of good cooking-apples* and peel them thinly with a sharp knife.

**2.** Take a knife and cut them in *slices*, and take out the *core*.

**3.** Put these sliced apples into a stewpan, with sufficient sugar to sweeten them, and one gill of water.

10

**4.** Take a *lemon,* wipe it clean in a cloth, and peel it very thin.

**5.** Take the rind of the lemon and tie it together with a piece of twine, and put it in the stewpan with the apples.

**6.** Put the stewpan on the fire, and stir well with a wooden spoon until it boils, and the apples are reduced to about half the quantity. It will take from one hour to one hour and a half.

**7.** Take the stewpan off the fire and stand it on a piece of paper on the table, and take out the lemon-peel.

**8.** Take a plain round tin mould (about one pint and a half).

**9.** Cut a slice of the crumb of bread, one-eighth of an inch in thickness, and round to the size of the mould.

**10.** Put a quarter of a pound of butter in a stewpan to melt and clarify.

**11.** Cut the round of bread into quarters, dip them in the clarified butter, and place them at the bottom of the mould.

**12.** Now cut slices of the crumb of bread one-eighth of an inch in thickness, and the depth of the mould in length.

**13.** Cut these slices into strips an inch wide.

**14.** Dip these strips into the clarified butter, and place them round inside the mould, allowing them to lie half over each other.

**15.** Now pour the apples into the middle of the mould.

**16.** Cover the apples with a round of bread dipped in the clarified butter.

**17.** Put the mould into a good oven (the *heat* of the oven should be about 220°), to bake for *three-quarters of an hour.*

N. B.—The bread should be quite brown and crisp.

**18.** For serving, turn it carefully out of the mould on to a hot dish.

LESSON FOURTH.

PANCAKES.

**Ingredients.**—Three ounces of flour. Two eggs. Half a pint of milk. Half a salt-spoonful of salt. Three ounces of lard. The juice of one-quarter of a lemon. Two ounces of moist sugar.

*Time required, about twenty minutes.*

To make *Pancakes* (this quantity will make about eight):

1. Take three ounces of flour and put it in a basin.
2. Add a salt-spoonful of salt, and mix it well into the flour.
3. Break two eggs into the flour, and add a dessert-spoonful of milk, and mix all well together with a wooden spoon.
4. Stir in gradually half a pint of milk, making the mixture very smooth.

> N.B.—If possible, it is better to let this mixture stand before frying it into pancakes.

5. Put a frying-pan on the fire and put into it a piece of lard the size of a chestnut, and let it get quite hot, but it must not burn.
6. Then pour into the frying-pan two large table-spoonfuls of the batter, and let it run thinly all over the pan.
7. When the pancake has become a light-brown on one side, shake the pan, and toss the pancake over, to brown the other side the same.
8. Stand a plate on the hot plate, or in the front of the fire, to heat.

**9.** When the pancake is fried, turn it on to this heated plate.

**10.** Squeeze a few drops of lemon-juice, and sprinkle a little moist sugar over it.

**11.** Now roll it up and place it on the edge of the plate, so as to leave room for the remainder of the pancakes.

> N. B.—Fry all the pancakes in this manner, adding each time a piece of lard the size of a chestnut.

**12.** For serving, arrange the pancakes on a hot dish, placing one on the top of the other.

---

### LESSON FIFTH.

#### RICE PUDDING.

**Ingredients.**—One and a half ounce of rice. Butter. One tablespoonful of moist sugar. One pint of milk.

*Time required, about two hours.*

To make a plain *Rice Pudding :*

**1.** Take a *pint dish* and *butter* it well inside.

**2.** Take *one ounce and a half of rice* and wash it well in *two* or *three waters.*

**3.** Put the rice into a buttered dish and sprinkle over it a tablespoonful of moist sugar.

**4.** Fill up the dish with new milk.

> N. B.—Nutmeg may be grated, or pounded cinnamon be sifted, over the top of the pudding before it is put in the oven.

**5.** Put the dish into a moderate oven (the *heat* should be about 220°) to bake for *two hours.*

**6.** Watch it occasionally, and as the rice soaks up the milk, more milk should be added (carefully lifting up the skin and pouring the milk in at the side), so as to keep the dish always full.

## LESSON SIXTH.

### CUSTARD PUDDING.

**Ingredients.**—Four eggs. One pint of milk. Grated nutmeg. One table-spoonful of powdered sugar. Butter and flour for paste.

*Time required, about thirty-five minutes.*

To make a *Custard Pudding :*

1. Take a pint-and-a-half dish, butter it well inside, and line the edge with paste. (*See* "Pastry," Lesson Second.)

2. Break *four eggs* and put the *yolks* into a basin. (Put two whites of eggs on a plate, the others put aside.)

3. Stir one pint of milk in with the eggs.

4. Add a *tablespoonful of castor sugar.*

5. Whip the whites of the two eggs with a knife to a stiff froth and add it to the basin, mixing it all lightly.

6. Pour this custard into the buttered dish lined with paste.

7. Grate half a teaspoonful of nutmeg over the top.

8. Put the dish into a moderate oven (the heat should rise to 220°) to bake for half an hour. It is then ready for serving.

---

## LESSON SEVENTH.

### PLUM PUDDING.

**Ingredients.**—One-half pound of beef-suet. Half a pound of currants. Half a pound of sultanas, or raisins. One-quarter of a pound of mixed candied peel, viz., citron, lemon, and orange. One-quarter of a pound of bread-crumbs. One-quarter of a pound of flour. Half a pound of moist sugar. One lemon. Four eggs. One gill of milk. One wineglassful of brandy. Two ounces of almonds. One-quarter of a teaspoonful of salt. Half a nutmeg.

**Ingredients** (for wine or brandy sauce).—Three eggs.   One gill of cream or milk.   One wineglassful of brandy or sherry.   One dessertspoonful of sugar.

*Time required, about five hours and a half.*

### To make a *Plum Pudding :*

**1.** Put a saucepan of *warm water* on the fire to boil.

**2.** Take *half a pound of beef-suet,* put it on a board, cut away all the *skin,* and chop up the *suet* as finely as possible with a sharp knife.

**3.** Take *half a pound of currants,* wash them clean in water, and rub them dry in a cloth.

**4.** Take up the currants in handfuls, and drop them, a few at a time, on to a plate, so as to find out if there are any stones with them.

**5.** Take half a pound of sultana raisins and pick them over.

N. B.—If large *raisins* are used, they should be stoned.

**6.** Place a wire sieve over a piece of paper.

**7.** Take some crumb of bread and rub it through the sieve.   (There should be a quarter of a pound of bread-crumbs.)

**8.** Take a quarter of a pound of mixed peel—citron, lemon, and orange—and cut it up into small pieces.

**9.** Put a quarter of a pound of flour into a kitchen-basin, and add to it the chopped suet and half a teaspoonful of salt.

**10.** Rub the suet well into the flour with your hands.

N. B.—Be careful not to leave any lumps.

**11.** Now add the bread-crumbs, the currants and raisins, half a pound of moist sugar, and the pieces of candied peel, and mix all well together.

**12.** Take a *lemon*, wipe it clean in a cloth, and grate the *rind* of it into the basin.

**13.** Grate *half a nutmeg* into the basin, and add *two ounces of almonds* (previously blanched and chopped up finely).

**14.** Break *four eggs* into a basin, and add to them one gill of milk and a wineglassful of brandy.

**15.** Stir this into the ingredients in the basin, mixing them all together.

**16.** Take a strong pudding-cloth, sprinkle about a teaspoonful of flour over it, and lay it in a basin.

**17.** Turn the mixture from the basin into the centre of the floured cloth.

**18.** Tie up the pudding tightly in the cloth with a piece of string.

> N. B.—If preferred, the pudding might be put into a buttered mould, and a cloth tied over the top.

**19.** When the water in the saucepan is quite boiling, put in the pudding, and let it boil for *five hours*.

**20.** For serving, take the pudding out of the cloth and turn it on to a hot dish.

> N. B.—*Brandy* or *wine* sauce (*see* below) can be served with the pudding, if liked, either poured over it or served separately in a sauceboat.

### FOR BRANDY OR WINE SAUCE.

**1.** Put *three yolks of eggs* into a small stewpan.

**2.** Add a *dessertspoonful of pulverized sugar, one gill of cream* or *milk*, and a *wineglassful of brandy* or *sherry*, and whisk all well together with a whisk.

**3.** Take a saucepan, fill it half full of hot water, and put it on the fire.

**4.** Stand the stewpan in the saucepan of hot water and whisk the *sauce* well for about *six or eight minutes.*

N. B.—Be careful that the sauce does not boil, or it will curdle.

**5.** After that time take the stewpan out of the saucepan.

**6.** Pour the sauce over the plum pudding (*see* above), or into a sauce-boat.

------

LESSON EIGHTH.

VENNOISE PUDDING.

**Ingredients.**—Five ounces of crumb of bread. Two ounces of candied peel. Three ounces of powdered sugar. One ounce of lump sugar. One lemon. Four eggs. Half a pint of milk. One gill of cream. Three ounces of sultana raisins. One wineglassful of sherry.

*Time required, about two hours.*

To make a *Vennoise Pudding :*

**1.** Take a piece of stale *crumb of bread* (about five ounces), put it upon a board, and cut it up in the shape of dice.

**2.** Put the *bread* into a basin with three ounces of *powdered sugar* and three ounces of *sultana raisins.*

**3.** Take a *lemon,* wipe it clean with a cloth, and grate the *rind* of it into the basin.

**4.** Chop up *two ounces of candied peel* and put it into the basin.

**5.** Pour in a *wineglassful of sherry.*

**6.** Put a saucepan of warm water on the fire to boil.

**7.** Put *one ounce of lump sugar* into a stewpan and put it on the fire to brown.

**8.** When it has become a dark-brown color, add to it half a pint of milk, and stir it until the *milk* is sufficiently colored.

N. B.—Be careful that the sugar is quite dissolved, and no lumps left.

**9.** Then stand the stewpan on a piece of paper on the table.

**10.** Put the yolks of four eggs into a basin (the whites should be put aside, as they are not required for present use).

**11.** Pour the colored milk into the eggs, stirring well all the time.

**12.** Stir the milk and eggs into the ingredients in the basin.

**13.** Also add *one gill* of *cream*.

**14.** Take a *pint-and-a-half mould* and butter it inside.

**15.** Pour the pudding into the mould.

**16.** Butter a piece of kitchen-paper and lay it over the top of the mould.

**17.** When the water in the saucepan is quite boiling, place in the mould to steam (the water should only reach half-way up the mould, or it will boil over and get into the pudding).

**18.** Let the pudding steam for *one hour and a half.*

**19.** For serving, take the buttered paper off from the top of the mould, and turn the pudding out carefully on to a hot dish.

> N. B.—*German sauce* (*see* "Puddings," Lesson Tenth) can be served with the *pudding*, if liked, either poured round it or served separately in a sauce-boat.

---

LESSON NINTH.

AMBER PUDDING.

**Ingredients.**—Six apples.  Three ounces of moist sugar.  One lemon. Two ounces of butter.  Three eggs.  Puff-paste.

*Time required, about one hour and one-quarter.*

To make an *Amber Pudding :*

**1.** Take *six large apples,* peel them, cut out the core, and cut them up into slices.

2. Put the apples into a stewpan, with three ounces of moist sugar and two ounces of butter.

3. Take a *lemon*, wipe it clean with a cloth, and peel it as thin as possible with a sharp knife.

4. Cut the lemon in half and squeeze the juice through a strainer into the stewpan.

5. Also add the lemon-peel.

6. Put the stewpan on the fire and let it stew till the apples are quite tender (it will take about *three-quarters of an hour*).

7. Place a hair sieve over a large basin.

8. When the apples are sufficiently stewed, pour them on to the sieve and rub them through into the basin with a wooden spoon.

9. Stir the yolks of three eggs into the basin.

10. Take a pie-dish (about *one pint*), and line the edge with *puff-paste* (*see* "Pastry," Lesson First).

> N. B.—If you have no puff-paste, short paste (*see* "Pastry," Lesson Second) will do.

11. Pour the mixture into the pie-dish, and put it in the oven (the heat should be 240°) for *twenty minutes*.

12. Whip the whites of the eggs to a stiff froth.

13. When the pudding is a light-brown, take it out, spread the whipped whites of the eggs over the top, and sift about a *dessertspoonful* of powdered sugar over it.

14. Put the dish back in the oven till the *icing* is a light-brown ; the pudding is then ready for serving.

## LESSON TENTH.

### BROWN-BREAD PUDDING.

**Ingredients.**—A loaf of brown bread. One lemon. Half a teaspoonful of essence of vanilla. One gill of milk. One gill of cream. Four eggs. Three ounces of powdered sugar.

**Ingredients** (of German sauce).—Two eggs. One wineglassful of sherry. One dessertspoonful of powdered sugar.

*Time required, about one hour and a half.*

To make a *Brown-Bread Pudding :*

1. Take a *stale brown loaf* and cut off all the crust.

2. Put a wire sieve over a plate and rub the *crumb of bread* through it.

3. Put one gill of milk into a stewpan, and put it on the fire to boil.

4. Put five ounces of the bread-crumb into a basin, with three ounces of powdered sugar.

5. Take a *lemon*, wipe it clean in a cloth, and grate the rind over the bread-crumbs.

6. Add *half a teaspoonful of essence of vanilla.*

7. Put a stewpan full of warm water on the fire to boil.

8. When the milk boils, pour it over the crumbs.

9. Put *one gill* of *cream* into a basin, and whip it to a stiff froth with a whisk.

10. Add the *cream* to the other *ingredients*, and also stir in, one at a time, the yolks of four eggs (the whites of two of the eggs put on a plate, the others put aside).

11. Whip the whites of the two eggs to a stiff froth with a knife, and then stir them lightly into the basin, mixing all the ingredients together.

12. Take a *pint mould* and butter it well inside.

**13.** Pour the mixture into the mould, butter a piece of kitchen-paper, and place it over the top.

**14.** When the water in the stewpan is quite boiling, stand the mould in it to steam the pudding (the water should only reach half-way up the mould, or it will boil over and spoil the pudding).

**15.** Let it steam for *one hour and a quarter.*

**16.** For serving, take off the buttered paper, and turn the pudding on to a hot dish.

### GERMAN SAUCE.

**1.** Put the *yolks of two eggs* into a stewpan, with a *wineglassful of sherry* and a *dessertspoonful of powdered sugar.*

**2.** Put the stewpan on the fire and mill it with a whisk till it comes to a thick froth.

N. B.—Be careful that the sauce does not boil, or it will curdle.

**3.** Pour the sauce round the pudding.

### LESSON ELEVENTH.
### CARROT PUDDING.

**Ingredients.**—Three or four carrots. Three ounces of bread-crumbs. Two ounces of butter. Half a gill of cream. Two eggs. Half a gill of sherry. One ounce of powdered sugar. One tablespoonful of orange-flower water. Puff-paste.

*Time required, about three-quarters of an hour.*

To make a *Carrot Pudding:*

**1.** Take *three or four carrots* (according to their size), wash them, and scrape them clean with a knife.

**2.** Take a grater and grate all the *red part* of the carrots into a basin. There should be about a quarter of a pound.

**3.** Stand a wire sieve over a plate.

**4.** Take some crumb of bread and rub it through the sieve. There should be about three ounces of bread-crumbs.

**5.** Put the bread-crumbs into the basin with the carrot; also add *one ounce of powdered sugar.*

**6.** Put *two ounces of butter* into a stewpan, and put it on the fire to melt.

**7.** When the butter is melted, take the stewpan off the fire and stand it on a piece of paper on the table.

**8.** Then stir into it *half a gill of sherry, half a gill of cream,* and a *tablespoonful of orange-flour water.*

**9.** Add the yolks of two eggs (put the whites on a plate).

**10.** Whip the whites of the two eggs to a stiff froth with a knife, and then stir them lightly into the stewpan, mixing all the ingredients together.

**11.** Then pour the contents of the stewpan into the basin with the carrot and bread-crumbs, and mix them well together.

**12.** Take a pie-dish (about *one pint*) and line the edge of it with puff-paste (*see* "Pastry," Lesson First).

**13.** Pour the pudding into the pie-dish, and put it into the oven (the *heat* should be 240°) to bake for *half an hour;* it is then ready for serving.

---

LESSON TWELFTH.

ALEXANDRA PUDDING.

**Ingredients.**—Ten eggs. Two ounces of powdered sugar. One gill of milk. Half a pint of good cream. A teaspoonful of essence of vanilla.

*Time required, about one hour and twenty minutes.*

To make an *Alexandra Pudding :*

**1.** Put a saucepan of warm water on the fire to boil.

**2.** Put the *yolks of ten eggs* into a basin. (The *whites of five of the eggs* should be put in another basin; put the others aside.)

**3.** Stir into the yolks of the eggs two ounces of powdered sugar.

**4.** Add one gill of milk and half a pint of good cream.

**5.** Whip the whites of the five eggs slightly with a whisk or knife.

**6.** Take a plain tin mould (about one pint) and butter it inside; cover the bottom with three rounds of buttered paper.

**7.** Add the *whipped whites of the eggs* and a *teaspoonful of essence of vanilla* to the *mixture* in the basin, and stir all lightly together.

**8.** Pour the mixture through a strainer into the mould, and tie over it a piece of stiff paper with a string.

**9.** When the water in the saucepan boils, stand in the mould. (The water should reach only half-way up the mould, or it will boil over and spoil the pudding.)

**10.** Let it simmer gently until the pudding is quite firm. (It will take about *one hour and a quarter*.)

N. B.—It must on no account boil fast.

**11.** After that time, take the pudding out of the saucepan and stand it in ice.

**12.** For serving, take off the buttered paper and turn the pudding carefully out on to a dish, and ornament it with red currant jelly according to taste.

## LESSON THIRTEENTH.

### BLANC-MANGE.

**Ingredients.**—Four tablespoonfuls of corn-starch. One quart of milk. Three ounces of loaf-sugar. One inch of the stick of cinnamon, or lemon-peel.

*Time required to make, about a quarter of an hour, and about three-quarters of an hour to get cold.*

To make *Blanc-Mange:*

**1.** Put *one quart of milk* into a saucepan, with *three ounces of loaf-sugar* and *one inch of stick of cinnamon*, or the peel of a *quarter of a lemon*, for flavoring.

**2.** Put the saucepan on the fire to boil.

**3.** Put four tablespoonfuls of corn-starch into a basin, and mix it smoothly with a *tablespoonful of cold milk*.

**4.** When the milk in the saucepan is quite boiling, stir in the corn-starch quickly, and let it boil for *two minutes*, stirring continually.

N. B.—Be careful not to let it get lumpy.

**5.** Take a quart basin, or a mould, and rinse it out in cold water.

**6.** Now take the piece of cinnamon or lemon-peel out of the corn-starch, and pour the corn-starch into the basin, and put aside to cool.

**7.** When it is quite cold, turn it out of the basin on to a dish, and it is ready for serving.

## LESSON FOURTEENTH.

### BOILED BATTER PUDDING.

**Ingredients.**—Half a pound of flour.　Salt.　Two eggs.　One pint of milk.

*Time required, about two hours and fifteen minutes.*

To make a *Boiled Batter Pudding :*

**1.** Put a saucepan of warm water on the fire to boil.

**2.** Put *half a pound of flour* into a basin, and mix *half a salt-spoonful of salt* with it.

**3.** Break two eggs into the flour, and beat them well together.

**4.** Now add, by degrees, one pint of milk, stirring smoothly all the time, until the batter is well mixed.

**5.** Let the batter stand for one hour.

**6.** Take a pudding-basin and grease it inside with *butter.*

**7.** Stir the batter, and then pour it into the basin.

**8.** Dip a pudding-cloth in boiling water, wring it out, and flour it well.

**9.** Place the cloth over the batter, and tie it on securely with a piece of string, just below the rim of the basin.　Pin or tie the four corners of the cloth over the top.

**10.** When the water in the saucepan is quite boiling, put in the pudding, and let it boil for one hour.

**11.** For serving, take the basin out of the saucepan, take off the cloth, and turn the pudding carefully out on a hot dish.

LESSON FIFTEENTH.

CORN-STARCH PUDDING.

**Ingredients.**—Two dessertspoonfuls of corn-starch. Half a pint of milk. Six lumps of sugar. One egg.

*Time required, about an hour.*

To make a *Corn-Starch Pudding* (in a cup, for infants or invalids):

**1.** Put a saucepan half full of warm water on the fire to boil.

**2.** Put *two dessertspoonfuls of corn-starch* into a saucepan.

**3.** Pour in, by degrees, *half a pint of milk*, mixing it very smoothly.

N. B.—Be careful that it does not get lumpy.

**4.** Now add to it *six lumps of sugar*, put the saucepan on the fire, and stir smoothly until it boils; it will take about *ten minutes.*

**5.** Then move the saucepan to the side of the fire.

**6.** Break *one egg* into the saucepan, and beat it up until it is all well mixed.

**7.** Take a cup (just large enough to hold the pudding) and grease it inside with a piece of butter.

**8.** Pour the mixture out of the saucepan into the cup.

**9.** Take a small cloth, wring it out in boiling water, flour it well, and tie it over the top of the cup with a piece of string.

N. B.—Tie the four corners of the cloth over the top of the cup.

**10.** When the water in the saucepan is quite boiling, put in the cup, and let it boil for *twenty-five minutes.*

**11.** For serving, take the cloth off the cup, and the *pudding* may be turned out or not, according to taste.

----

LESSON SIXTEENTH.

BATTER PUDDING.

**Ingredients.**—One egg.   One tablespoonful of flour.   One teacupful of milk.   Salt.

*Time required, about thirty-five minutes to make, and thirty minutes to stand.*

To make *Batter Pudding* (in a cup, for infants or invalids):

**1.** Put a saucepan half full of warm water on the fire to boil.

**2.** Put a *tablespoonful of flour* into a basin, with a *few grains of salt.*

**3.** Break *one egg* into the basin, and mix it well into the *flour.*

**4.** Now add, by degrees, a *teacupful of milk*, stirring vigorously with a wooden spoon.

**5.** Let the batter stand for *half an hour.*

**6.** After that time, take a cup (just large enough to hold the *batter*), and grease it well inside with a piece of *butter.*

**7.** Stir the batter, and then pour it into the cup.

**8.** Take a small cloth, wring it out in boiling water, *flour* it well, and tie it over the top of the cup with a piece of string.

N.B.—Tie the four corners of the cloth together over the top of the cup.

**9.** When the water in the saucepan is quite boiling, put in the cup, and let it boil for *half an hour.*

**10.** For serving, take the cloth off the cup, and the pudding may be turned out or not, according to taste.

### CORN-STARCH PUDDING.

**Ingredients.**—Four tablespoonfuls of corn-starch. One quart of milk. Three tablespoonfuls of pounded sugar. Two eggs. One inch of the stick of cinnamon, or a bay-leaf. Grated nutmeg.

*Time required, about half an hour.*

To make a *Corn-Starch Pudding :*

**1.** Put *four tablespoonfuls of corn-starch* into a basin, and mix it quite smooth with a *tablespoonful of cold milk*.

**2.** Put the remainder of the *quart of milk* into a saucepan, with three tablespoonfuls of powdered sugar and one inch of cinnamon or a bay-leaf.

**3.** Put the saucepan on the fire to boil.

**4.** When the *milk* boils, pour it on the mixture, stirring it smoothly all the time.

**5.** Break *two eggs* into the *corn-starch*, and beat it lightly.

**6.** Grease a quart pie-dish with butter.

**7.** Pour the mixture into the pie-dish, and grate *half a teaspoonful of nutmeg* over the top.

**8.** Put the dish into the oven (the heat should be 220°) to bake *half an hour*.

**9.** It will then be ready for serving.

---

### RICE PUDDING.

**Ingredients.**—Half a pound of rice. One quart of milk. Two eggs. Two ounces of moist sugar. Two ounces of suet. Grated nutmeg.

*Time required, from forty minutes to an hour.*

To make a *Rice Pudding :*

**1.** Wash *half a pound of rice* in two or three waters,

and then put it into a saucepan of *cold water*, and put it on the fire till it boils and swells.

**2.** Break *two eggs* into a basin.

**3.** Add to them two ounces of moist sugar and one quart of milk, and stir them together.

**4.** Put *two ounces of suet* on a board, cut away all the skin, and shred it as fine as possible.

**5.** Take a quart dish and grease it inside with clarified dripping or butter.

**6.** Drain off the *rice* on a colander as dry as possible, and lay it in the greased dish.

**7.** Pour the mixture of *milk* and *eggs* over the *rice*, and sprinkle the *shredded suet* over the top.

**8.** Take a grater and grate *half a teaspoonful of nutmeg* over the top.

**9.** Put the dish into an oven (the *heat* should be 220°) to bake for from *forty minutes* to *an hour*.

**10.** After that time, it is ready for serving.

---

LESSON NINETEENTH.

CURATE'S PUDDING.

**Ingredients.**—One pound of potatoes. Three eggs. One pint of milk. Sugar.

*Time required, about one hour.*

To make a *Curate's* (or *Sweet Potato*) *Pudding:*

**1.** Wash one pound of potatoes and boil them (*see* "Vegetables," Lesson First).

> N. B.—Any remains of cold boiled potatoes may be used instead of fresh ones.

**2.** Rub these boiled potatoes through a colander into a basin with a wooden spoon.

**3.** Break *three eggs* into another basin, and stir into them *one pint of milk*.

**4.** Stir the milk and eggs smoothly into the potatoes, and add *sugar* to taste.

**5.** Grease a quart pie-dish, and pour the mixture into it.

**6.** Put it in the oven (the heat should be 220°) and bake half an hour; it will then be ready for serving.

---

### LESSON TWENTIETH.

#### BREAD PUDDING.

**Ingredients.**—One pound of scraps of bread. One quart of milk. Two eggs. Two tablespoonfuls of moist sugar. Four ounces of raisins or currants.

*Time required, three-quarters of an hour.*

To make a *Bread Pudding:*

**1.** Put *one pound of scraps of bread* into a basin with plenty of *cold water*, to soak.

> N.B.—Any scraps of bread, either crumb or crust, however stale, so long as they are not mouldy or burnt, can be used for this pudding.

**2.** Put *one quart of milk* into a saucepan, and put it on the fire to boil.

**3.** Put into the milk a piece of butter the size of a nut, to prevent it from burning.

**4.** Take the bread out of the basin and squeeze out all the water.

**5.** Empty the water out of the basin and put back the bread.

**6.** When the milk boils, pour it over the bread, and let the bread soak until it is soft.

**7.** Break *two eggs* into a small basin, add to them *two tablespoonfuls of moist sugar*, and beat them lightly together.

**8.** Take *four ounces of large raisins* and stone them; or, if *currants* are preferred, wash them, dry them in a cloth, and pick them over, to see that there are no stones with them.

**9.** Now beat the bread up with a fork as smooth as possible.

**10.** Put in the raisins or currants and the eggs and sugar, and mix them all well together.

**11.** Take a pie-dish, or tin, holding two pints and a half, grease it well inside, and pour in the mixture.

**12.** Put it in the oven (the *heat* should be 220°) to bake for *half an hour;* it will then be ready for serving.

----

LESSON TWENTY-FIRST.

TREACLE PUDDING.

**Ingredients.**—One pound of flour. Quarter of a pound of suet. One teaspoonful of baking-powder. Salt. One teaspoonful of ground ginger. Quarter of a pound of treacle. Quarter of a pint of milk. One egg.

*Time required, two and a half hours.*

To make a *Treacle Pudding:*

**1.** Put a large saucepan of *warm water* on the fire to boil.

**2.** Take a *quarter of a pound of suet*, put it on a board, cut away the *skin*, and chop up the *suet* as fine as possible.

**3.** Put one pound of flour into a basin, with a little salt and one teaspoonful of baking-powder.

**4.** Add the chopped suet and one teaspoonful of ground ginger, and mix all well together with a spoon.

**5.** Put a quarter of a pound of treacle into a basin, with a quarter of a pint of milk and one egg, and mix them together.

N. B.—If liked, rather more treacle can be added.

**6.** Stir this into the mixture in the basin, and add more milk, if required to make the pudding moist.

N. B.—When the pudding is mixed, it should be rather stiff.

**7.** Take a *quart basin*, grease it well inside, and pour the mixture into it.

N. B.—Be careful that the basin is full ; for, if not quite full, the water will get into it and spoil the pudding.

**8.** Sprinkle some flour over the top of the pudding, put a cloth over it and tie it tightly down with a piece of string, just below the rim of the basin, and tie or pin the corners of the cloth together.

**9.** When the water in the saucepan is quite boiling, put in the pudding, and let it boil for *two hours*.

**10.** For serving, take the pudding out of the saucepan, take off the cloth, place a hot dish over the pudding, and turn it carefully out of the basin.

---

### LESSON TWENTY-SECOND.

#### PLUM PUDDING.

**Ingredients.**—Five ounces of bread-crumbs. Seven ounces of flour. One-quarter of a pound of suet. Quarter of a pound of raisins. Quarter of a pound of currants. Two ounces of moist sugar. Two ounces of candied peel. One teaspoonful of baking-powder. Two eggs. One gill of milk.

*Time required, two and a half hours.*

To make a *Plum Pudding :*

**1.** Put a large saucepan of *warm water* on the fire to boil.

**2.** Stand a grater on a piece of paper, and grate some *bread-crumbs.* There should be *five ounces.*

**3.** Take a quarter of a pound of suet and put it on a board.

**4.** Take a knife, cut away all the *skin*, and chop up the *suet* as fine as possible.

**5.** Sprinkle flour over the suet, to prevent it sticking to the board or knife.

**6.** Take a quarter of a pound of currants, wash them well in cold water, and rub them dry in a cloth.

**7.** Take up the currants in handfuls and drop them a few at a time on to a plate, so as to find out if there are any stones mixed with them.

**8.** Take a quarter of a pound of large raisins and stone them.

**9.** Take two ounces of mixed candied peel—i. e., citron, lemon, and orange—and cut them up into small pieces.

N. B.—If disliked, the candied peel may be omitted.

**10.** Put seven ounces of flour into a basin, and add to it the chopped suet, quarter of a salt-spoonful of salt, and a teaspoonful of baking-powder.

**11.** Rub the suet well into the flour with your hand.

N. B.—Be careful not to leave any lumps.

**12.** Now add the *bread-crumbs*, the *currants* and *raisins*, *two ounces of moist sugar*, the pieces of *candied peel*, and mix all well with a wooden spoon.

N. B.—If preferred, treacle may be used instead of sugar.

**13.** Break *two eggs* into a basin, add to them *one gill of milk*, and beat them up.

**14.** Now stir the *milk* and *eggs* into the *pudding*, and mix all well together.

**15.** Take a cloth, wring it out of hot water, flour it, and lay it over a quart basin.

N. B.—Be careful that the cloth is strong, and that there are no holes in it.

**16.** Turn the mixture from the basin into the centre of the floured cloth.

**17.** Hold up the four corners of the cloth, and tie up the pudding tightly with a piece of string.

**18.** When the water in the saucepan is quite boiling, put in the pudding, and let it boil for *two hours.*

N. B.—The lid should be on the saucepan.

**19.** For serving, take the pudding out of the cloth and turn it on to a hot dish.

---

### LESSON TWENTY-THIRD.

#### TAPIOCA AND APPLES.

**Ingredients.**—Two tablespoonfuls of tapioca. Six apples. Four cloves, and the peel of half a lemon. Two tablespoonfuls of sugar.

*Time required (after the tapioca has soaked twelve hours), about three-quarters of an hour.*

To make a Stew of *Tapioca and Apples:*

**1.** Put *two tablespoonfuls of tapioca* into a basin with *one pint of water*, and let it soak *twelve hours.*

N. B.—This should be done over night.

**2.** Peel, quarter, and core six apples.

**3.** Put in four cloves for flavoring.

**4.** Wipe a lemon with a cloth, and peel half of it very thin with a sharp knife.

N. B.—Be careful not to take any of the white, as it is very bitter.

**5.** Put the soaked tapioca into a large saucepan, with the lemon-peel and two tablespoonfuls of pounded white sugar.

**6.** Put the saucepan on the fire, and stir it well until it boils.

N. B.—Be careful not to let any stick to the bottom.

11

**7.** Let it boil *ten minutes*, until the tapioca has become clear.

**8.** After that, put the apples into the saucepan, arranging them at the bottom so that they are covered with the tapioca.

**9.** Move the saucepan to the side of the fire, and let the apples stew gently for from *fifteen* to *thirty minutes*, according to their size.

**10.** You must not let them boil, or they will break.

**11.** When they are stewed quite tender, take them out of the saucepan and put them on a dish.

**12.** Pour the tapioca over the apples.

N. B.—If liked, the tapioca sauce can be colored by stirring in about half a teaspoonful of cochineal.

---

### LESSON TWENTY-FOURTH.

#### INVALID PUDDING.

**Ingredients.**—Three tablespoonfuls of chopped suet. Three tablespoonfuls of bread-crumbs. Three tablespoonfuls of flour. Three tablespoonfuls of moist sugar. Three tablespoonfuls of milk. Two eggs.

*Time required, about one hour and three-quarters.*

To make an *Invalid Pudding :*

**1.** Take about a *quarter of a pound of mutton-suet*, put it upon a board, and chop it up as fine as possible.

**2.** When it is chopped, there should be about three tablespoonfuls.

N. B.—Mutton-suet is much lighter of digestion than beef-suet.

**3.** Put a saucepan half full of warm water on the fire to boil.

**4.** Take a piece of *bread* and a grater, and grate some

*bread-crumbs* on to a piece of paper. There should be about *three tablespoonfuls of bread-crumbs.*

5. Put the bread-crumbs and the chopped suet into a basin, with three tablespoonfuls of flour and three table-spoonfuls of moist sugar.

6. Mix all these well together.

7. Now break in *two eggs,* and add *three tablespoonfuls of milk,* and stir all well together with a spoon.

8. Take a half-pint pudding-basin and grease it well inside.

9. Pour the mixture into the basin.

10. Take a cloth, dip it in hot water, and flour it.

11. Put this cloth over the top of the basin, and tie it on with a piece of string, just under the rim of the basin.

12. Tie the four corners of the cloth together loosely over the top of the basin.

13. Put this basin into the saucepan of boiling water; but you must be very careful that the water only reaches half-way up the basin, or it will boil over and get into the pudding.

14. Let the pudding steam for *one hour and a half.*

N. B.—Keep a kettle of water boiling, to add to the water in the saucepan as it boils away.

15. After that time, take the basin out of the saucepan, take off the cloth, and carefully turn the pudding out on to a warm dish.

### LESSON TWENTY-FIFTH.

#### SEMOLINA PUDDING.

**Ingredients.**—Half a pint of milk.  One tablespoonful of crushed semolina.  One egg.  One dessertspoonful of moist sugar.  Butter and nutmeg.

*Time required, about twenty-five minutes.*

To make a *Semolina Pudding :*

1. Put *half a pint of milk* and *one tablespoonful of
semolina* into a saucepan.

2. Put the saucepan on the fire, and stir occasionally
until it boils and swells ; then set it by the side of the fire.

3. Break one egg into a basin and add to it one dessertspoonful of moist sugar, and beat them lightly together.

4. Take a three-quarters-of-a-pint pie-dish and grease
it inside with a piece of butter.

5. When the semolina is sufficiently cooled, stir in
lightly the sweetened egg.

6. Pour this mixture into the pie-dish.

7. Take a grater and a *nutmeg* and **grate** a *quarter of
a teaspoonful* over the *mixture.*

8. Put the dish into the oven (the *heat* should be 220°)
to bake for a *quarter of an hour.*

N. B.—Puddings can be made in the same way with sago, tapioca, or
rice.

---

### LESSON TWENTY-SIXTH.

#### BATTER AND FRUIT.

**Ingredients.**—Quarter of a pound of flour.  Salt.  Half a pint of milk.
Two eggs.  Quarter of a pound of fruit.  Half an ounce of butter.  Sugar.

*Time required, about forty minutes.*

To make a *Batter Pudding* with *fruit* in it :

1. Put a quarter of a pound of flour in a basin.

**2.** Add a quarter of a teaspoonful of salt.

**3.** Stir in gradually half a pint of milk.

**4.** When it has become sufficiently liquid, you should beat it with a spoon, instead of stirring it, as that will make it lighter.

**5.** Break an egg into a cup, and then add it to the batter, beating it up lightly all the time, until it is thoroughly mixed.

**6.** Then break a second egg into the cup, and add it to the batter, mixing it thoroughly as before.

> N. B.—Eggs should always be broken separately into a cup, to see if they are good, before cooking.

> N. B.—The more the batter is beaten the lighter it becomes.

**7.** Take a pint-and-a-half pie-dish and grease it well inside with butter.

**8.** Pour the batter into the pie-dish.

**9.** Take a *quarter of a pound of damsons* (or any other fruit) and wipe them with a cloth, to be sure that they are quite clean.

**10.** Sprinkle the fruit into the batter, and put two or three bits of butter on the top, to prevent its being dry.

**11.** Put the pie-dish into the oven (the *heat* should be 220°) to bake for *half an hour*.

**12.** After that time, take the pie-dish out of the oven and sprinkle some sugar over the top.

> N. B.—Sugar should, of course, be eaten with the batter pudding.

> N. B.—If sugar were added to the batter before it was baked, it would make it heavy.

### COLD CABINET PUDDING.

**Ingredients.**—Six sponge finger-biscuits. Two ounces of ratafias. Half a pint of milk. Half an ounce of best gelatine. The yolks of four eggs. Two ounces of dried cherries. Two or three pieces of angelica. Half a gill of cream. One teaspoonful of essence of vanilla. One tablespoonful of powdered sugar.

*Time required, about half an hour.*

## To make a *Cold Cabinet Pudding:*

**1.** Take a *pint mould* and ornament the bottom of it (according to taste) with the *dried cherries* and *pieces of angelica.*

**2.** Split the *sponge-biscuits* in half and line the inside of the tin with them and the *ratafias* in the mould.

N. B.—Place the *biscuits* only round the sides of the tin (not over the bottom), arranging them alternately back and front next the tin.

**3.** Break four eggs, put the yolks in a basin (the whites put aside, as they are not required for present use), and beat them well with a wooden spoon.

**4.** Stir half a pint of milk into the eggs, and pour the mixture into a jug.

**5.** Take a saucepan, fill it half full of hot water, and put it on the fire to boil; when the water boils, remove the saucepan to the side of the fire.

**6.** Stand the jug in the saucepan, and stir the custard very smoothly until it thickens to the consistence of cream; but it must not boil, or it will curdle.

**7.** Put half an ounce of gelatine in a small stewpan or gallipot, with a tablespoonful of water, and stand it near the fire to melt.

8. When the custard is sufficiently thick, take the jug out of the saucepan and stand it aside to cool.

N. B.—Place a piece of paper over the mouth of the jug, to prevent the dust getting in.

9. Stir the gelatine until it is quite melted.

10. Pour the melted gelatine through a strainer into the custard.

11. Also add *half a gill of cream,* a *teaspoonful of essence of vanilla,* and a *tablespoonful of powdered sugar.*

12. Pour it all on the cakes in the mould.

13. Stand the mould in a cold place to set; in summertime it should be placed on ice.

14. When the pudding is quite cold and set, turn it out carefully on to a dish, and it is ready for serving.

---

LESSON TWENTY-EIGHTH.

SUET PUDDING.

**Ingredients.**—Half a pound of suet. One pound of flour. One teaspoonful of baking-powder.

*Time required, about one hour and three-quarters.*

To make a *Suet Pudding :*

1. Put a saucepan of *warm water* on the fire to boil.

2. Take *half a pound of suet,* put it on a board, cut away all the skin, and chop the suet up as fine as possible with a sharp knife.

3. Put *one pound of flour* into a basin with *one teaspoonful of baking-powder.*

4. Add the *chopped suet,* and rub it well into the *flour* with your hands.

N. B.—Be careful not to have any *lumps.*

5. Now add enough *cold water* to mix it into a stiff *paste*.

6. Take a strong pudding-cloth, wring it out in boiling water, and sprinkle flour over it.

7. Turn the paste out on to the cloth, hold up the ends of the cloth, and tie it tightly round the pudding with a piece of string, leaving room for the pudding to swell.

8. When the water in the saucepan is quite boiling, put in the pudding, and let it boil gently for *one hour and a half*.

N. B.—Keep a kettle of boiling water, and fill up the saucepan as the water in it boils away.

9. For serving, take the pudding out of the saucepan, take off the cloth, and turn it on to a hot dish.

N. B.—This *pudding* can be eaten with *meat*, or with *sugar*, *jam*, or *treacle*.

----

### LESSON TWENTY-NINTH.

#### YORKSHIRE PUDDING.

**Ingredients.**—Eight ounces of flour.  One pint of milk.  Half a teaspoonful of baking-powder.  Salt.  Two eggs.

*Time required, one hour.*

To make a *Yorkshire Pudding :*

1. Put *eight ounces* of flour into a basin, and mix into it *half a teaspoonful of baking-powder* and *half a salt-spoonful of salt*.

2. Break two eggs into the flour, and stir it well.

3. Now add, by degrees, a *pint of milk*, beating all the time with a wooden spoon, to make the batter as smooth and light as possible.

**4.** Place a pint pudding-tin under the meat that is roasting in front of the fire, to catch some dripping to grease the tin.

**5.** Then pour the batter into the tin, and let it cook under the meat *half an hour*, or bake it twenty minutes in the oven.

**6.** Turn the tin so that the pudding will not get burned.

N. B.—It is better to make batter some time before it is wanted, so that it may rise.

N. B.—A plainer and more substantial Yorkshire pudding can be made, in the same way as above, with six ounces of flour, one egg, one pint of milk, and one tablespoonful of chopped suet, sprinkled over the batter when it is poured into the tin.

**7.** When the pudding is done, turn it out of the tin on to a hot dish, and it is ready for serving with roast meat.

# CHAPTER XV.

## *DUMPLINGS.*

---

### HARD DUMPLINGS.

**Ingredients.**—Half a pound of flour. Salt.

*Time required, about twenty-five minutes.*

- To make *Hard Dumplings :*

1. Put a saucepan of warm water on the fire to boil.

2. Put *half a pound of flour* into a basin, and mix in *half a salt-spoonful of salt.*

3. Add cold water enough to make it into a firm dough.

4. Flour your hands and divide the dough into pieces about the size of an egg, and roll each piece into a smooth ball, without a crack in it.

5. When the water in the saucepan is quite boiling, drop in the dumplings, and let them boil twenty minutes.

N. B.—They are best boiled with meat—either salt beef or pork.

6. Then take them out of the saucepan, put them on a hot dish, and they are ready for serving.

LESSON SECOND.

## NORFOLK DUMPLINGS.

**Ingredients.**—One pound of patent flour.   Water.

*Time required, about half an hour.*

To make *Norfolk Dumplings:*

1. Put a saucepan of warm water on the fire to boil.

2. Put one pound of patent flour into a basin.

3. Add to it enough cold water to make it into a smooth dough (it must not be too stiff).

4. Form this dough into round balls about the size of a large egg.

N. B.—This quantity will make about ten dumplings.

5. When the water in the saucepan is quite boiling, put in the dumplings, and let them boil for twenty minutes.

6. After that time, take them out of the saucepan, and they are then ready for serving.

# CHAPTER XVI.

## *JELLIES.*

### LESSON FIRST.

#### WINE JELLY.

**Ingredients.**—Two calves' feet. Two lemons. Two eggs. Two ounces of loaf-sugar. One inch of the stick of cinnamon. Four cloves. One wineglass of sherry. Half a wineglass of brandy.

*Time required (the jelly-stock should be made the day before required for use) to finish making it, about an hour.*

To make about one quart of *Wine Jelly* from *calves' feet*:

1. Take two calves' feet and put them on a board.

2. Chop each foot in four pieces with a chopper.

3. Put these pieces in a basin of clean cold water and wash them well.

4. Take them out of the basin and put them in a stewpan with sufficient cold water to cover them.

N. B.—This is to blanch them.

5. Put the stewpan on the fire to boil.

6. When the water boils, take the stewpan off and stand it on a piece of paper on the table.

7. Take the pieces of the feet out of the stewpan with

a fork, and put them in a basin of cold water and wash them well.

8. Empty the water out of the stewpan.

9. Wash the stewpan well.

10. Take the pieces of the feet out of the basin, and put them in the stewpan with *five pints of cold water*.

> N. B.—This stock will be reduced to about *one pint and a half* when it is sufficiently boiled.

11. Put the stewpan on the fire to boil.

12. Watch it, and skim it often with a skimming-spoon.

13. Let it boil very gently for *five hours*.

14. After that time strain off the liquor through a hair sieve into a basin.

15. Put this basin in a cool place for some hours, until the stock is perfectly cold and is in a jelly.

16. Now take this basin of jelly-stock and skim off all the fat carefully with a spoon.

17. Take a clean cloth and put it in hot water.

18. Take this damp cloth and dab it over the jelly-stock, so as to remove every particle of grease.

19. Take a clean dry cloth and rub lightly over the jelly-stock, to dry it.

20. Take *two lemons*, wipe them clean in a cloth, and peel them very thinly with a sharp knife.

> N. B.—Be careful, in peeling the lemons, not to cut any of the white skin, as it would make the jelly bitter.

21. Put the lemon-peel into a stewpan.

22. Squeeze the juice of the two lemons, through a strainer, into the stewpan.

23. Take two eggs, and put the yolks in one basin and the whites in another.

24. Whip the whites of the eggs slightly, but not very stiff.

**25.** Put the whipped white of the egg into the stewpan, and the crushed egg-shell.

**26.** Put in also two ounces of loaf sugar, one inch of the stick of cinnamon, and four cloves.

**27.** Whip all these together with a whisk.

**28.** Now add the jelly-stock.

**29.** Put the stewpan on the fire, and whisk well till it boils.

**30.** Now put the lid on the stewpan and stand it by the side of the fire for *twenty minutes*, to form a crust.

**31.** Place the jelly-bag stand in front of the fire and hang the jelly-bag in it (you must put a basin on the stand underneath the jelly-bag).

N.B.—Be sure that the *jelly-bag* is quite clean.

**32.** Take a jug of *boiling* water and pour it through the jelly-bag.

**33.** Do this *four or five times*, always using *boiling* water until the bag is quite warm.

**34.** Look at the jelly in the stewpan, and when the crust is formed it is ready to be strained.

N.B.—Be sure that there is no water left in the bag before passing the jelly through; and the basin in the stand should be quite dry.

N.B.—The pouring of the jelly into the bag forces the water (the few drops that remain) out first into the basin; these first few drops should be thrown away, and a clean basin put in its place immediately.

**35.** Now take the stewpan off the fire and pour the jelly carefully into the bag, to pass into the basin.

**36.** Repeat this two or three times, until the jelly runs through quite clear.

N.B.—Be careful, in pouring the jelly through the bag, that you do not disturb the sediment at the bottom of the bag, which will serve as a filter.

**37.** Add a *wineglassful of sherry* and *half a wineglassful of brandy*, or any other *wine* or *liqueur*, according to taste.

**38.** Take a *quart mould*, scald it with *boiling* water, and then rinse it in *cold water*.

**39.** Place the mould in ice.

N. B.—Be careful that the mould stands quite straight and firm.

**40.** Pour in enough of the jelly just to cover the bottom of the mould.

**41.** When this jelly has set slightly, garnish the mould with grapes, strawberries, etc., according to taste.

**42.** Then pour the remainder of the *jelly* into the mould, and let it stand in the ice until it is firmly set.

**43.** When the jelly is required for use, dip the mould into a basin of hot water.

**44.** Shake the mould to loosen the jelly, place a dish over the top of the mould, and turn the jelly carefully out, so as not to break it.

----

### LESSON SECOND.

#### ASPIC JELLY.

**Ingredients.**—Two calves' feet. Two pounds of knuckle of veal. Salt. Thirty pepper-corns. Two blades of mace. One clove of garlic. Two shallots. One sprig of thyme. Two or three sprigs of parsley. One onion, stuck with four cloves. One leek. Half a head of celery. Two carrots. One turnip. One sprig of tarragon. One sprig of chervil. Two bay-leaves. The rind of one lemon. The juice of three lemons. The whites of two eggs. One pound of lean veal. One gill of chablis or sherry. Two tablespoonfuls of French vinegar.

*Time required (the jelly-stock should be made the day before) to finish making it, if not decorated, about an hour.*

To make one quart of savory *Aspic Jelly :*

**1.** Take *two calves' feet* and put them on a board.

2. Chop the feet in eight pieces with a chopper.

3. Put these pieces in a basin of clean *cold* water and wash them well.

4. Take them out of the basin, and put them in a stewpan with enough *cold* water to cover them.

5. Put the stewpan on the fire to boil.

N. B.—This is to blanch them.

6. When the water boils, take the stewpan off and stand it on a piece of paper on the table.

7. Take the pieces of feet out of the stewpan with a fork, put them in a basin of cold water, and wash them well.

8. Empty the water out of the stewpan.

9. Wash the stewpan well.

10. Take the pieces of feet out of the basin and put them back into the stewpan.

11. Take two pounds of knuckle of veal and put it on a board.

12. Take a sharp knife and cut the meat from the bone.

13. Put the meat and the bone into the stewpan with the feet.

14. Pour in *five pints of water*, put the stewpan on the fire, and just bring it to the boil.

15. Watch it, and skim it with a spoon.

16. Now add half a teaspoonful of salt, thirty peppercorns, two blades of mace, one clove of garlic, two shallots, one sprig of thyme, and two or three sprigs of parsley.

17. Take an onion, peel it, and stick *four cloves* in it.

18. Take one leek and half a head of celery, and wash them in *cold* water.

**19.** Wash two carrots and scrape them clean.

**20.** Wash a turnip and peel it.

**21.** Put all these vegetables into the stewpan.

**22.** Add one sprig of tarragon, one sprig of chervil, and two bay-leaves.

**23.** Let all these boil gently for *five hours.*

**24.** Then strain off the liquor, through a hair sieve, into a basin.

**25.** Put this basin in a cool place for some hours, until the stock is perfectly cold and in a jelly.

**26.** Now take the basin of jelly and skim off all the *fat* carefully with a spoon.

**27.** Take a clean cloth and put it in hot water.

**28.** Take this damp cloth and dab it over the jelly-stock, so as to remove every particle of grease.

**29.** Take a clean dry cloth and rub lightly over the jelly-stock, to dry it.

**30.** Take one lemon, wipe it clean in a cloth, and peel it very thinly with a sharp knife.

> N. B.—Be careful, in peeling the lemon, not to cut any of the pith, as it would make the jelly bitter.

**31.** Put the lemon-peel into a stewpan.

**32.** Squeeze the juice of three lemons, through a strainer, into the stewpan.

**33.** Whip the whites of two eggs slightly, but not very stiff.

**34.** Put the whipped whites of the eggs into the stewpan, also the *egg-shells.*

**35.** Take *one pound of lean veal*, put it on a board, and chop it up fine.

**36.** Put this chopped veal in the stewpan.

**37.** Pour in *one gill of chablis* or *sherry,* and two table-spoonfuls of *French vinegar.*

**38.** Add salt and pepper to taste, and whip all together with a whisk.

**39.** Put in the jelly-stock.

**40.** Put the stewpan on the fire, and whisk well until it boils.

**41.** Now take a large spoon and skim it carefully, if necessary.

**42.** Put the stewpan by the side of the fire, and let it stand for *half an hour* to form a crust.

**43.** Take a clean soup-cloth, or a jelly-bag, and fix it on the stand.

**44.** Take a large basin and place it below the cloth.

**45.** Take the stewpan off the fire and pour the contents into the cloth, and let it all pass into the basin.

N. B.—The chopped veal acts as a filter to the jelly.

**46.** After the jelly has all passed through, remove the basin, and put a clean one in its place.

**47.** Take a soup-ladle and pour a ladleful of the *jelly* at a time over the meat in the cloth, and let it pass for the second time very slowly into the basin.

N.B.—Be careful not to disturb the deposit of chopped veal which settles at the bottom of the cloth.

**48.** If a border-mould of aspic jelly is required, scald the mould with boiling water, and then rinse it in cold water.

N. B.—If the aspic jelly is only required for garnishing cold meats, stand the basin of jelly on ice, or in a cool place, until it is firmly set; then cut the jelly into fancy shapes, or chop it up finely with a knife.

**49.** Place the mould in ice.

N. B.—Be careful that it stands straight and firm.

**50.** Pour in enough of the *jelly* just to cover the bottom of the mould.

**51.** When this jelly has slightly set, garnish the mould with *fish* or *vegetables*, etc., according to taste or to what it is to be served with.

**52.** Then pour the remainder of the *jelly* into the mould, and let it stand in the *ice* until it is firmly set.

**53.** When the jelly is required for use, dip the mould into a basin of *hot* water for about a second.

**54.** Shake the mould to loosen the *jelly*, and place a dish over the top of the mould and turn the *jelly* carefully out, so as not to break it.

N. B.—The centre of the mould can be filled with a salad of mixed vegetables (*see* No. 13 in "Entrées," Lesson Fifth).

---

### LESSON THIRD.

#### ICELAND MOSS.

**Ingredients.**—One ounce of Iceland moss. One quart of milk or water. Two tablespoonfuls of powdered loaf sugar.

*Time required (after the Iceland moss has soaked all night), for "Water Jelly," about one hour ; for "Milk Jelly," about two hours.*

To make *Jelly* with *Iceland Moss :*

**1.** Wash *one ounce of Iceland moss* well in cold water.

**2.** Then put it in a basin of cold water and let it soak all night.

**3.** After that time take it out of the water and squeeze it dry in a cloth.

**4.** Then put it in a saucepan, with *one quart of cold water*.

**5.** Put the saucepan on the fire and let it boil for *one hour ;* you must stir it frequently.

**6.** Then strain it through a sieve into a basin, and sweeten it with loaf sugar.

**7.** It can be taken with either *wine* or *milk*, according to taste.

For *Milk Jelly :*

**1.** Boil the *moss* in the same quantity of *milk*, instead of *water* (after it has been soaked), as above, only for *two hours* instead of *one hour*.

**2.** Then strain it into a basin, and sweeten with loaf sugar according to taste.

**3.** When it is cold, turn the jelly out of the basin on to a dish, and it is ready for use.

---

LESSON FOURTH.

MILK JELLY FROM COW-HEEL, AND THE MEAT SERVED WITH ONION-SAUCE.

**Ingredients** (for Milk Jelly).—One cow-heel. One quart of milk. Two inches of the stick of cinnamon. Sugar.

To make a *Milk Jelly* from *Cow-Heel :*

**1.** Buy a dressed cow-heel from a tripe-shop.

**2.** Put the *cow-heel* on a board and cut it up into small pieces.

**3.** Put these pieces into an earthen jar or a saucepan, with *one quart* of *milk* and *two inches* of *the stick of cinnamon*.

**4.** Put the lid on the top of the jar; put a piece of paper over the lid, and tie it tightly down.

**5.** Put the jar into a very slow oven, to stew for at least three hours.

**6.** If there is no oven to the stove, stand the jar by the side of the fire to stew.

N. B.—It reduces less if stewed in the oven.

7. When the stew is finished, take the jar out of the oven, take off the lid, strain the milk into a basin, and sweeten it according to taste.

8. Put the basin aside till the jelly is set. It may be eaten hot or cold, according to taste.

## FOR ONION-SAUCE.

**Ingredients.**—Three or four onions. Half a pint of milk. Half an ounce of flour. Half an ounce of butter.

For serving the *Cow-Heel* with *Onion-Sauce:*

1. Take three or four onions, peel them, and cut them in quarters.

2. Put them into a saucepan with half a pint of milk.

3. Put the saucepan on the fire to boil till the onions are quite tender; it will take about *one hour*.

4. After that time strain off the milk into a basin, put the *onions* on a board, and chop them up small.

5. Put *half an ounce of butter* into the saucepan, and put it on the fire to melt.

6. When the butter is melted, add half an ounce of flour, and mix them smoothly together with a wooden spoon.

7. Pour the milk in gradually, stirring it till it boils and thickens.

8. Then add the onions, season with *pepper* and *salt* according to taste, and move the saucepan to the side of the fire.

9. Put the pieces of cow-heel into the sauce, and let them warm through.

10. For serving, put the pieces of cow-heel on a hot dish, and pour over them the onion-sauce.

N. B.—The meat from the cow-heel might be served as a curry. The curry should be made in the same way as described in "Cooked Meat," Lesson Fourth.

N. B.—The bones of the cow-heel should be put into the stock-pot.

———

LESSON FIFTH.

JELLY AND STEW FROM OX-FOOT.

**Ingredients** (for Jelly).—One ox-foot.  Quarter of a pound of lump sugar. One egg.  Two lemons.  Spices.

**Ingredients** (for Stew).—One carrot.  One turnip.  One onion.  Half an ounce of dripping.  Half an ounce of butter.  Flour and seasoning.

To make a *Jelly* from *Ox-Foot:*

1. Take a scalded *ox-foot*, put it in cold water, and wash it well.

2. Take it out of *water*, dry it with a cloth, and put it on a board.

3. Cut the *foot* with a sharp knife across the *first joint* and down between the *hoofs*, and chop the long piece in half.

4. Put these pieces into a saucepan, with enough cold water to cover them.

5. Put the saucepan on the fire and just bring it to the boil.

6. Then take the pieces out and wash them thoroughly in a basin of *cold water*.

7. Empty the water out of the saucepan, and wash it out well.

8. Put the pieces of foot back in the saucepan, covering them well with cold water (about *two quarts* will be enough for a moderate-sized foot).

9. Put the saucepan on the fire, and when it boils

move it to the side of the fire and let it stew gently for
*six hours*.

**10.** Watch it, and skim it carefully with a spoon from
time to time.

**11.** After that time strain off the stock into a basin, and
put it aside to cool.

N. B.—The foot should be put aside until required for use.

**12.** When the stock is quite cold, take an iron spoon,
dip it in hot water, and carefully skim off the fat.

**13.** Take a clean cloth, dip it in hot water, and wipe
over the top of the jelly, so as to remove every particle of
fat.

N. B.—For "Porter Jelly," *see* below.

**14.** Take two lemons, wipe them with a cloth to be sure
that they are quite clean, and peel them very thinly with
a sharp knife.

N. B.—Be careful, in peeling the lemons, not to cut any of the white
skin, as it would make the jelly bitter.

**15.** Put the *peel of one lemon* into the stewpan or saucepan.

**16.** Cut the lemons in halves, and squeeze the juice of
the two into the saucepan.

N. B.—Be careful to remove all the pips.

**17.** Take one egg, put the yolk in one basin and the
white in another.

**18.** Whip up the white of the egg slightly.

**19.** Put the whipped white of the egg and the egg-shell
into the saucepan.

**20.** Put in a quarter of a pound of lump sugar, half an

inch of the stick of cinnamon, four cloves, and about a quarter of an inch of saffron.

**21.** Now add the jelly-stock.

**22.** Put the saucepan on the fire, and stir the contents well with a whisk or iron spoon until it boils.

**23.** Now put the lid on the saucepan and stand it by the side of the fire for *twenty minutes* or *half an hour*.

**24.** If there is no jelly-bag, you should take a clean cloth, folded over cornerwise, and sew it up one side, making it the shape of a jelly-bag.

**25.** Place two chairs back to back in front of the fire.

**26.** Hang the sewn-up cloth between the two chairs, by pinning it open to the top bar of each chair.

**27.** Place a basin underneath the bag.

**28.** Look at the *jelly* in the saucepan; and when there is a good crust formed over, it is ready to be strained.

**29.** Then take the saucepan off the fire, and pour the jelly into the bag, to pass into the basin.

**30.** Repeat this two or three times, until the jelly runs through quite clear.

N. B.—A glass of wine may be added now, if desired.

**31.** Take a *quart basin*, or a mould, scald it with hot water, and rinse it out with cold water.

**32.** Pour the *jelly* into the basin and stand it aside to cool and set, until it is required for use.

N. B.—If Porter Jelly is required, put the jelly-stock into a saucepan, with a quarter of a pound of lump sugar, half a teaspoonful of mixed spice, and half a pint of porter; put it on the fire and let it boil for an hour and a half, stirring occasionally; then strain it in the same way as for lemon jelly.

To make a *Stew of the meat of the foot:*

**1.** Take one carrot, wash it, scrape it clean, and cut it in slices with a sharp knife.

**2.** Take a small turnip and an onion, peel them, and cut them in slices.

**3.** Put these vegetables into a saucepan with half an ounce of clarified dripping.

**4.** Put the saucepan on the fire and let the vegetables fry a light-brown. Be careful they do not burn.

**5.** Cut the meat off the bones of the foot, cut it up into nice pieces, and season them with *pepper* and *salt* according to taste.

**6.** Put these pieces of meat into the saucepan with the vegetables.

**7.** Then pour in one pint of cold water, just bring it to the boil, and remove the saucepan to the side of the fire to stew gently one hour, or till the vegetables are tender.

**8.** Then strain off the liquor, and put the vegetables and meat on a dish.

**9.** Put the dish near the fire, to keep warm.

**10.** Put half an ounce of butter into the saucepan and put it on the fire to melt.

**11.** When the butter is melted, add half an ounce of flour, and mix them well together with a wooden spoon.

**12.** Stir in the liquor gradually, and stir it till it boils and thickens.

**13.** Then remove the saucepan to the side of the fire.

N.B.—The sauce can be colored with burnt sugar or a browned onion.

**14.** Now place in the meat and the vegetables, and let them just warm through.

**15.** Serve this stew on a hot dish with *boiled potatoes*, or *rice* (*see* "Vegetables," Lessons First and Thirteenth).

N.B.—The bones of the foot should be put in the stock-pot.

12

LESSON SIXTH.

APPLE JELLY.

**Ingredients.**—One pound of apples.  One lemon.  Three ounces of lump sugar.  One ounce of gelatine.  Half a teaspoonful of cochineal.

*Time required, about one hour.*

To make *Apple Jelly* :

**1.** Peel one pound of apples with a sharp knife, cut them in half, take out the core, and then cut the apples in small pieces.

**2.** Put them in a stewpan, with three ounces of lump sugar and half a pint of water.

**3.** Wipe a lemon with a clean cloth.

**4.** Take a grater and grate the rind of a lemon over the apples.

> N. B.—Be very careful to grate only the yellow peel of the lemon, as the white rind is very bitter.

**5.** Cut the lemon in half, and squeeze the juice through a strainer on the apples.

**6.** Put the stewpan on the fire to boil, and cook the apples quite tender.

**7.** Stir the apples occasionally, to prevent them from sticking to the bottom of the pan and burning.

**8.** Put *one ounce of gelatine* in a gallipot or small saucepan, with *half a gill* of *cold water*, and stand it by the side of the fire to dissolve.

**9.** When the apples are cooked to a pulp, place a hair sieve over a basin and rub the apples through with a wooden spoon.

**10.** Now stir the melted gelatine into the apple.

N. B.—Be very careful that the gelatine is quite smoothly dissolved; there should be no lumps.

N. B.—If liked, part of the apple might be colored by stirring in half a teaspoonful of cochineal.

**11.** Take a pint-and-a-half mould, rinse it out in boiling water, and then in cold water.

**12.** Ornament the bottom of the mould with *pistachio nuts* cut in small pieces, or preserved cherries, according to taste.

**13.** Now pour the apple in the mould, and if part of the apple is colored, you should fill the mould with alternate layers of colored and plain apple.

**14.** Stand the mould aside in a cool place, to set the apple.

**15.** For serving, dip the mould in boiling water for a second, and then turn out the apple jelly carefully on to a dish.

N. B.—Half a pint of double cream, whipped to a stiff froth, should be served with the apple jelly, either put round the edge of the dish or in the centre of the mould.

# CHAPTER XVII.

## *CREAMS.*

LESSON FIRST.

### VANILLA CREAM.

**Ingredients.**—Three eggs. Half a pint of milk. Half an ounce of best gelatine. Half a pint of double cream. A tablespoonful of powdered sugar. Half a teaspoonful of essence of vanilla.

*Time required for making, about three-quarters of an hour.*

To make a *Vanilla Cream :*

1. Take the *yolks of three eggs* and *one white*, put them into a basin, and beat them well with a wooden spoon.

2. Stir in *half a pint of milk.*

3. Pour this mixture into a jug.

4. Take a saucepan half full of hot water and put it on the fire to boil.

5. When the water is quite boiling, move the saucepan to the side of the fire.

6. Stand the jug of custard in the saucepan of boiling water, and stir the mixture very smoothly, until it thickens to the consistence of cream.

> N.B.—Stir it very carefully, and watch it continually, that it does not curdle.

**7.** When the custard is sufficiently thick, take the jug out of the water and stand it aside to cool.

**8.** Put *half an ounce of the best gelatine* in a small stewpan, with *half a gill of cold water*, to soak and swell.

**9.** Then put the stewpan on the fire, and stir the gelatine until it is quite melted.

**10.** Pour this melted gelatine through a strainer and stir it into the custard.

**11.** Pour *half a pint of double cream* into a basin, and whip it to a stiff froth with a whisk.

**12.** Add to it a tablespoonful of powdered sugar and half a teaspoonful of essence of vanilla.

> N. B.—If any other flavoring be preferred, it should now be added, instead of the essence of vanilla.

**13.** When the custard is sufficiently cooled, stir it lightly into the whipped cream.

**14.** Take a pint-and-a-half mould, scald it with hot water, and then rinse it out with cold water.

**15.** Pour the cream into the mould, and stand it in ice until required for use.

**16.** For serving, dip the mould into boiling water for a second, shake it to loosen the cream, and then turn it out carefully on to a dish.

> N. B.—This is an economical receipt for making cream; but if made entirely of cream, instead of cream and milk, it would, of course, be richer.

LESSON SECOND.

STRAWBERRY CREAM.

**Ingredients.**—One pint of fresh strawberries. Two and a half ounces of powdered sugar. Half an ounce of the best gelatine. The juice of one lemon. Half a pint of good cream.

*Time required, about half an hour.*

To make a *Strawberry Cream :*

1. Take a *pint of fresh strawberries* and put them on a board.

2. Pick them over, and put aside any that are not quite good.

3. Stalk them, and put them in a basin.

4. Sprinkle over them *half an ounce of white powdered sugar*, which will help to draw out the juice.

5. Take a silk sieve and place it over a basin.

N. B.—A hair sieve could be used instead.

6. Pass the fruit through the sieve with a wooden spoon.

7. Put *half an ounce of the best gelatine* into a small stewpan, with *half a gill of cold water,* to soak and to swell.

8. Then put the stewpan on the fire, and stir the gelatine until it is quite melted.

9. Add two ounces of powdered sugar, and squeeze the juice of one lemon, through a strainer, into the stewpan.

10. Pour this mixture through a strainer, and stir it into the strawberries in the basin, and mix them well together.

11. Pour half a pint of good cream into a basin, and whip it to a stiff froth with a whisk.

**12.** Now add this cream to the strawberries in the basin, and stir them lightly together.

**13.** Take a pint mould, scald it with hot water, and then rinse it out with cold water.

**14.** Pour the strawberry cream into the mould, and stand it in *ice* until required for use.

**15.** For serving, dip the mould into boiling water for a second, shake it to loosen the cream, and then turn it out carefully on to a dish.

---

### LESSON THIRD.

#### CHARLOTTE RUSSE.

**Ingredients.**—Twelve sponge finger-biscuits. Half an ounce of the best gelatine. One gill of milk. Half a pint of double cream. One dessertspoonful of sifted sugar. Thirty drops of essence of vanilla.

*Time required for making, about half an hour.*

To make a *Charlotte Russe:*

**1.** Take a *pint tin* and line it inside with *sponge finger-biscuits.*

> N. B.—Be careful to fit the biscuits close to each other, so that they form a wall of themselves.

**2.** Take a knife and cut off the tops of the *finger-biscuits* that stand above the tin.

**3.** Put *half an ounce of the best gelatine* in a small stewpan, with *one gill of cold milk,* to soak and swell.

**4.** Pour *half a pint of double cream* into a basin and whip it to a stiff froth with a whisk.

**5.** Add to it a dessertspoonful of sifted powdered sugar and thirty drops of essence of vanilla.

**6.** Put the stewpan on the fire, and stir the gelatine until it is quite melted.

**7.** Stir the melted gelatine into the cream, pouring it through a strainer.

**8.** Pour this cream into the tin.

> N.B.—Be careful, in pouring in the cream, not to disarrange the finger-biscuits.

**9.** Stand this tin in ice until it is required for use.

**10.** For serving, dip the tin into hot water for a second, shake the tin to loosen the cream, and turn it carefully on to a dish.

> N.B.—A more economical Charlotte Russe might be made by using a quarter of a pint of custard to a quarter of a pint of cream (as in " Creams," Lesson First).

# CHAPTER XVIII.

## SOUFFLES.

___

### LESSON FIRST.

### VANILLA SOUFFLÉ.

**Ingredients.**—Four eggs. One and one-quarter ounce of butter. A dessertspoonful of sugar. One ounce of flour. Half a teaspoonful of essence of vanilla. Salt. One gill of milk.

**Ingredients** (for Wine-Sauce).—One ounce of sugar. One tablespoonful of jam. Wineglassful of sherry. Half a teaspoonful of lemon-juice.

**Ingredients** (for Custard-Sauce).—One egg. Sugar, and six drops of vanilla. One gill of milk.

*Time required, about three-quarters of an hour.*

To make a *Steamed Vanilla Soufflé Pudding :*

**1.** Prepare the tin for the soufflé pudding—thus :

**2.** Take a pint-and-a-half tin and butter it well inside, using your fingers for the purpose.

**3.** Fold a piece of paper so as to make a band round the tin, allowing about two inches of paper to stand up above the tin.

**4.** Butter the part of paper above the tin with a knife.

**5.** Put the paper round the outside of the tin, and tie it on with a string.

**6.** Take a stewpan and just melt *one ounce of butter* in it over the fire.

**7.** Take the stewpan off the fire and stand it on a piece of paper on the table.

**8.** Add *one ounce of flour* to the *melted butter*, and mix them both well together.

**9.** Then add rather more than a dessertspoonful of powdered sugar.

**10.** Add one gill of milk.

**11.** Put the stewpan on the fire, and stir smoothly with a wooden spoon until it thickens.

**12.** Then take the stewpan off the fire again.

**13.** Add to the mixture the yolks of three eggs, one at a time, and beat all well together.

**14.** Take the three whites and put them in a basin, with one more white to make four, adding half a salt-spoonful of salt, and then whip the whites quite stiff.

**15.** Add the whites to the above mixture, and stir it lightly.

**16.** Now add the flavoring—half a teaspoonful of vanilla essence.

> N. B.—If the essence is very strong, or the bottle newly opened, so much is not required.

**17.** Mix all together, and pour it into the buttered tin.

**18.** Have ready a saucepan half filled with hot water, and put it on the fire to boil.

**19.** When the water boils, stand the tin in it, but be careful that the water does not reach the paper round the tin, for it is only the steam which cooks the pudding.

**20.** Move the saucepan to the side of the fire, and let the pudding steam from twenty to thirty minutes.

**21.** Watch it, not letting the water boil too fast, or the saucepan will get dry and the pudding will burn.

**22.** When it is sufficiently steamed, take the mould out of the saucepan of water.

> N. B.—To test if the pudding is done, touch the centre of it with your finger; it should feel firm.

**23.** Shake the tin and turn the *soufflé pudding* out on a hot dish, and pour the sauce round it, which you must prepare while the soufflé is being steamed.

> N. B.—If a baked vanilla soufflé pudding is required, put the tin in a quick oven (the heat should be 240°) to bake for half an hour, instead of putting it in the boiling water. No sauce is then wanted.

To make the *Sauce* for the *Steamed Vanilla Soufflé Pudding:*

For *Wine-Sauce:*

**1.** Take a small saucepan and put in it one ounce of loaf sugar and one gill of cold water.

**2.** Put the saucepan on the fire and stir the sugar and water with a spoon, until the sugar has quite melted and it has become a smooth syrup, reduced in quantity.

**3.** Put into it a tablespoonful of apricot jam.

**4.** Stir it all together over the fire, to melt the jam.

**5.** Add a wineglassful of sherry and a few drops of lemon-juice, and stir it all again.

**6.** Take the stewpan off the fire, and pour the sauce round the soufflé pudding.

> N. B.—Pour the sauce around very carefully, so as not to drop any of it on the side of the pudding.

You can make a *Custard-Sauce*, if preferred—thus:

**1.** Break a whole egg in a basin and whip it well.

**2.** Add half a teaspoonful of pounded sugar.

**3.** Add one gill of milk and six drops of vanilla essence.

4. Pour all the mixture into a jug or gallipot.

5. Get a large saucepan of hot water and put it on the fire.

6. Stand the gallipot in the saucepan of hot water.

N. B.—The water must only come half-way up the gallipot.

7. Stir the mixture in the gallipot with a wooden spoon.

8. As soon as the mixture has thickened, take the gallipot out of the saucepan.

9. Pour the custard round the *soufflé pudding*.

---

LESSON SECOND.

### CHEESE SOUFFLÉ.

**Ingredients.**—One ounce of butter and one ounce of flour. One teaspoonful of mignonette or white pepper. Salt, pepper, and Cayenne pepper. One gill of milk. Three eggs. Three ounces of Parmesan cheese.

*Time required, about forty minutes.*

To make a *Cheese Soufflé :*

1. Take a stewpan and put into it *one ounce of butter.*

2. Add one teaspoonful of mignonette pepper.[1]

3. Put the stewpan on the fire and let the pepper fry in the butter (to extract its flavor) for two or three minutes.

4. Take the stewpan off the fire, and strain the butter into a basin; as the pepper is only for flavoring, the grains must not be left in the butter.

5. Wash out the stewpan, to prevent any of the grains remaining.

6. Pour the flavored butter back in the stewpan.

7. Add one ounce of flour, a teaspoonful of salt, half

[1] White pepper-corns.

a teaspoonful of pepper, and Cayenne pepper according to taste, and stir well together with a wooden spoon.

8. Add one gill of milk.

9. Put the stewpan on the fire, and stir the mixture smooth until it thickens.

10. Take the stewpan off the fire and stand it on a piece of paper on the table.

11. Add one by one the yolks of two eggs, and beat them well together.

12. Take three ounces of Parmesan cheese.

13. Grate the cheese with a grater on to a plate or piece of paper.

14. Add the three ounces of grated cheese to the above mixture in the stewpan, and mix it all well together.

15. Whip the whites of four eggs with a little salt in a basin, until quite stiff.

16. Add the whites to the above mixture, and stir it lightly.

17. Take a plain pint tin mould and prepare it in the same way as for the *Vanilla Soufflé Pudding* (*see* Lesson First).

18. Pour the mixture into the buttered tin mould.

> N. B.—This same mixture, if poured into Ramaquin papers and baked, will make cheese Ramaquins.

19. Put the tin in a hot oven to bake from twenty minutes to half an hour. Look at it once or twice to see that it does not burn; but the door of the oven should not be opened too often while the soufflé is inside, lest it should check the soufflé from rising properly.

> N. B.—To serve a baked soufflé, it should be kept in the tin, the buttered paper taken off, and a clean napkin folded round the tin. It can also be baked in a mould, which slips inside a plated-silver dish sold for the purpose. This is the more elegant way of serving a soufflé or fondu.

LESSON THIRD.

POTATO SOUFFLÉ.

**Ingredients.**—Four potatoes. One ounce of butter. Half a gill of milk. Four eggs. Seasoning.

*Time required, about an hour.*

To make *Potato Soufflé:*

1. Take *four good-sized potatoes,* and wash and scrub them with a brush in a basin of *cold water.*

2. Take them out of the water and dry them with a cloth.

3. Put them in the oven (the heat should rise to 230°) to bake ; they will take from *half an hour* to *three-quarters of an hour,* according to the heat of the oven and the size of the *potatoes.*

4. Take a steel fork or skewer and stick it into the potatoes, to see if they are done. They must be soft inside.

N. B.—This should be carefully done, so as not to spoil the *potato-skins.*

5. When they are done, take them out and cut them (with a sharp knife) in half, so that each half of the potato will stand—because you will want to use the skins to put the potatoes into them again.

6. Take a small spoon and carefully scoop out all the inside of the potatoes. Take care not to make holes, or spoil the skins in any way.

7. Take a wire sieve and put it over a plate, and take the inside of the potatoes and rub it through with a wooden spoon.

8. Put *one ounce of butter* and *half a gill of milk* in a stewpan, and put it on the fire to boil.

9. Add *salt* and *pepper* according to taste.

**10.** Then add three ounces of the sifted potatoes, and stir it smoothly.

**11.** Now take the stewpan off the fire, and stand it on a piece of paper or wooden trivet on the table.

**12.** Take three eggs and add, one by one, only the yolks, beating all well together with a wooden spoon.

**13.** Take the three whites and add another white to make four, and put them in a basin; add a quarter of a salt-spoonful of salt to them, and whip them to a stiff froth.

**14.** Add the whites to the above mixture, and stir the whole lightly.

**15.** Now stand the eight half-potato skins on a baking-sheet.

**16.** Pour the mixture carefully into each potato-skin (they should be only half full).

**17.** Put the sheet into the oven (the heat should rise to 240°) for *ten minutes*, until they have risen well and become a pale-brown color.

**18.** Fold a table-napkin, and arrange them on it for serving.

----

LESSON FOURTH.

OMELET SOUFFLÉ.

**Ingredients.**—Two eggs. Half an ounce of butter. Jam. Sugar and salt. Teaspoonful of orange-flower water.

*Time required, about ten minutes.*

To make an *Omelet Soufflé of two eggs:*

**1.** Break two eggs; put the whites in one basin and the yolks in another.

**2.** Put one teaspoonful of orange-flower water and one tablespoonful of powdered sugar into a stewpan.

3. Put the stewpan on the fire and let it boil quickly for three minutes, stirring occasionally.

4. Then pour it into a cup to cool, add it to the yolks of egg, and beat them to a cream.

5. Add a quarter of a salt-spoonful of salt to the whites of egg, and whip them to a stiff froth.

6. Add the whites to the mixture in the basin, and mix them together very lightly.

7. Put half an ounce of butter into a frying-pan.

8. Put the pan on the fire and let the butter get quite hot, but not burn.

9. When the butter is quite hot, pour in the mixture.

10. Let it stay on a slow fire for two, but not more than three, minutes.

11. Then take the pan off the fire and put it in a brisk oven (the heat should rise to 240°).

12. Let it stay for about three or four minutes in the oven.

13. Take rather more than a dessertspoonful of jam.

14. Put the jam into a stewpan on the fire and stir it until it has melted.

15. Take the pan out of the oven.

16. Take a knife and pass it round the edge of the omelet soufflé, to ease it from the pan.

17. Give the pan a shake, to loosen the omelet soufflé.

18. Turn the omelet soufflé on to a hot dish.

19. Spread the jam on the omelet soufflé, and fold it over like a sandwich.

20. Sprinkle a little white powdered sugar over it.

## LESSON FIFTH.

### SAVORY OMELET.

**Ingredients.**—Two eggs. Salt, pepper, and parsley. One ounce of butter.

*Time required, about four minutes.*

To make a *Savory Omelet* of *two eggs :*

**1.** Break *two eggs* in a basin.

**2.** Add a *quarter of a teaspoonful of salt*, and *pepper* to taste.

**3.** Take a *sprig of parsley*, wash it, dry it, and chop it up finely on a board (there should be about a *teaspoonful*).

**4.** Add the chopped parsley to the eggs.

**5.** Beat the eggs lightly for two seconds with a fork.

> N. B.—The omelet could be flavored with chopped herbs or mush-rooms, with bacon or kidney cut in small pieces, or with grated cheese, according to taste.

**6.** Take *one ounce of butter* and put it in an omelet or frying pan.

**7.** Put the pan on the fire to melt the butter.

> N. B.—The fire should be bright and clear.

**8.** Wait till the butter is quite hot, taking care that it does not burn.

**9.** Pour the mixture of the egg into the pan.

**10.** Stir the mixture quickly with a wooden spoon.

**11.** Do not let it burn, or stick to the pan. Shake the pan, to prevent the omelet sticking or burning.

**12.** Spread it over the bottom of the pan and let it cook through.

**13.** Watch it very carefully.

**14.** Take a knife and put it under the omelet, and fold it over.

**15.** When the omelet has become a pale-brown, turn it out of the pan on to a hot dish.

----

### CHEESE STRAWS.

**Ingredients.**—Two ounces of butter. Two ounces of flour. Two ounces of grated Parmesan cheese. One ounce of Cheddar cheese. One egg. Salt, and Cayenne pepper.

*Time required, about twenty minutes.*

To make *Cheese Straws :*

**1.** Put two ounces of flour on a board, and mix into it half a salt-spoonful of salt and a quarter of a salt-spoonful of Cayenne pepper.

**2.** Take *two ounces of Parmesan cheese* and *one ounce of Cheddar* or some strong *cheese,* and grate them on a grater.

**3.** Rub the cheese and two ounces of butter into the flour.

**4.** Now mix all the ingredients, together with the yolk of an egg, into a smooth, stiff paste.

**5.** Flour the board and the rolling-pin, and roll out the *paste* into a strip one-eighth of an inch in thickness and five inches wide (the length the cheese straws are to be).

**6.** Now take a sharp knife, dip it in flour, and cut the paste into strips *one-eighth of an inch* wide, so that they will be *five inches* long and *one-eighth of an inch* in thickness.

**7.** Take two round cutters, dip them in flour, and cut little rings of paste.

**8.** Take a baking-sheet and grease it with butter.

**9.** Put the cheese straws and the rings on the baking-sheet, and put them into a hot oven (the heat should rise to 240°) for *ten minutes*.

**10.** Look at the cheese straws occasionally, and see that they do not burn; they should be of a pale-brown color when done.

**11.** For serving, take the cheese straws off the baking-sheet, and put them through the rings of paste, like a bundle of sticks.

# CHAPTER XIX.

## PICKLES FOR MEAT AND CABBAGE.

### PICKLE FOR MEAT.

**Ingredients.**—One and one-half pound of salt. Six ounces of brown sugar. One ounce of saltpetre. One gallon of water.

*Time required, about half an hour.*

To make *Pickle for Meat:*

**1.** Put one pound and a half of salt, six ounces of brown sugar, one ounce of saltpetre, and one gallon of water, into a large saucepan.

**2.** Put the saucepan on the fire to bring it to the boil, and then let it boil for five minutes. Keep it well skimmed.

**3.** Then strain it into a tub or large basin.

**4.** When the *pickle* is quite cold, meat can be put into it.

N. B.—The meat should be kept well covered with the pickle nine days.

N. B.—This pickle will keep for three weeks in summer and three months in winter.

N. B.—When the pickle is required again after it has once been used, it should be boiled up again, skimmed, strained, and allowed to get cold, before the fresh meat is put into it.

N. B.—If used for pig's head, it should be thrown away, and not used again.

LESSON SECOND.

PICKLED CABBAGE.

**Ingredients.**—A red cabbage.  A gallon of vinegar.  Mace, cloves, all-spice, whole pepper.  Salt and ginger.

*Time required, about three days.*

To *Pickle a Cabbage:*

**1.** Take a *red cabbage*, cut it in half and cut out the stalk, and wash it well in salt and cold water.

> N. B.—A white-heart cabbage will do to pickle, but green cabbages cannot be used.

**2.** Put it on a board and cut it in thin slices.

**3.** Lay the slices in a large pan, sprinkle a handful of salt over each layer of slices, cover the top well with salt, and leave them for two days.

> N. B.—Turn the slices every morning and evening, and sprinkle a handful of salt over the layers each time you turn them.

**4.** Then drain the slices on a hair sieve for one day.

**5.** Put a gallon of vinegar, two blades of mace, twenty-four cloves, twenty-four allspice berries, and twenty-four pepper-corns, into a saucepan, with three pieces of ginger an inch long.

**6.** Put the saucepan on the fire, and let it boil up.

**7.** Then turn the vinegar and spices out of the saucepan into a broad pan, to cool.

> N. B.—They must on no account be allowed to cool in the saucepan.

**8.** Put the cabbage into a stone jar, and pour the vinegar and spices over it.

**9.** The cabbage must be quite covered with *vinegar*, and as it soaks it up more vinegar must be poured over it.

N. B.—This quantity of vinegar is sufficient for a large cabbage; a smaller one will take less.

**10.** Tie the jar over with wash-leather, brown paper, or a bladder.

# CHAPTER XX.

## CAKES.

### LESSON FIRST.

#### SULTANA CAKE.

**Ingredients.**—Half a pound of flour. Quarter of a pound of butter. Quarter of a pound of sugar. Quarter of a pound of sultana raisins. One ounce of candied peel. Two eggs. One teaspoonful of baking-powder. Half a gill of milk. One lemon.

*Time required, about one hour and a half.*

To make a *Sultana Cake :*

1. Put *half a pound of flour* into a basin.

2. Rub a *quarter of a pound of butter* into the flour with your hands.

3. Now add a *quarter of a pound of powdered sugar,* a *teaspoonful of baking-powder,* and a *quarter of a pound of sultana raisins.*

4. Take a *lemon,* wipe it clean in a cloth, and grate the rind of it into the basin.

5. Cut up *one ounce of candied peel* into small pieces, and add it to the other ingredients.

6. Put half a gill of milk into a small basin, and add to it the yolks of two eggs. (Put the whites on a plate.)

7. Stir the milk and the eggs together and then pour it into the other ingredients, and mix all together.

8. Butter a cake-tin.

9. Whip the whites of the eggs into a stiff froth with a knife, and stir it lightly into the mixture.

10. Now pour it into the tin, and put it into the oven (the heat should rise to 240°) to bake for *one hour and a quarter*.

11. After that time, turn the *cake* out of the tin and stand it on its side, or on a sieve, to cool.

N. B.—This will prevent its getting heavy.

LESSON SECOND.

### GERMAN POUND-CAKE.

**Ingredients.**—Ten ounces of flour. Eight ounces of fresh butter. Eight ounces of powdered sugar. Two ounces of candied peel. One lemon. Quarter of a pound of sultana raisins. Four eggs.

*Time required, about two hours and a quarter.*

To make a *German Pound-Cake :*

1. Stand a wire sieve over a plate, and rub through it *ten ounces of flour.*

2. Put *eight ounces of fresh butter* into a basin, and work it to a *cream* with your hand.

3. Add a *tablespoonful of the sifted flour*, a *tablespoonful of powdered sugar*, and *one egg*, and mix them well into the *butter*.

4. Continue to mix in, by degrees, the flour, sugar, and eggs, until they are all used up.

5. Take a *lemon*, wipe it clean in a cloth, and grate the *rind* of it into the basin.

6. Add a quarter of a pound of sultana raisins and two ounces of candied peel (cut up in small pieces).

7. Stir all the ingredients together with a spoon.

**8.** Line a cake-tin with buttered foolscap paper, and put three rounds of buttered paper at the bottom of the tin.

**9.** Pour the mixture into the tin, and put it into the oven (the heat should rise to 240°) to bake for *two hours*.

**10.** After that time, turn the cake out of the tin and stand it on its side, or on a sieve, to cool.

---

LESSON THIRD.

PLAIN CAKE.

**Ingredients.**—One pound of flour. Four ounces of dripping. Baking-powder, allspice, and salt. Quarter of a pound of currants. Half a pint of milk. Quarter of a pound of sugar.

To make a *Plain Cake:*

**1.** Take *one pound of flour* and put it in a pan or large basin.

**2.** Mix into the *flour* a *teaspoonful of baking-powder* and *half a salt-spoonful of salt.*

**3.** Take *four ounces of clarified dripping,* and rub it well into the flour with your fingers until there are no lumps remaining.

**4.** Take a *quarter of a pound of currants,* put them in a cloth, and rub them clean.

**5.** Add the currants to the flour; also *half a teaspoonful of ground allspice* and a *quarter of a pound of brown sugar.*

**6.** Mix these ingredients together with a wooden spoon.

**7.** Now pour in half a pint of milk, and mix it all well together.
13

**8.** Take a half-a-quartern tin and grease it inside with a piece of dripping.

**9.** Pour this mixture into the tin.

**10.** Put the tin into the oven (the heat should rise to 240°) to bake for *one hour*.

**11.** After that time, take the tin out of the oven.

**12.** Turn the cake out of the tin and stand it on its side, to cool.

------

### LESSON FOURTH.

#### SEED CAKE.

**Ingredients.**—Ten ounces of flour. Two ounces of sugar. One teaspoonful of baking-powder. One teaspoonful of caraway seeds. Two ounces of clarified dripping. Half a gill of milk. One egg. Salt.

*Time required, one hour and a half.*

To make a *Seed Cake:*

**1.** Take *ten ounces of flour* and put it in a basin.

**2.** Mix into the *flour one teaspoonful of baking-powder* and *half a salt-spoonful of salt.*

**3.** Take *two ounces of clarified dripping* and rub it well into the flour with your hands, until there are no lumps remaining.

**4.** Add *two ounces of powdered sugar* and *one teaspoonful of caraway seeds.* .

**5.** Mix these well together with a wooden spoon.

**6.** Break one egg into a cup, and beat it up with half a gill of milk.

 · **7.** Pour this into the basin, and mix all quickly together into a stiff paste—stiff enough to allow a spoon to stand up in it.

**8.** Take a cake-tin and grease it inside with a piece of dripping.

**9.** Pour the mixture into the tin, and put it at once in the oven (the heat should rise to 240°) to bake for *one hour.*

**10.** To know when the cake is sufficiently baked, run a clean knife into it; if it comes out perfectly bright and undimmed by steam, the cake is done.

**11.** Turn the cake out of the tin and stand it on its side, to cool.

LESSON FIFTH.

PLUM CAKE.

**Ingredients.**—One pound of flour. Half a pound of fruit (plums or currants). Quarter of a pound of dripping. Quarter of a pound of sugar. One egg. Half a gill of milk. A teaspoonful of baking-powder. Salt. Two ounces of candied peel.

*Time required, about one hour and a quarter.*

To make a *Plum Cake :*

**1.** Put *one pound of flour* into a basin, with a *teaspoonful of baking-powder* and *half a salt-spoonful of salt.*

**2.** Take a *quarter of a pound of clarified dripping* and rub it well into the *flour* with your hands until there are no lumps remaining.

**3.** Take half a pound of plums or currants, or a quarter of a pound of each, and add them to the flour.

> N. B.—If currants are used, they should be well washed and dried in a cloth, and picked over, to see that there are no stones in them. Large plums should be stoned before they are used.

**4.** Take *two ounces of candied peel,* cut it in small pieces, and put it in the basin. Also add a *quarter of a pound of sugar.*

> N. B.—If peel is disliked, it may be omitted.

**5.** Break one egg into a basin, and add to it half a gill of milk, and beat them up.

**6.** Stir this into the ingredients in the basin, mixing them all well together.

**7.** Take a tin and grease it inside with dripping.

**8.** Pour the mixture into the tin and put it into the oven (the heat should rise to 240°) to bake for about an *hour.*

**9.** After that time, turn the cake out of the tin and stand it on its side, slanting against a plate, till it is cold.

---

## LESSON SIXTH.

### CORN-STARCH CAKE.

**Ingredients.**—Quarter of a pound of corn-starch. Quarter of a pound of loaf sugar. Two ounces of butter. One teaspoonful of baking-powder. Two eggs.

*Time required, about one hour.*

To make a *Corn-Starch Cake :*

**1.** Put *two ounces of butter* into a basin and beat it to a cream.

**2.** Add to the butter a quarter of a pound of pounded loaf sugar, and mix it well.

**3.** Break in two eggs, and beat all well together.

**4.** Now stir lightly into the mixture a quarter of a pound of corn-starch and a teaspoonful of baking-powder, and beat it well together for five minutes.

**5.** Grease a cake-tin inside with butter or dripping.

**6.** Pour the mixture into the tin and put it immediately into the oven (the heat should rise to 240°) to bake for *half an hour.*

**7.** After that time, turn the cake out of the tin and slant it against a plate, until it is cold.

N. B.—If preferred, the mixture could be baked in small tins instead of one large one, in which case it would take only fifteen minutes to bake.

LESSON SEVENTH.

DOUGH CAKE.

**Ingredients.**—Half a quartern of dough. Two eggs. Half a pound of sugar. One pound of currants.

*Time required, about an hour and a half.*

To make a *Dough Cake:*

**1.** Put *half a quartern of dough* (made as for *bread—see* "Bread," Lesson First) into a basin.

**2.** Take *one pound of currants*, wash them, dry them in a cloth, and pick them over, to see that there are no stones mixed with them.

**3.** Add the currants and half a pound of moist sugar to the dough.

N. B.—If liked, half a teaspoonful of mixed spice might be added.

**4.** Now break two eggs into the basin, and beat all the ingredients well together.

**5.** Take a quartern tin and grease it well inside with dripping.

**6.** Turn the mixture into the greased tin.

**7.** Put the tin into the oven (the heat should rise to 240°) until the cake is sufficiently baked; it will take about *forty minutes.*

N. B.—To test if the cake is done, run a clean knife into it; and if it comes out clean, the cake is sufficiently baked.

8. Then turn the cake out of the tin and place it on its side, leaning against a plate, until it is cold.

LESSON EIGHTH.

SHREWSBURY CAKES.

**Ingredients.**—Quarter of a pound of butter. Quarter of a pound of castor sugar. Six ounces of flour. One teaspoonful of pounded cinnamon and mace. One egg.

*Time required, about half an hour.*

To make *Shrewsbury Cakes:*

1. Put a quarter of a pound of butter and a quarter of a pound of castor sugar into a basin, and beat them together till the mixture is of the same consistence as cream.

N.B.—If the butter is very hard, it might be beaten over hot water.

2. Add to the mixture one egg and about a teaspoonful of pounded cinnamon and mace (mixed together), and beat all well together.

3. Now stir in smoothly, by degrees, six ounces of flour.

N.B.—Be careful not to let it get lumpy.

4. Flour a board and turn the paste out on to it.

5. Flour a rolling-pin and roll out the paste as thin as possible.

6. Dip a cutter, or wineglass, in flour, and cut the paste into biscuits or cakes.

7. Grease a baking-tin with dripping or butter, and put the cakes on it.

8. Put the tin into the oven (the heat should rise to 240°) to bake for about twenty minutes. They should be a light-brown when baked.

9. The cakes are then ready for use.

## LESSON NINTH.

### ROCK CAKES.

**Ingredients.**—Half a pound of flour. Quarter of a pound of currants. Quarter of a pound of sugar. Two ounces of candied peel. Two teaspoonfuls of baking-powder. One teaspoonful of grated nutmeg or ginger. Quarter of a pound of clarified dripping. One egg. Half a gill of milk.

*Time required, half an hour.*

To make *Rock Cakes:*

**1.** Put *half a pound of flour* into a basin.

**2.** Stir *two teaspoonfuls of baking-powder* into the *flour.*

**3.** Take a quarter of a pound of clarified dripping and rub it well into the flour with your hands until there are no lumps remaining.

**4.** Take a quarter of a pound of currants, put them in a cloth, rub them clean, and pick them over to see that there are no stones with them.

**5.** Add the *currants* to the *flour*, also one teaspoonful of ground ginger or grated nutmeg, and a quarter of a pound of crushed loaf sugar.

**6.** Take two ounces of candied peel, cut it in pieces, and add it to the other ingredients.

**7.** Mix all these ingredients together with a wooden spoon.

**8.** Break one egg into a cup, and beat it up with about half a gill of milk.

**9.** Pour this into the basin, and mix all well together into a very stiff paste.

**10.** Take a tin and grease it with dripping.

**11.** Divide the paste into small portions with two forks, and lay them in rough heaps on the tin.

**12.** Put them into the oven (the heat should rise to 240°) to bake for about *fifteen minutes.*

**13.** After that time, take them out of the oven, and the cakes are then ready for use.

----

LESSON TENTH.

GINGER-BREAD NUTS.

**Ingredients.**—One pound of flour. Half a pound of treacle. Four ounces of butter. Half an ounce of ground ginger. Allspice. One teaspoonful of carbonate of soda. Salt.

*Time required, about twenty-five minutes.*

To make *Ginger-Bread Nuts :*

**1.** Put *one pound of flour* into a basin with about *half a salt-spoonful of salt.*

**2.** Add *half an ounce of ground ginger, one teaspoonful of carbonate of soda,* and *allspice.*

**3.** Put *half a pound of treacle* and *four ounces of butter* into a saucepan, and melt them together over the fire.

**4.** Mix the ingredients together, and then add the melted treacle and the four ounces of butter, and mix all well together into a firm paste.

> N. B.—Be very careful that all the ingredients are well mixed, and that there are no lumps left.

**5.** Flour a board, and turn the paste out on to it.

**6.** Flour your hands and knead the paste.

**7.** Now divide the paste into about twenty-four pieces.

**8.** Roll each piece into a ball, like a walnut, and put them two inches apart on a greased tin.

**9.** Put them into the oven (the heat should rise to 240°) for *fifteen minutes.*

**10.** After that time, turn the ginger-bread nuts off the tin and set them aside to cool.

# CHAPTER XXI.

## *BUNS, BISCUITS, ROLLS, BREAD, ETC.*

---

### LESSON FIRST.

#### BUNS.

**Ingredients.**—Half an ounce of German yeast.   One and a half pound of flour.   Three gills of milk.   One ounce of butter.   Quarter of a pound of moist sugar.   Quarter of a pound of sultana raisins or currants.

*Time required, about two hours and a half.*

To make *Buns:*

**1.** Put *one gill and a half of milk* into a saucepan, and put it on the fire.

**2.** Put *half an ounce of German yeast* into a basin.

**3.** When the *milk* is just warm, pour it by degrees on to the *yeast*, mixing them well together with a spoon.

**4.** Put one pound of flour into a large basin, and stir into it the milk and yeast, mixing it into a dough.

**5.** Cover the basin with a cloth and stand it on the fender, and let it rise for about *one hour*.

**6.** Put one gill and a half of milk into a saucepan with one ounce of butter, and put it on the fire to warm.

**7.** Put half a pound of flour into a basin, and stir into it the milk and butter.

**8.** When the dough is sufficiently risen, turn it into this mixture, and work them well together.

**9.** Now add a *quarter of a pound of sultana raisins* or *currants* and a *quarter of a pound of moist sugar*, and mix all well together.

> N. B.—If currants are used, they should be well washed, dried in a cloth, and carefully picked over, to see if there are any stones mixed with them.

**10.** Cover the basin with a cloth and stand it near the fire, to rise again for *one hour*.

**11.** After that time, take a tin and grease it with dripping or butter.

> N. B.—If there is no tin, the shelf from the oven should be greased and used instead.

**12.** Flour a paste-board and turn the dough out on it.

**13.** Take a knife, dip it in flour, and cut the dough into pieces.

**14.** Flour your hands, and form the dough into balls.

> N. B.—This quantity of dough will make about twenty-seven ordinary-sized buns.

**15.** Put the buns on the tin.

**16.** Put the tin into the oven (the heat should rise to 240°), to bake the buns for about *half an hour*.

**17.** When they are half done, take the tin out of the oven, brush the buns over with water, and sprinkle white sugar over them.

**18.** Now put the tin back into the oven.

**19.** When the buns are sufficiently baked, take them off the tin, and slant them against a plate, until they are cold.

> N. B.—This will prevent their getting heavy.

## LESSON SECOND.

### RICE BUNS.

**Ingredients.**—Quarter of a pound of ground rice.   Quarter of a pound of sugar.   Two ounces of butter.   Two eggs.   Half a teaspoonful of baking-powder.

*Time required, half an hour.*

To make *Rice Buns :*

1. Put a *quarter of a pound of ground rice* into a basin, with *half a teaspoonful of baking-powder.*

2. Add a *quarter of a pound of pounded loaf sugar* and *two ounces of butter*, and mix all together with a wooden spoon.

3. Break in two eggs, and beat all lightly together.

> N. B.—Be careful to see that the eggs are good before adding them to the mixture.

4. Take some small tins, or patty-pans, and grease them well with a piece of dripping or butter.

5. Fill these tins two-thirds full with the mixture.

> N. B.—This quantity will make about eight or ten buns.

> N. B.—If there are no small tins, the mixture could be put into a cake-tin, which should be previously greased inside.

6. Put the tins into the oven (the heat should rise to 240°) to bake for *fifteen minutes.*

7. After that time, turn the buns out of the tins and lean them against a plate, until they are cold.

## LESSON THIRD.

### MILK BISCUITS.

**Ingredients.**—One gill of milk. One ounce of butter. Half a pound of flour. Teaspoonful of baking-powder.

*Time required, about half an hour.*

To make *Milk Biscuits :*

**1.** Put *one gill of milk* into a saucepan; add to it *one ounce of butter*, and put it on the fire to warm.

**2.** Put half a pound of flour into a basin, with a teaspoonful of baking-powder.

**3.** When the milk is hot, pour it into the flour, and stir it into a smooth, stiff paste.

**4.** Flour a board and turn the paste on to it.

**5.** Flour a rolling-pin, and roll the paste into as thin a sheet as possible.

**6.** Flour a docker or tumbler, and cut the paste into rounds the size of a teacup.

**7.** Grease a tin with dripping or butter, and place the biscuits on it.

**8.** Put the tin into the oven (the heat should rise to 240°) to bake for *twenty minutes.*

**9.** After that, turn the biscuits off the tin and set them aside to cool.

LESSON FOURTH.

### OATMEAL BISCUITS.

**Ingredients.**—Seven ounces of flour. Three ounces of oatmeal. Three ounces of powdered sugar. Three ounces of lard or butter. Quarter of a teaspoonful of carbonate of soda. One egg.

*Time required, about half an hour.*

To make *Oatmeal Biscuits:*

1. Put *three ounces of lard* or *butter* into a saucepan, and put it on the fire to melt.

2. Put *seven ounces of flour* into a basin, with *three ounces of oatmeal, three ounces of powdered sugar,* and a *quarter of a teaspoonful of carbonate of soda,* and mix all together with a spoon.

3. Now stir in the melted lard.

4. Put about a tablespoonful of cold water into a tea-cup; break one egg into the water, and beat them slightly together.

5. Add this to the mixture in the basin, and mix all well and smoothly together with a spoon.

6. Flour a board and turn the paste out on it.

7. Take a rolling-pin, flour it, and roll out the paste as thin as possible.

8. Flour a tumbler and cut the paste into biscuits, according to taste.

9. Grease a baking-tin with dripping or butter, and place the biscuits on it.

10. Put the tin into the oven (the heat should rise to 240°) to bake for *twenty minutes.*

SCONES.

**Ingredients.**—One pound of flour.   Quarter of a pint of milk.   Quarter of a pound of butter.   One dessertspoonful of baking-powder.

*Time required, about forty minutes.*

To make *Scones :*

**1.** Put one pound of flour into a basin, and mix into it a dessertspoonful of baking-powder.

**2.** Take a quarter of a pound of butter and rub it well into the flour with your hands.

**3.** Now turn it out on to a floured board.

**4.** Flour a rolling-pin and roll it out, to make sure that the butter is well mixed with the flour.

**5.** Mix it into a smooth *paste* with rather less than a quarter of a pint of milk.

N. B.—The paste must not be moist.

**6.** Flour the rolling-pin and roll out the paste to a thin sheet, about one-third of an inch in thickness.

**7.** Take a knife, dip it in flour, and cut the paste into triangular pieces, each side about *four inches* long.

**8.** Flour a tin, put the scones on it, and bake them directly in the oven (the heat should rise to 240°) for *thirty* to *forty minutes.*

**9.** When the scones are half done, brush them over with milk.

## LESSON SIXTH.

### SHORT-BREAD.

**Ingredients.**—Quarter of a pound of flour. Two ounces of butter. One ounce of castor sugar.

*Time required, about half an hour.*

To make *Short-Bread :*

1. Put two ounces of butter in a saucepan, and put it on the fire to melt.

2. Put a quarter of a pound of flour into a basin, with one ounce of castor (pounded lump) sugar and the melted butter.

3. Mix these ingredients well together.

4. Flour a board and turn the paste on to it.

5. Flour your hands, and knead the paste well.

6. Flour a rolling-pin, and roll out the paste to about one-third of an inch in thickness.

7. Flour a knife, and cut the paste into oval shapes.

8. Grease a baking-tin with dripping or butter.

9. Put the short-bread on the tin, and put it in the oven (the heat should rise to 240°) to bake till a pale-brown.

---

## LESSON SEVENTH.

### MILK-ROLLS.

**Ingredients.**—One pound of self-raising flour. Two ounces of butter. Milk.

*Time required, about half an hour.*

To make *Milk-Rolls :*

1. Put *one pound of self-raising flour* into a basin, and rub *two ounces of butter* into it with your hands.

**2.** Add sufficient *milk* to make it into a lithe, firm *dough*.

**3.** Sprinkle flour over a board, and turn the dough out on it.

**4.** Take a knife, dip it in flour, and cut the dough into twelve pieces.

> N.B.—Keep your hands floured, to prevent the dough from sticking to them.

**5.** Form each piece into a small roll.

**6.** Flour a baking-tin.

**7.** Put these rolls on to the tin, and put the tin in the oven (the heat should rise to 240°) to bake for *twenty minutes*.

**8.** The milk-rolls will then be ready for use.

---

LESSON EIGHTH.

YORKSHIRE TEA-CAKES.

**Ingredients.**—Three-quarters of a pound of flour. One and one-half a gill of milk. One ounce of butter. One egg. Half an ounce of German yeast.

*Time required, about one hour and a half.*

To make *Yorkshire Tea-Cakes:*

**1.** Put *one and one-half a gill of milk* into a small saucepan, and put it on the fire.

**2.** Put *half an ounce of German yeast* into a basin; and when the *milk* is just warm, pour it on to the *yeast*.

**3.** Put *three-quarters of a pound of flour* into a large basin, and rub into it *one ounce of butter*.

**4.** Beat up one egg in a cup, and then add it to the *flour*.

5. Now pour the yeast and milk through a strainer into the basin, and mix all well together with a wooden spoon.

6. Flour a board and turn the dough out on it.

7. Flour your hands, and knead the dough for a minute or two.

8. Take a knife, dip it in flour, and divide the dough into *cakes*.

9. Take some cake-tins (as many as are required) and grease them inside with dripping.

10. Put the cakes into the tins.

N. B.—The tins should be only three-quarters full, so as to allow for the cakes to rise.

11. Stand the tins near the fire, and allow the cakes to rise for *one hour*.

12. After that time, put the tins into the oven (the heat should rise to 240°) to bake for a *quarter of an hour*.

13. Then turn the cakes out of the tins and place them on a sieve, or on the cane-seat of a chair, to cool.

N. B.—This will prevent their getting heavy.

---

### LESSON NINTH.

#### BREAD.

**Ingredients.**—Three and one-half pounds of flour.   One ounce of German yeast.   Half a salt-spoonful of salt.

*Time required, quarter of an hour for making, two or three hours for rising, and one hour and a half for baking.*

To make *Bread:*

1. Take three and a half pounds of seconds flour, put three pounds of it into a large pan, and make a hole in the centre of the flour.

N. B.—Half a pound is reserved, with which to work up the bread.

**2.** Put one ounce of German yeast into a basin.

**3.** Add about a gill of tepid water, and stir the yeast into a stiff paste.

**4.** Then fill the basin with lukewarm water, and stir the yeast smoothly, making in all about one pint and three gills.

**5.** Add to the flour half a teaspoonful of salt, and then by degrees pour in the yeast, mixing the flour lightly into a dough with your hands.

**6.** Add more lukewarm water, if the dough is too stiff.

N. B.—Be sure to mix up all the flour into dough. ·

**7.** Sprinkle about a tablespoonful of dry flour over the dough, and cover the pan with a cloth.

**8.** Place the pan near the fire for at least two hours, to let the dough rise.

**9.** When it has risen sufficiently, take up the pan and work in more flour, if necessary, to make the dough stiff enough to turn out of the pan.

N. B.—Keep your hands well floured all through the process of bread-making.

**10.** Turn the dough out on a well-floured board, and knead it well, using up a good deal more flour.

**11.** Divide the dough into six equal pieces, knead each piece separately, and make it into a loaf.

N. B.—If the bread is to be baked in tins, form each loaf into a dumpling or ball (with a smooth surface, and no cracks in it), either long or round, according to the shape of the tin.

**12.** Put the bread into the tins, which should be well floured.

**13.** Cut a slit in the top of the dough, or prick it with a fork.

N. B.—If the bread is to be made into cottage loaves :

**14.** Divide each piece into two, one rather larger than the other.

**15.** Make each into a ball, put the smaller one on the top of the other, and press your forefinger into the middle of the top.

N. B.—Cottage loaves are baked on floured tins.

N. B.—If there are no tins, the oven-shelf should be washed and floured, and then a tin is not necessary.

**16.** Let the loaves rise *half an hour* in a warm place, before putting them into the oven.

**17.** Then put them into the oven (the heat should rise to 280°, and after a *quarter of an hour* be reduced to 220°) for about *one hour and a half.*

N. B.—To test if the bread is sufficiently baked, run a clean knife into the loaves ; and if it comes out perfectly bright, the bread is done.

**18.** When you take the bread out of the oven, stand each loaf up on its side to cool.

---

LESSON TENTH.

UNFERMENTED BREAD.

**Ingredients.**—One pound of flour. One teaspoonful of baking-powder. Salt.

*Time required, about three-quarters of an hour.*

To make *Unfermented Bread :*

**1.** Put *one pound of flour* into a basin, and mix into it *one teaspoonful of baking-powder* and *half a salt-spoonful of salt.*

**2.** Add sufficient water to make it into a light, firm dough (not too stiff).

N. B.—It will take about half a pint of water.

**3.** Sprinkle flour over a board, and turn the dough out on it.

> N. B.—Keep your hands floured, to prevent the dough from sticking to them.

**4.** Knead it with your hands, and make it up quickly into small loaves.

> N. B.—Small loaves do better than large ones for unfermented bread; and the quicker the bread is made and put into the oven, the better.

**5.** Put the loaves on a floured baking-sheet, and put them in the oven (the heat should rise to 240°) to bake for *half an hour*.

> N. B.—To see if bread is sufficiently baked, run a clean knife into it; and if it comes out bright and untarnished, the bread is done.

**6.** Take the bread out of the oven, and stand each loaf on its side to cool.

# CHAPTER XXII.

## *SICK-ROOM COOKERY.*

### CHICKEN PANADA.

**Ingredients.**—Half a chicken.  A tablespoonful of cream.

*Time required, about four hours.*

To make *Chicken Panada:*

**1.** Take a *chicken* and clean it in the same way as in " Roasting a Fowl " (*see* " Trussing a Fowl for Roasting ").

**2.** Cut the chicken in half, dividing it down the middle of the back with a sharp knife.

**3.** Take all the flesh off the bones of half the chicken, and cut it into small pieces with a sharp knife.

**4.** Put the pieces of *chicken* into a gallipot, and sprinkle over them half a salt-spoonful of salt.

**5.** Take a piece of paper and tie it over the top of the gallipot.

**6.** Take a saucepan half full of boiling water and put it on the fire.

**7.** Stand the gallipot in the saucepan, and let it simmer for two hours.  The water must not cover the gallipot.

**8.** After that time, take the gallipot out of the saucepan.

**9.** Take the pieces of chicken out with a spoon, and be careful not to lose any of the liquor.

**10.** Take the pieces of chicken and put them into a mortar, and pound them well to a pulp.

**11.** Take a tammy-sieve and stand it over a basin.

**12.** Pass the pounded chicken through the sieve, rubbing it with a wooden spoon. Pour a little of the chicken-liquor into the pulp on the sieve, to make it pass through more easily.

**13.** When all the chicken-pulp has been passed through into the basin, stir in one tablespoonful of cream.

Use the bones for *Chicken Broth:*

**1.** Take the chicken-bones and put them in a saucepan with one pint of cold water.

**2.** Put the saucepan on the fire, and let it boil for three hours.

**3.** Watch it, and skim it occasionally.

**4.** When required for use, take a strainer and strain the chicken broth into a basin.

**5.** Flavor it with pepper and salt, according to the taste of the patient.

N. B.—Some of this broth is required to help to pass the chicken through the sieve.

---

LESSON SECOND.

BEEF ESSENCE.

**Ingredients.**—One pound of gravy-beef.

*Time required, about two hours.*

To make *Beef Essence:*

**1.** Take *one pound of gravy-beef*, and cut off all fat and gristle with a sharp knife.

2. Cut the *lean* up into small pieces, and put them into a jar.

3. Put the cover over the jar, and tie a piece of paper over it.

4. Take a saucepan half full of *boiling water* and stand it on the fire.

5. Stand the jar in the saucepan of boiling water, to steam for two hours. The water must not cover the jar.

6. When it is done, take a strainer and put it over a basin.

7. Strain off the liquor into the basin, and flavor it with *pepper* and *salt*, according to the patient's complaint.

N. B.—The *meat* can be put aside, and used again for second stock.

---

### LESSON THIRD.

#### CREAM OF BARLEY.

**Ingredients.**—Half a pound of veal cutlet. Half an ounce of barley. Half a gill of cream.

*Time required, about four hours.*

To make *Cream of Barley :*

1. Take half a pound of veal cutlet, and cut off all the fat with a sharp knife.

2. Cut the lean into small pieces, and put it in a saucepan with one pint of cold water.

3. Add half an ounce of barley, previously well washed and soaked an hour or two in cold water, and half a salt-spoonful of salt.

4. Put the saucepan on the fire, and let it boil for two hours.

5. Strain off the liquor into a basin, and put the meat and barley in a mortar, and pound them together.

**6.** Take a hair sieve and put it over a basin.

**7.** Turn the pounded meat and barley on to the sieve, and rub them through with a wooden spoon.

**8.** Pour the liquor on to the sieve, to help the pulp to pass through.

**9.** When it has all passed through the sieve into the basin, stir in smoothly two tablespoonfuls of cream.

---

## LESSON FOURTH.

### A CUP OF ARROW-ROOT, AND ARROW-ROOT PUDDING.

**Ingredients.**—A dessertspoonful of arrow-root.    Half a pint of milk. Powdered sugar.    Two eggs.

*Time required, about a quarter of an hour.*

To make a *Cup of Arrow-root:*

**1.** Take a *dessertspoonful of arrow-root* and put it into a small basin.

**2.** Add a *dessertspoonful of cold milk,* and stir it smoothly into a *paste* with a spoon.

**3.** Add a *small teaspoonful of powdered sugar,* according to taste.

**4.** Take a small saucepan and put in it half a pint of cold milk.

**5.** Put the saucepan on the fire, and watch the milk carefully until it boils.

**6.** When it is quite boiling, pour it on to the arrow-root paste, stirring all the time to get it quite smooth.

N. B.—If the patient prefers an *Arrow-root Pudding* :

**7.** Add to the mixture described above the yolks of two eggs, whipping it all well together.

N. B.—The eggs should not be added till the mixture has cooled a little, for they would curdle.

**8.** Put the whites of the same eggs into another basin, and whisk them to a stiff froth.

**9.** Add the whites of the eggs to the arrow-root mixture, stirring them lightly together.

**10.** Pour the mixture into a buttered dish, and put it into the oven (the heat should rise to 240°) to bake for *ten minutes.*

---

LESSON FIFTH.

R I C E - W A T E R .

**Ingredients.**—Three ounces of rice. One inch of cinnamon-stick. Sugar. *Time required, about one hour.*

To make *Rice-Water:*

**1.** Take *three ounces of rice* and wash it well in two or three waters.

**2.** Take a stewpan with *one quart of warm water.*

**3.** Put the stewpan on the fire to boil.

**4.** When the water is quite boiling, put in the rice, and one inch of the stick of cinnamon, and let it boil for one hour, until the rice has become a pulp.

**5.** Then take the stewpan off the fire and strain the *rice-water* into a basin, and sweeten it according to taste.

N. B.—When cold, it is ready for use.

14

## LESSON SIXTH.

### BARLEY-WATER.

**Ingredients.**—Two ounces of pearl barley. The rind of a quarter of a lemon. Two lumps of loaf sugar.

**Ingredients** (for making Thick Barley-Water).—Two ounces of pearl barley. The rind of half a lemon. Sugar.

*Time required, about two hours.*

To make two kinds of *Barley - Water—Clear Barley Water* and *Thick Barley - Water.*

For *half a pint of Clear Barley - Water :*

**1.** Take *two ounces of pearl barley* and wash it well in two or three waters.

**2.** Put a kettle of water on the fire to boil.

**3.** Take a *quarter of a lemon*, wipe it clean in a cloth, and peel it very thin.

> N. B.—Be careful, in peeling the lemon, not to cut any of the white skin, as it would make it bitter.

**4.** Put the washed barley into a jug.

**5.** Put in the lemon-peel, and two lumps of loaf sugar.

**6.** When the water in the kettle is quite boiling, pour one pint of it on to the barley in the jug.

**7.** Cover over the top of the jug, and let it stand on ice, or in a cool place, until it is perfectly cold.

**8.** Then strain the water into a clean jug for use.

> N. B.—The barley can be used again, with the addition of *one ounce* of fresh.

For *one pint of Thick Barley - Water :*

**1.** Take *two ounces of pearl barley* and wash it well in two or three waters.

2. Put the barley into a stewpan, with *one quart of cold water.*

·3. Put the stewpan on the fire, and let it boil gently for *two hours.*

4. Take *half a lemon,* wipe it clean in a cloth, and peel it very thin.

5. Put the lemon-peel into a jug.

6. When the barley-water is sufficiently boiled, strain it into the jug over the lemon.

7. Put the jug into a cool place; when it is perfectly cold, take out the lemon-peel, and sweeten the water according to taste.

———

### LESSON SEVENTH.

### APPLE-WATER.

**Ingredients.**—Six apples.   The rind of half a lemon.   Sugar.

*Time required for making, about eight minutes.*

To make *Apple - Water :*

1. Take six apples, peel them, and cut out the cores.

> N. B.—When the apples are juicy, six will be sufficient; but more may be required, according to the season of the year.

2. Put a kettle of water on the fire to boil.

3. Cut up the apples in slices.

4. Take half a lemon, wipe it clean in a cloth, and peel it very thin.

5. Put the slices of apple and the lemon-rind into a jug.

6. When the water is quite boiling, pour one quart of it on to the apples in the jug.

7. Sweeten it according to taste.

8. Stand the jug of apple-water aside to cool.

9. When the water is quite cold, strain it into another jug, and it is then ready for use.

## LESSON EIGHTH.

### LEMONADE.

**Ingredients.**—Two lemons.  Loaf sugar.

*Time required, about one hour.*

To make *Lemonade :*

1. Put a kettle of water on the fire to boil.

2. Take *two lemons*, wipe them clean in a cloth, and peel them very thin.

> N.B.—Be careful, in cutting the lemons, not to cut any of the pith, or white skin, as it would make the lemonade bitter.

3. Now cut off all the pith.

4. Cut up the lemons into thin slices, take out all the pips, and put the slices and half the rind of the lemons into a jug.

5. Add loaf sugar according to taste—about one ounce.

6. When the water is quite boiling, pour one pint and a half on to the lemons in the jug.

7. Cover over the jug, and stand it aside to cool.

8. When the lemonade is quite cold, strain it into another jug, and it is then ready for use.

---

### LESSON NINTH.

### TOAST AND WATER.

**Ingredients.**—One crust of bread.  One quart of water.

*Time required, half an hour.*

To make *Toast and Water :*

1. Take a *crust of bread* and toast it quite brown on all sides, in front of the fire.

> N.B.—Crumb should not be used, as it would turn sour.

2. Put the toasted crust of bread into a jug, and pour on it *one quart of cold water.*

3. Cover the jug with a cloth, and stand it aside for *half an hour.*

N. B.—This is a pleasant drink, and considered more refreshing than when made with boiling water.

---

LESSON TENTH.

GRUEL.

**Ingredients.**—Two dessertspoonfuls of patent groats.   Sugar.   A small piece of fresh butter.   Half a gill of rum.

*Time required, about fifteen minutes.*

To make *Gruel:*

1. Put a stewpan with one pint of water on the fire to boil.

2. Take two dessertspoonfuls of patent groats and put them in a basin.

3. Add, by degrees, two tablespoonfuls of cold water to the groats, and stir it into a smooth paste.

4. When the water in the stewpan is quite boiling, pour in the mixed gruel and stir it well with a wooden spoon, until it has boiled for ten minutes (it must not be lumpy); then pour it into a basin, and it is ready for use.

N. B.—If the gruel is required for a cold:

5. Stir in a piece of fresh butter the size of a chestnut, and sweeten it according to taste.

6. Also add two tablespoonfuls of rum.

N. B.—If the patient is feverish, spirits should not be added.

## LESSON ELEVENTH.

### WHITE-WINE WHEY, OR TREACLE POSSET.

**Ingredients** (for White-Wine Whey).—Half a pint of milk. Four lumps of sugar. One wineglassful of wine.

**Ingredients** (for Treacle Posset).—Half a pint of milk. Half a gill of treacle.

*Time required, about ten minutes.*

To make *White - Wine Whey :*

1. Put *half a pint of milk* into a saucepan, and *four lumps of sugar.*

2. Put the saucepan on the fire to boil.

3. When it boils, pour in a *wineglassful of wine* (*sherry* or *cowslip*, according to taste).

> N. B.—If the milk is not quite boiling, the wine will not curdle it.

4. Move the saucepan to the side of the fire, and let it stand for about *one minute.*

5. Then strain the whey into a glass.

> N. B.—The curds are not digestible.

> N. B.—Treacle Posset is made in the same way, except that no sugar should be added to the milk, and the same quantity of treacle is used instead of wine.

---

## LESSON TWELFTH.

### BRAN TEA.

**Ingredients.**—Three tablespoonfuls of bran. Sugar or honey.

*Time required, about twenty minutes.*

To make *Bran Tea :*

1. Put a kettle of warm water on the fire to boil.

**2.** Take *three tablespoonfuls of bran* (not too coarse, for that is greasy) and put it into a large jug.

> N. B.—Bran is the husk of the grain, which is sifted from the flour after the wheat is ground by the miller.

**3.** When the *water* is quite boiling, pour *one quart* into the jug.

**4.** Cover the jug, and let it stand for a *quarter of an hour* to draw.

**5.** When it is drawn, strain off the *tea* through a piece of muslin, and sweeten it according to taste with either *sugar* or *honey*.

> N. B.—When wine is good for the patient, it may be added to the tea, or a little lemon-juice, but it is very good without.

> N. B.—This is an invaluable drink for softening the throat.

---

### LESSON THIRTEENTH.

#### MUTTON BROTH.

**Ingredients.**—Four pounds of the scrag end of the neck of mutton. Two knuckles from the legs of mutton. A salt-spoonful of salt. Two ounces of rice.

*Time required for making : The stock should be made the day before, and then the broth can be finished in about half an hour.*

To make two quarts of *Mutton Broth :*

**1.** Take *four pounds of the scrag end of the neck of mutton,* wash it well, put it on a board, cut away all the *fat,* and chop it up in large pieces.

**2.** Put these pieces into the stewpan, with two knuckle-bones from the legs of mutton.

**3.** Pour in five pints of cold water, and add a salt-spoonful of salt.

**4.** Put the stewpan on the fire, just bring it to the boil, and then let it simmer for *four hours*.

**5.** Watch it, and skim it very often.

**6.** After that time, strain the stock into a basin, and put it aside until it is quite cold and in a stiff jelly.

**7.** Then take the *stock* and remove all the fat from the top with a spoon.

**8.** Take a clean cloth and dip it in hot water, and dab over the top of the stock so as to remove every particle of grease.

**9.** Now take a clean dry cloth and wipe the top of the stock dry.

**10.** Take *two ounces of rice* and wash it well in two or three waters.

**11.** Put the stock into a stewpan.

**12.** Put the stewpan on the fire to boil.

**13.** When the stock is quite boiling, stir in the *rice*, and let it boil for *twenty-five minutes*, to cook the *rice*.

N. B.—See that the rice is quite tender.

**14.** Season it with pepper and salt, according to the patient's complaint.

**15.** For serving, pour the broth into a basin.

N. B.—The *bones* should be put in the stock-pot.

## LESSON FOURTEENTH.

### MUTTON BROTH.

**Ingredients.**—Two pounds of the scrag end of the neck of mutton. One ounce of pearl barley or rice. Half a salt-spoonful of salt. Half an ounce of butter. Half an ounce of flour. Two sprigs of parsley.

*Time required, about two hours and forty minutes.*

To make *Mutton Broth :*

1. Take *two pounds of the scrag end of the neck of mutton* and wash it well until it is quite clean.

2. Put the meat into a large saucepan with *three pints of cold water*, and put it on the fire to boil.

3. Take *one ounce of pearl barley* or *rice* and wash it well in cold water.

4. When the water boils, put in the *pearl barley* or *rice*, and *half a salt-spoonful of salt*, to help the scum to rise.

5. Now draw the saucepan to the side of the fire, and let it simmer gently for *two hours and a half.*

6. Watch it, and skim it occasionally with a spoon.

7. If the meat is required for immediate use, make sauce to pour over it.

8. Take a sprig or two of parsley, wash it and clean it in a cloth, put it on a board, and chop it up fine with a knife.

9. Put half an ounce of butter into a saucepan, and put it on the fire.

10. When the butter is melted, stir in smoothly half an ounce of flour with a wooden spoon.

11. Take one gill of broth from the mutton, pour it on to the butter and flour, and stir smoothly until it boils and thickens.

12. Now add the chopped parsley to the sauce, and move the saucepan to the side of the fire, to keep warm till required for use.

13. When the mutton is sufficiently cooked, take out the meat and put it on a hot dish.

14. Pour the parsley-sauce all over the mutton.

15. Pour the broth into a basin to cool.

16. When it is cold, remove all the fat before warming it up for use.

N.B.—If the broth is required for immediate use, remove the *grease* with blotting-paper or whity-brown paper.

---

### LESSON FIFTEENTH.

#### BEEF TEA.

**Ingredients.**—One pound of gravy-beef.

*Time required, about six hours.*

To make *Beef Tea* :

1. Take *one pound of gravy-beef*, put it on a board, and cut it up very fine, removing all the *skin* and *fat*.

2. Put the *meat* into a saucepan, with *one pint and a half of cold water, half a salt-spoonful of salt*, and *two* or *three pepper-corns*, if allowed.

3. Put the saucepan on the fire, and just bring it to the boil.

4. Then move it to the side of the fire to simmer gently for *five* or *six hours*, but do not let it reduce too much.

N.B.—The lid should be on the saucepan.

5. After that time, pour off the beef tea, or strain it through a coarse cloth into a basin, and let it get cold.

**6.** Remove all fat from the beef tea before warming it up for use.

> N.B.—Fat can be taken off hot beef tea with blotting-paper or whity-brown paper.

> N.B.—It is better not to strain beef tea, as it removes all the little brown particles, which are most nutritious.

### LESSON SIXTEENTH.

#### BEEF TEA.

**Ingredients.**—Half a pound of gravy-beef.

*Time required, about three hours and a quarter.*

To make *Beef Tea :*

**1.** Take half a pound of gravy-beef, put it on a board, and cut it up very fine, removing all the skin and fat.

**2.** Put the meat into a stone jar with half a pint of water.

> N.B.—In making this beef tea, the quantity of meat and water should be of equal weight—i. e., one pint to the pound.

**3.** Put the lid on the jar, and tie a piece of paper over it.

**4.** Stand the jar in a saucepan of boiling water on the hob for three hours, or in the oven for one hour and a half.

> N.B.—If the jar is put into the saucepan of boiling water, you should be careful that the water does not cover the jar, or it would get inside.

**5.** After a time, take out the jar and pour off the beef tea into a cup.

> N.B.—If allowed, add salt according to taste.

## LESSON SEVENTEENTH.

### LIEBIG'S QUICK BEEF TEA.

**Ingredients.**—Half a pound of gravy-beef.

*Time required, about a quarter of an hour.*

To make *Baron Liebig's Quick Beef Tea :*

**1.** Take half a pound of gravy-beef, put it on a board, and cut it up very fine, removing all the skin and fat.

**2.** Put it into a saucepan with its equal weight in water—i. e., half a pint.

**3.** Put the saucepan on the fire and bring it quickly to the boil.

**4.** Let it boil for *five minutes,* and then pour it off into a cup.

---

### LESSON EIGHTEENTH.

### SAVORY CUSTARD.

**Ingredients.**—Two eggs.   Salt.   One gill of beef tea.

*Time required, about twenty minutes.*

To make *Savory Custard :*

**1.** Take the yolks of *two eggs* and the white of *one,* and put them in a small basin.

**2.** Add *one gill of beef tea* and a *quarter of a salt-spoonful of salt.*

**3.** Whisk up the *eggs* and the *beef tea* well together.

**4.** Take a small gallipot and butter it inside.

**5.** Pour the mixture into the gallipot.

**6.** Take a piece of whity-brown paper and butter it.

**7.** Put this buttered paper over the top of the gallipot, and tie it on with a piece of string.

**8.** Take a saucepan of hot water and put it on the fire.

**9.** When the water is quite boiling, stand the little gallipot in it.

> N. B.—The water must not quite reach the paper with which the gallipot is covered.

**10.** Draw this saucepan to the side of the fire, and let it simmer for a *quarter of an hour*.

> N. B.—It must not boil, or the custard will be spoiled.

**11.** Take the gallipot out of the saucepan, take off the buttered paper, and the custard is ready for serving.

# CHAPTER XXIII.

## CANNED MEATS.

Note.—In the English edition of this work, the present chapter appeared under the title of "Australian Meat," which consists of cooked and canned meats that are brought into England in large variety, and are coming into such general use there that it was found desirable to give them some attention at the training-school. "Australian Meat," however, is not to be obtained in the American market; but as we have its equivalent in the canned meats put up in this country, the title of the chapter has been changed, to prevent misapprehension and inconvenience.

The directions in the following lessons are not so much for cooking canned meats—which are indeed already cooked—as for using them as ingredients of various complex dishes, such as soups, stews, curries, fricassees, and hashes, and for these purposes the American canned preparations answer just as well as the Australian. For such uses canned meats deserve more attention than they generally receive.[1] Everybody now understands the value of having fruits and vegetables—such as peaches, cherries, pears, tomatoes, corn, beans, peas, and asparagus—ready at hand, as they not only give an agreeable and healthy variety to diet, but are easily and quickly prepared, and thus save labor and trouble to the house-keeper. The advantages are the same with canned meats, especially in the country, where markets are not near by. And even in competition with butcher's meat, canned beef and mutton do not make a bad showing in point of economy; for when beef and mutton are procured from the market, there is not only a loss by the removal of bone, fat, and gristle, but also a loss of weight in the operation of cooking, so that the meat upon the table should properly be estimated at nearly double the market-price. As the canned meats consist of the pure muscular fibres, with

---

[1] Yet their use is rapidly extending. We were informed by Mr. Alexander Wiley, the intelligent superintendent of the department of "canned goods" in the establishment of H. K. & F. B. Thurber, of New York, that this trade has doubled in a comparatively short time, while the saving to the country through this preservation of perishable food-products is probably not less than fifty million dollars annually.

their contained nutritive juices, these sources of loss are avoided; and while the expense is no greater, the trouble of preparation is saved.

In purchasing canned meats, much depends upon the character of the articles, and the buyer will consult his interest by purchasing only well-known brands. Among these are Thurber & Co., Wilson, Libby, Underwood, and Richardson & Robbins. Almost everything in the way of meat is to be had thus preserved, but different establishments confine themselves more or less to special preparations. As an example of the variety of animal products that are furnished in this manner, the following are selected from Thurber's Price-List of June 6, 1878: Corned beef, beef tongue, mutton, ham, lamb's tongue, pig's feet, tripe, sausage, pork and beans, turkey, duck, chicken, clams, clam broth, lobster, oysters, green turtle, salmon, shrimps, codfish-balls, julienne, mock-turtle and ox-tail soups, condensed milk. Most of these articles are, moreover, prepared in a variety of forms.—EDITOR.

---

### LESSON FIRST.

#### MULLIGATAWNY.

**Ingredients.**—Two-pound tin of canned calf's-head. Two pounds of canned mutton or chicken. Two apples. Two leeks. Two carrots. One turnip. Two good-sized onions. Two tablespoonfuls of flour. One table-spoonful of curry-powder. Salt and sugar. A bunch of herbs.

*Time required, three hours.*

To make *Mulligatawny Soup:*

1. Take *two pounds of canned mutton* or *chicken* out of the tin; put it in a basin with *two quarts of warm water.*

2. Peel *two apples*, and put them on a plate.

3. Cut the *apples* in *quarters*, cut out the *core*, and then cut the quarters into slices, and put them into a saucepan with *two ounces of the clarified fat.*

4. Take *one turnip* and *two good-sized onions*, peel them, cut them in pieces, and put them in the saucepan.

5. Put the saucepan on the fire, and give one stir to the *vegetables* with a wooden spoon.

**6.** Take *two leeks*, wash them well in cold water, and cut off the green tops of the leaves.

**7.** Cut up the *leeks* and put them in the saucepan.

**8.** Take *two carrots*, wash them, scrape them with a knife, cut them in pieces, and put them in the saucepan.

**9.** Give one stir with a wooden spoon, to mix the *vegetables* together, and let them fry for *ten minutes*.

**10.** Also add a *sprig of parsley*, a *sprig of thyme*, a *sprig of marjoram*, and *two bay-leaves*, tied tightly together with a piece of string.

**11.** When the *vegetables* have fried for *ten minutes*, take *half a pint of the liquor* (in which the meat is soaking), pour it into the saucepan, and let it boil and reduce to a quarter of a pint.

**12.** Stir the *vegetables* occasionally.

**13.** Put *two tablespoonfuls of flour* and *one tablespoonful of curry-powder* into a basin, and mix them into a smooth *paste* with *one gill* of the *liquor*.

**14.** Stir this mixture into the saucepan with the *vegetables*.

**15.** Now put the *meat* or *fowl* and the remaining *liquor* into the saucepan, put the lid on, and let it come to the boil.

**16.** When it boils, put one *salt-spoonful of salt* and *half a salt-spoonful of moist sugar* into the saucepan.

**17.** Now move the saucepan to the side of the fire and let it simmer for *two hours and a half*.

**18.** Watch it, and skim it occasionally with a spoon.

**19.** After that time strain off the *soup* through a strainer into a basin.

**20.** Pour the soup back into the saucepan.

**21.** Open the *two-pound tin of calf's-head*, remove all the *fat* from the top, and stir the contents of the tin into the soup in the saucepan.

**22.** For serving, pour the soup into a hot soup-tureen.

## LESSON SECOND.

### BROWN PURÉE.

**Ingredients.**—One pound of canned mince-meat. Two carrots and a small turnip. Two leeks. Two sticks of celery. One onion stuck with four cloves. A bouquet garni (two bay-leaves, thyme, and marjoram). A sprig of parsley. One teaspoonful of Liebig's Extract.

*Time required, about two hours.*

To make *Brown Purée:*

1. Open a tin of *canned mince-meat,* and put the *meat* in a mortar.

2. Pound the *meat* well with a pestle.

3. Put *two quarts of water* into a saucepan and put it on the fire to boil.

4. Wash *two carrots* and scrape them with a knife.

5. Cut off the outside green leaves of *two leeks,* wash them thoroughly in cold water, and cut them in quarters.

6. Take *two sticks of celery,* wash them, and scrape them clean with a knife.

7. Tie these *vegetables* into a small bundle with a string.

8. Take *one small turnip* and peel it.

9. Take an *onion,* peel it, and stick *four cloves* in it.

10. When the *water* in the saucepan is quite boiling, put in all these *vegetables.*

11. Add a *bouquet garni,* consisting of *two bay-leaves* and a *sprig of thyme* and *marjoram,* tied tightly together.

12. Take a *sprig of parsley,* wash it in cold water, wring it in a cloth, and put it in the saucepan.

13. Take the *jelly* which came from the *meat,* and a little more out of the tin, and put it in the saucepan.

14. Stir in *one teaspoonful* of *Liebig's Extract,* or ten or twelve drops of caramel (see note below), for coloring.

**15.** Let the *vegetables* boil gently for an hour and a half.

N. B.—The lid should be on the saucepan.

**16.** After that time stir in the *pounded meat*, and season according to taste.

**17.** Take a colander and strain the *purée* through on to a hot dish.

N. B.—To make caramel (browned sugar) for coloring gravies, etc.: Put a quarter of a pound of moist or loaf sugar into an old saucepan, and put it on the fire and let it burn until it has become quite a dark-brown liquid; add to it half a pint of boiling water, and let it boil for five minutes, stirring it occasionally; then strain it and pour it into a bottle, and it is ready for use at any time.

---

LESSON THIRD.

### IRISH STEW.

**Ingredients.**—One and a half pound of canned meat. One and a half pound of potatoes. Half a pound of onions.

*Time required, about one hour.*

To make an *Irish Stew:*

**1.** Wash *one and a half pound* of *potatoes* well in cold water, and scrub them clean with a scrubbing-brush.

N. B.—If the potatoes are not very good, or are in any way diseased, take a sharp knife, peel them, and cut out the eyes and any black specks about them; but it is much better to steam or boil them in their skins.

**2.** Fill a saucepan with hot water and put it on the fire to boil.

**3.** Peel *half a pound* of *onions*.

**4.** When the water is quite boiling, put the *potatoes* in a steamer and sprinkle them over with salt.

N. B.—As the onions are to be eaten with the potatoes, put them in the saucepan of boiling water, and they can be boiled while the potatoes are being steamed.

**5.** Place the steamer on the saucepan of boiling water, and cover it down tight to keep the steam in.

**6.** Let the *potatoes* steam and the *onions* boil for half an hour.

**7.** Now open a tin of *canned meat*.

**8.** Take *one and a half pound of meat* out of the tin and cut it in slices.

**9.** Take a fork and put it in the *potatoes* and the *onions*, to feel if they are quite tender.

**10.** When they are sufficiently cooked, take the *potatoes* out of the steamer, put them on a board, peel them carefully, and cut them in slices.

**11.** Take the *onions* out of the saucepan, put them on a board, and cut them in slices.

**12.** Take a large saucepan, put in a layer of *potatoes*, then a layer of *onions*, and then a layer of *meat*.

**13.** Sprinkle a little *pepper* and *salt* over each layer of *meat* for seasoning.

**14.** Pour *half a pint of warm water* into the saucepan, put it on the fire, and let the *meat* and *vegetables* simmer until they are thoroughly warmed through.

**15.** For serving, turn the *Irish stew* out on to a hot dish.

----

### LESSON FOURTH.

#### SAUSAGE ROLLS.

**Ingredients.**—Half a pound of mince-meat. Half a pound of flour. Half a pound of dripping. One teaspoonful of baking-powder. Salt and pepper. Four sage-leaves. One egg.

*Time required, half an hour.*

To make *Sausage Rolls :*

**1.** Take a tin of *canned mince-meat* and open it carefully.

**2.** Take *half a pound* of the *mince-meat* out of the tin, put it in a basin, and season it well with *pepper and salt.*

**3.** Take *four sage-leaves*, put them on a board, and chop them up as finely as possible with a knife.

**4.** Mix the *chopped sage* well into the *mince-meat* with a spoon.

**5.** Put *one pound of flour* into another basin.

**6.** Add to it *one teaspoonful of baking-powder, a pinch of salt,* and *half a pound of clarified dripping.*

**7.** Rub the *dripping* well into the *flour* with your hands.

N. B.—Mix it thoroughly, and be careful not to leave any *lumps.*

**8.** Add enough *water* to the *flour* to make it into a stiff *paste.*

**9.** Flour the paste-board and turn the *paste* out on it.

N. B.—Divide the *paste* in two, so as not to handle it too much.

**10.** Take a rolling-pin, flour it, and roll out *each portion* into a thin sheet, about *one-eighth of an inch* in thickness.

**11.** Cut the *paste* into pieces about *six inches* square.

**12.** Collect all the scraps of *paste* (so that none will be wasted), fold them together, and roll them out and cut them into squares.

N. B.—There should be about *two dozen squares* of paste.

**13.** Put about a *tablespoonful* of the *mince-meat* into the centre of each square of *paste.*

**14.** Fold the *paste* round the *meat*, joining it smoothly down the centre, and pressing the *ends* of the *paste* together with your finger and thumb.

**15.** Take a baking-tin, grease it well, and place the *sausage rolls* on it.

**16.** Break *one egg* on to a plate, and beat it slightly with a knife.

**17.** Take a paste-brush, dip it in the *egg*, and paint over the tops of the *rolls*.

**18.** Place the tin in a hot oven to bake for *fifteen minutes*.

> N. B.—Look at them once or twice, and turn them if necessary, so that they shall be equally baked.

**19.** For serving, take the *rolls* off the tin and place them on a hot dish.

----

LESSON FIFTH.

CURRIED RABBIT.

**Ingredients.**—Two-pound tin of canned rabbit. Two ounces of butter or dripping. Two moderate-sized onions. One good-sized apple. One dessertspoonful of curry-powder. Salt and flour. Rice served with the curry.

*Time required, half an hour.*

To make a *Curry* of *Canned Rabbit* or *Chicken :*

**1.** Take a *two-pound tin* of *rabbit* and open it carefully.

> N. B.—Chicken or any other meat can be used for the curry instead of rabbit.

**2.** Put *two ounces* of *butter* or *clarified fat* into a stew-pan.

**3.** Put the stewpan on the fire to heat the *fat*.

**4.** Peel *two* medium-sized *onions* and cut them in slices.

**5.** When the *fat* is quite hot, put in the *onions* to fry brown.

> N. B.—Watch it, and stir the onions occasionally, so as not to let them burn, or stick to the bottom of the pan.

**6.** Turn the *rabbit* out of the tin on to a plate.

**7.** Take a *good-sized apple*, peel it, take out the core, and chop it up as finely as possible.

**8.** When the *onions* are sufficiently browned, take all the pieces carefully out of the stewpan with a perforated spoon, and put them on a plate.

**9.** Take the pieces of *rabbit*, dry them in a cloth, and sprinkle them over well with *flour*.

**10.** Now put the pieces of *rabbit* into the stewpan to fry a nice brown.

**11.** Turn the pieces occasionally so as to let them brown on both sides alike.

**12.** Put a *dessertspoonful of curry-powder* into a cup, and mix it into a smooth paste with a little *cold water*.

**13.** When the *rabbit* is browned, put the *chopped apple* and the *fried onions* into the stewpan.

**14.** Stir in smoothly the curry-paste, and then add *half a pint of cold water* or *stock*, and *salt* according to taste.

**15.** Give one stir with a spoon, and mix it all together.

**16.** Now put the lid on the stewpan, draw it rather to the side of the fire, and let it stew very gently for about *a quarter of an hour*, until the apple is quite tender.

**17.** Boil the *rice* as directed. (*See* Lesson on "Rice.")

**18.** For serving, turn the *curry* on to a hot dish. The *rice* can be put as a border on the same dish as the *curry*, or served on a separate dish.

LESSON SIXTH.

MEAT PIE.

**Ingredients.**—One and a half pound of canned mutton or beef. Half a pound of canned kidneys. Three-quarters of a pound of flour. One-quarter of a pound of dripping. One teaspoonful of baking-powder. Pepper and salt.

*Time required, about three-quarters of an hour.*

To make *Meat Pie:*

1. Open a *tin of canned mutton* or *beef*.

2. Take *one and a half pound* of the *meat* out of the tin and cut it neatly into nice-sized pieces, and season with *pepper* and *salt*.

3. Take *half a pound* of the *kidneys* and cut them up in pieces.

4. Put *three-quarters of a pound of flour* into a basin with a small *teaspoonful of baking-powder* and a pinch of *salt*.

5. Take a *quarter of a pound of clarified dripping* and rub it well into the *flour* with your hands.

N. B.—Be careful not to leave any lumps.

6. Add sufficient *water* to make it into a stiff *paste;* it will take rather less than *one gill*.

7. Take a board, flour it, and put the *paste* on it.

8. Take a *quart* pie-dish and fill it with the pieces of *meat* and *kidney*.

9. Take a little of the *jelly* out of the tin and put it in the dish with the *meat*, to make the *gravy*.

10. Take a rolling-pin, flour it, and roll out the *paste* to the shape of the top of the pie-dish, only rather larger.

N. B.—Keep your hands floured, to prevent the paste sticking.

**11.** Take a knife, dip it in the *flour*, and cut off a strip of the paste about *one inch* wide.

> N. B.—This strip should be cut off from round the edge of the *paste*, leaving the centre piece the size of the top of the pie-dish.

**12.** Wet the edge of the pie-dish with *water*, and place the strip of *paste* round the edge.

**13.** Now wet the strip of *paste* on the pie-dish.

**14.** Take the piece of *paste*, lay it over the top of the pie-dish, pressing the edges together with your thumb.

**15.** Flour a knife and trim off the rough edges of the *paste*.

**16.** Take the knife, and with the back of the blade make little notches in the edge of the paste, pressing it with your thumb, to keep it in its proper place.

**17.** Make a small hole in the *centre* of the *paste*, to let out the steam while it is baking.

**18.** Ornament the top of the pie with the remains of the *paste*, according to taste.

**19.** Put the *pie* into a quick oven to bake for *half an hour*.

**20.** Look at it occasionally, to see that it does not burn.

----

### LESSON SEVENTH.

#### FRICASSEE OF MUTTON.

**Ingredients.**—Two pounds of canned mutton. Two ounces of butter. One and a half ounce of flour. Pepper and salt. One dozen mushrooms. Bread. About a pint of milk.

*Time required, about half an hour.*

To make *Fricassee of Mutton :*

**1.** Put *two ounces of butter* into a saucepan, and put it on the fire.

**2.** When the *butter* is melted, stir in *one and a half ounce of flour*, and a little *pepper* and *salt* according to taste.

**3.** Now pour in *three-quarters of a pint of cold milk*, and stir smoothly with a wooden spoon until it boils and thickens.

**4.** Peel *one dozen mushrooms*, and cut off the ends of the stalks.

**5.** Add these *mushrooms* to the *sauce*, and let them stew gently until they are quite tender.

**6.** Wash the *peel* and *stalks* of the *mushrooms* in cold water, and put them in a small saucepan with about a gill of milk.

**7.** Put the saucepan on the fire and let it stew gently, to extract the *flavor* of the *mushrooms*.

**8.** Take a *two-pound* tin of *mutton*, open it carefully, and remove all the *fat* from the top of the *meat* with a spoon.

**9.** Turn the *meat* out of the tin and cut it in small pieces.

**10.** Cut a thin slice of *crumb of bread*, put it on a board, and cut it up in small square pieces.

**11.** Cut these square pieces in half cornerwise, making them into triangles.

**12.** Put *three ounces of clarified dripping* into a frying-pan, and put it on the fire to heat the *fat*.

**13.** Take a piece of kitchen-paper and put it on a plate.

**14.** When the *fat* is quite hot and smoking, throw in the *sippets of bread* and let them fry a pale-brown.

**15.** Then take them out of the frying-pan and put them on the piece of paper, to drain off the grease.

**16.** Sprinkle a little *salt* over the *sippets*, and keep them warm till required for use.

15

**17.** When the *mushrooms* are sufficiently cooked, strain the *milk* (in which the mushroom peelings were stewed), and stir it smoothly into the sauce.

**18.** Draw the saucepan to the side of the fire, and when the *sauce* is a little cooled, put in the *slices of mutton* and let them just warm through.

N. B.—Be careful that the *meat* does not boil, or it will be hardened.

**19.** Now take out the pieces of *meat* and put them on a hot dish.

**20.** Pour the *sauce* over the *meat*, and arrange the *mushrooms* in the centre.

**21.** Place the fried *sippets of bread* round the edge of the dish.

---

### LESSON EIGHTH.

#### RISSOLES.

**Ingredients.**—Half a pound of canned meat. Half a pound of flour. Four ounces of dripping. Salt and pepper. A few sprigs of dried herbs. One egg. Two ounces of vermicelli, or some bread-crumbs. Clarified dripping (for frying).

*Time required, one hour.*

To make *Rissoles* of *Canned Meat:*

**1.** Put *one pound of clarified dripping* in a saucepan, and put it on the fire to heat.

N. B.—Watch it, and be careful that it does not burn.

**2.** Put *half a pound of flour* into a basin with a *pinch of salt* and *four ounces of clarified dripping.*

**3.** Rub the *dripping* well into the *flour* with your hands, until it is quite a powder.

**4.** Add a little *cold water*, and mix it into a stiff paste.

**5.** *Flour* a board and turn the *paste* out on it.

**6.** Take a tin of *canned meat*, open it carefully, and with a spoon remove all the *fat* from the part of the meat required for immediate use.

**7.** Take *half a pound of meat* out of the tin and scrape off as much of the *jelly* as possible.

**8.** Put the *meat* on a board and chop it up as fine as possible.

N. B.—*Minced meat* might be used, which, of course, would not require chopping up.

**9.** Take a small bunch of *dried herbs* and rub the *leaves* into a powder.

N. B.—The *stalks* of the *herbs* need not be thrown away, as they can be used in soups for flavoring.

**10.** Sprinkle the *herbs* over the *meat;* also a little *pepper* and *salt* and a little *flour.*

**11.** Take a rolling-pin and roll out the paste as thin as possible.

**12.** Cut the paste into *rounds* with a *cutter* (which should be dipped in *flour*); the *rounds* should be rather larger than the top of a teacup.

**13.** Put some *meat* into the *centre* of each *round* of *paste.*

**14.** Break an *egg* on a plate and beat it up slightly with a knife.

**15.** Take a *paste-brush*, dip it in the *egg*, and just wet the edges of the paste with the *egg.*

**16.** Fold the paste carefully over the *meat*, pressing the edges together with your thumb.

**17.** Take *two ounces of vermicelli* and rub it between your hands, crushing it up as fine as possible.

**18.** Put this crushed *vermicelli* on a piece of paper.

**19.** Put the *rissoles* into the plate of *egg*, and *egg* them well all over with the brush.

**20.** Then turn them into the crushed *vermicelli*, and cover them well with it, but not too thickly.

N. B.—Be careful to finger them as little as possible, so as not to rub off any of the *egg* or *vermicelli*, or the *rissoles* will burst while frying.

N. B.—Bread-crumbs might be used instead of vermicelli.

**21.** Take a frying-basket and put in the *rissoles ;* you must be careful that they do not touch each other.

**22.** When the *fat* in the saucepan is quite hot and smoking, put in the frying-basket and let the rissoles fry a minute or two, until they become brown.

**23.** Put a piece of kitchen-paper on a plate.

**24.** As the *rissoles* are fried, turn them from the frying-basket on to the piece of paper, to drain off the grease.

**25.** Put them on a hot dish, and they are ready for serving.

———

LESSON NINTH.

SAVORY HASH.

**Ingredients.**—A pound and a half of canned meat. One ounce of butter. Half an ounce of flour. Half an onion. A teaspoonful of vinegar. A dessertspoonful of chopped herbs. Pepper and salt. One dessertspoonful of mushroom catchup.

*Time required, about ten minutes.*

To make a *Savory Hash :*

**1.** Put one ounce of *butter* in a saucepan, and put it on the fire to melt.

**2.** Peel *half an onion* and cut it in slices.

**3.** Put the *onion* into the *butter.*

**4.** Stir in *half an ounce of flour*, and let all fry for a *minute or two* to brown.

**5.** Take a tin of *canned mutton* or *beef*, open it carefully, and remove the *fat* from the part of the *meat* required for immediate use.

**6.** Take *one and a half pound* of the *meat* out of the tin.

**7.** If all the *meat* is required for present use, turn it all out of the tin, and then rinse out the tin with *half a pint of warm water*, to make the *gravy* for the *hash*.

> N. B.—If all the meat has not been taken out of the tin, take some of the jelly out of the tin, and melt it in half a pint of warm water, to make the gravy.

**8.** Pour this *gravy* into the saucepan with the *flour* and *butter*, and stir well until it boils and thickens.

**9.** Now move the saucepan to the side of the fire to keep warm.

**10.** Take a *penny's worth of mixed pickles* and chop them up finely.

**11.** Stir the *chopped pickles*, or a *teaspoonful of vinegar*, into the *sauce*.

> N. B.—If the flavor of the pickles or the vinegar is disliked, they might be omitted.

**12.** Take a *sprig or two of parsley* (wash it and dry it in a cloth) and a *sprig of marjoram* and *thyme*, take away the stalks, and chop up the leaves finely on a board. (There should be about a dessertspoonful.)

**13.** Cut up the *meat* into neat pieces, and sprinkle over each piece some of the *chopped herbs* and a little *pepper* and *salt*.

**14.** Put the *meat* into the saucepan of *sauce* and let it just warm through for about *five minutes*.

**15.** Now pour into the *sauce* a *dessertspoonful of mushroom catchup*.

**16.** For serving, put the *meat* on a hot dish and strain the *sauce* over it.

## LESSON TENTH.

### MINCE-MEAT.

**Ingredients.**—One pound of canned mince-meat. A pound and a half of potatoes. One ounce of butter. One gill of milk. One tablespoonful of mushroom catchup. Salt and pepper.

*Time required, about forty minutes.*

To make a *Mince* served with *Mashed Potatoes:*

**1.** Wash *one and a half pound of potatoes* in cold water, and scrub them clean with a scrubbing-brush.

**2.** Peel them with a sharp knife; cut out the eyes and any black specks.

**3.** Put them into a saucepan of cold water—enough to cover them—and sprinkle over them one teaspoonful of salt.

**4.** Put the saucepan on the fire to boil the *potatoes* for from *twenty minutes* to *half an hour.*

**5.** Take a fork and put it into the potatoes, to feel if the centre is quite tender.

**6.** When they are sufficiently boiled, drain off all the water, and stand the saucepan by the side of the fire with the lid half on, to steam the *potatoes.*

**7.** Put *one ounce of butter* and *one gill of milk* into a small saucepan, and put it on the fire to boil.

**8.** When the *potatoes* have become quite dry, take the saucepan off the fire and stand it on a piece of paper on the table.

**9.** Mash them up smoothly with a spoon or fork.

N.B.—The best way to mash potatoes is to rub them through a wire sieve; you can then be sure there are no lumps left.

**10.** When the *milk* boils, pour it into the *mashed potatoes*, and stir it till it is quite smooth.

11. Add *pepper* and *salt* according to taste.

12. Stand the saucepan of *mashed potatoes* by the side of the fire, to keep warm until required for use.

13. Open a can of *mince-meat*.

14. Take *one pound* of the *mince* out of the tin, put it in a saucepan with *one tablespoonful of mushroom catchup*, and stir it into a paste.

15. Put the saucepan on the fire and let the *mince* just warm through.

> N. B.—Be very careful that it does not boil, or the meat will get hardened.

16. For serving, make a wall of the *mashed potatoes* round the edge of a hot dish, and pour the *mince* in the centre; stand the dish in front of the fire, to color the *potato* a pale-brown.

THE

# PRINCIPLES OF DIET

IN

## HEALTH AND DISEASE.

BY

THOMAS K. CHAMBERS, M.D.

[A REPRINT OF THE ARTICLE "DIETETICS" IN THE NEW EDITION OF
THE "ENCYCLOPÆDIA BRITANNICA."]

# THE PRINCIPLES OF DIET IN HEALTH AND DISEASE.

THE application of science to the regulation of the continuous demands of the body for nutriment aims mainly at three objects: Health, Pleasure, and Economy. They are rarely inconsistent with one another, but yet require separate consideration, as, under varying circumstances, each may claim the most prominent place in our thoughts.

## INFLUENCE OF DIET UPON HEALTH.

The influence of diet upon the health of a man begins at the earliest stage of his life, and, indeed, is then greater than at any other period. It is varied by the several phases of internal growth and of external relations, and in old age is still important in prolonging existence and rendering it agreeable and useful.

*Diet in Infancy.*—No food has as yet been found so suitable for the young of all animals as their mother's milk. And this has not been from want of seeking. Dr. Brouzet ("Sur l'Éducation Médicinale des Enfants," i., p. 165) has such a bad opinion of human mothers, that he expresses a wish for the State to interfere and prevent them from suckling their children, lest they should communicate immorality and disease! A still more determined pessimist was the famous chemist, Van Helmont, who thought life had been reduced to its present shortness by our inborn propensities, and proposed to substitute bread boiled in beer and honey for milk, which latter he calls "brute's food." Baron Liebig has followed the lead with a "food for infants," in the prescription for which half-ounces and quarter-grains figure freely, and which has to be prepared on a slow fire, and after a few minutes boiled well. And after all, not nearly such a close imitation of human milk is made as by the addition to fresh cow's milk of half its bulk of soft water, in each pint of which has been mixed a heaped-up teaspoonful of powdered "sugar of milk" and a pinch of phosphate of lime.   Indeed, in default of these cheap chemicals, the milk and water alone, when fresh and pure, are safer than an artificial compound which requires cooking.   And experience shows that the best mode of administering food to the young is also that which is most widely adopted throughout warm-blooded nature—namely, in a fresh, tepid, liquid state, frequently, and in small quantities at a time.

Empirical observation is fully supported in these deductions by physiological and chemical science.   Milk contains of

| | |
|---|---|
| Water.................................................................88 | per cent. |
| Oleaginous matter (cream or butter)............................... 3 | " |
| Nitrogenous matter (cheese and albumen)........................... 4 | " |
| Hydrocarbon (sugar)............................................... 4⅓ | " |
| Saline matter (phosphate of lime, chloride of sodium, iron, etc.)..... ⅓ | " |

These are at once the constituents and the proportions of the constituents of food suited to a weakly, rapidly-growing animal.   The large quantity of water makes it pass easily through the soft, absorbent walls of the digestive canal; and the complete suspension, in an alkaline fluid, of the finely-divided fat and nitrogenous matter introduces more of them than could be effected were they in a solid form.   The fat is the germ of new cellular growth, and the nitrogenous matter is by the new cells formed into flesh, which is doubling its bulk monthly.   The phosphate of lime is required for the hardening bones, the chloride of sodium and the iron for the daily-increasing amount of blood in circulation.   Milk may be said to be still alive as it leaves the breast fresh and warm, and quickly becomes living blood in the infant's veins.   A very slight chemical change is requisite.   Its frequent administration is demanded by the rapid absorption, and the absence of regular meals prevents the overloading of the delicate young stomach with more than it can hold at once.

The wholesomest nutriment for the first six months is milk alone. A vigorous baby can, indeed, bear with impunity much rough usage, and often appears none the worse for a certain quantity of farinaceous food; but the majority do not get habituated to it without an exhibition of dislike, which indicates rebellion of the bowels.

To give judicious diet its fair chance, the frame must be well protected from the cold; and just in proportion as the normal temperature of the body is maintained, so does growth prosper, as is satisfactorily proved by experiments on the young of the lower animals.

It is only when the teeth are on their way to the front, as shown by dribbling, that the parotid glands secrete an active saliva capable of digesting bread-stuffs. Till then, anything but milk must be given tentatively, and considered in the light of a means of education for its future mode of nutrition. Among the varieties of such means, the most generally applicable are broth and beef-tea, at first pure, and then thickened with tapioca and arrow-root. Chicken-soup, made with a little cream and sugar, serves as a change. Baked flour, biscuit-powder, tops and bottoms, should all have their turn. Change is necessary in the imperfect dietary which art supplies, and for change the stomach should be prepared by habit.

The consequences of premature weaning are insidious. The external aspect of the child is that of health; its muscles are strong, but the bones do not harden in proportion; and if it tries to walk, its limbs give way, and it is said to be suffering from rachitis, or "rickets."

These consequences follow in other animals as surely as in the human race; and in them it was possible to make the experiment crucial. A gentleman named Guérin set himself to find if he could produce rickets at will. He took a number of puppies in equally good condition, and, having let them suckle for a time, he suddenly weaned half of them and fed them on raw meat—a fare which on first thought would seem the most suitable for carnivorous animals. Nevertheless, after a short time those which continued to take the mother's milk had grown strong and hearty, while those which had been treated with a more substantial dietary pined, and frequently threw up their victuals, then their limbs bent, and at the end of about four months they showed all the symptoms of confirmed rickets. From these experiments we must conclude that the rachitis depended mainly on the derangements of nutrition brought on by improper diet. A diet which is taken at the wrong season may fairly be called improper. For carnivora, it is flesh before the age of suckling has passed; for herbivora (and an experiment bearing on the point has been made on pigs), it is vegetable feeding begun when they ought to be at the teat.[1]

[1] Trousseau, "Clinique Médicale," vol. iii., p. 484, third edition.

The time for weaning should be fixed partly by the child's age, partly by the growth of the teeth. The troubles to which children are subject at this crisis are usually gastric, such as are induced by summer weather; therefore at that season the weaning should be postponed, whereas in winter it should be hurried forward. The first group of teeth, nine times out of ten, consists of the lower central front teeth, which may appear any time during the sixth and seventh month. The mother may then begin to diminish the number of suckling times; and by a month she can have reduced them to twice a day, so as to be ready, when the second group makes its way through the upper front gums, to cut off the supply altogether. The third group—the lateral incisors and first grinders—usually after the first anniversary of birth give notice that solid food can be chewed. But it is prudent to let dairy-milk form a considerable portion of the fare till the eye-teeth are cut, which seldom happens till the eighteenth or twentieth month. At this period children are liable to diarrhœa, convulsions, irritation of the brain, rashes, and febrile catarrhs. In such cases it is often advisable to resume a complete milk-diet, and sometimes a child's life has been saved by its reapplication to the breast. These means are most feasible when the patient is accustomed to milk; indeed, if not, the latter expedient is hardly possible.

*Diet in Childhood and Youth.*—At this stage of life the diet must obviously be the best which is a transition from that of infancy to that of adult age. Growth is not completed, but yet entire surrender of every consideration to the claim of growth is not possible, nor indeed desirable. Moreover, that abundance of adipose tissue, or reserve new growth, which a baby can bear, is an impediment to the due education of the muscles of the boy or girl. The supply of nutriment needs not to be so continuous as before, but at the same time should be more frequent than for the adult. Up to at least fourteen or fifteen years of age the rule should be four meals a day, varied indeed, but nearly equal in nutritive power and in quantity—that is to say, all moderate, all sufficient. The maturity the body then reaches involves a hardening and enlargement of the bones and cartilages, and a strengthening of the digestive organs, which in healthy young persons enables us to dispense with some of the watchful care bestowed upon their diet. Three full meals a day are generally sufficient, and the requirements of mental training may be allowed to a certain extent to modify the attention to nutrition, which has hitherto been paramount.  But it must not be forgotten that the changes in figure and in internal organs are not completed till several years have passed, and that they involve increased growth and demand full supplies.  As less bulky food is used, care should be taken that it is sufficiently nutritious, and habits should be acquired which conduce to making the most of it for the maintenance of strength.

The nutritiousness of food depends on *digestibility* and *concentration*.  Food is digestible when it yields readily its constituents to the fluids destined for their reduction to absorbable chyme.  It is more or less concentrated, according as a given weight contains more or less matter capable of supporting life.  The degree in which they possess these qualifications united constitutes the absolute nutritive value of alimentary matters.

The degree of cohesion in the viands influences digestibility. Tough articles incapable of being completely ground up by the teeth remain unused, while fluids and semifluids lead the van of digestibles.  The tissues of young vegetables and young animals are, for this reason, more digestible than old specimens.  It is desirable also that the *post-mortem* rigidity, which lasts several days in most instances, should have merged into softness before the meat is cooked, or should have been anticipated by cooking before the flesh is cold.  In warm climates and exceptionally warm weather, the latter course is the preferable.  The dietician, especially when the feeding of the young is in question, will prefer those methods of culinary preparation which most break up the natural cohesion of the viands.  And it may be noticed that the force of cohesion acts in all directions, and that it is no advantage for an article to be laterally friable if it remains stringy in a longitudinal direction.

Fat interposed between the component parts of food diminishes its digestibility.  It is the interstitial fat, between the fasciculi of muscular fibre in beef, which renders it to young persons, and to dyspeptics, less digestible than mutton.

A temperature above that of the body retards digestion.  Meat, which is digested by the gastric juice in the stomach, has time to cool before it gets there; but farinaceous food, which depends for its conversion into chyme on the salivary glands, suffers a serious loss if, by reason of being too hot, it cannot avail itself of the saliva supplied by the mouth.  It should also be borne in mind that a temperature much above that of the body cracks the enamel of the teeth.

Excessive concentration impairs digestibility. The principal medium by which nutriment is carried through the absorbent membrane of the digestive canal is water. There is no doubt it passes more rapidly by endosmosis than anything else. The removal, then, of water is an injury to viands; and drying, salting, over-frying, over-roasting, and even over-boiling, renders them less soluble in the digestive juices, and so less nutritious. A familiar illustration of this may be taken from eggs. Let an egg be lightly boiled, poached in water, custarded, or raw, and the stomach even of an invalid can bear it; but let it be baked in a pudding which requires a hot oven, or boiled hard, or otherwise submitted to a high temperature for a prolonged period, and it becomes a tasteless, leathery substance, which can be of no more use in the stomach than so much skin or hair. It is obvious, then, that it is mainly in a commercial point of view that articles of diet can be called nutritious in proportion to their concentration. About this there can be no question; milk adulterated from the pump is worth so much less than pure milk, and a pound of beef-steak sustains a man longer than a pint of veal-broth.

The attainment of nutritiousness by concentration is of considerable importance to travelers and in military medicine. There are not a few strategists who attribute the success of the Germans in the war of 1870 to the easily-carried and easily-prepared food supplied to them by the sausage-makers of Berlin. Concentration of viands carried to excess, so as to be likely to affect the health, is usually made manifest by a diminution in the secretion of urine and its condensed condition; while, on the other hand, if dilution is needlessly great, the action of the kidneys is excessive. Now, the urine of young persons is naturally of lower specific gravity—that is, more aqueous—than that of adults. If it is found to equal in density the excretion of full growth, or if it is observed to be voided but rarely, the meals should be made more bulky, or, better still, more frequent, so as not to overload the stomach.

An over-concentrated diet often induces costiveness. This should be counteracted by green vegetables and other dilute appetizing dishes, and never by purgative drugs. The habit of taking a considerable quantity and variety of fresh green vegetables has the further advantage of preventing that tendency to minor developments of scurvy which is not uncommonly found in youths nourished mainly on animal food. A softness or friability of the gums is one of the first signs of this. If the mouth bleeds after the application of a tooth-brush, the use of fresh vegetables at every meal should be enforced.

The young are peculiarly liable to be affected by poisons conveyed in fluids. Their sensitive frames absorb quickly, and quickly turn to evil account such substances, even when diluted to an extent which makes them harmless to adults. The water, therefore, with which families, and still more with which schools, are supplied, should be carefully subjected to analysis. Wherever a trace of lead is found, means should be adopted to remove the source of it; and organic products should have their origin clearly accounted for, and all possibility of sewage contamination excluded. These precautions are essential, in spite of the grown-up portion of the household having habitually used the water without injury.

Fresh milk has long had a bad popular reputation as occasionally conveying fever, and in some parts of Ireland the peasantry can hardly ever be got to take it "raw." This is quite irrespective of the state of the cattle which furnish it; no cases of disease thus communicated have ever been traced home to sick cows. It is probably always due either to adulteration with dirty water, or to the vessels being washed in that dangerous medium, or to their being exposed to air loaded with elements of contagion.

Up to the period of full development, the daily use of wine should be allowed only during illness and the express attendance of a medical adviser. Its habitual consumption by healthy children hastens forward the crisis of puberty, checks growth, and habituates them to the artificial sensations induced by alcohol.

*Diet for Bodily Labor.*—It seems certain that the old theory of Liebig, which attributed the whole of the force exhibited in muscular movements to the oxidation of muscular tissue, is untenable. There is not enough of the material oxidized—that is to say, destroyed and carried away as urea and other nitrogenous excretions—to generate so much force, as measured by the method of Joule. On the other hand, Traube goes too far when he would make out that in the performance of muscular work the metamorphosis of the organized constituents of contractile tissue is not involved, and that non-nitrogenous substances alone are consumed. The prolonged feats of walking performed by the pedestrian Weston in 1876 vastly increased the amounts excreted of those elements of the urine which are derived from the oxidation of muscle and nerve.[1] The urea formed by the destructive assimilation of contractile fibre, and the phosphates whose main source is nervous tissue, were each nearly doubled during and shortly after the extraordinary strain upon those parts of the body. As might be expected, the machinery wears away quicker when it is harder worked, and requires to be repaired immediately by an enhanced quantity of new material, or it will be worn beyond the power of repair. The daily supply, therefore, of digestible nitrogenous food—meat *par excellence*—must be increased whenever the muscular exercise is increased. In making the recent extension of railways in Sicily, the progress was retarded by the slack work done by the Sicilian navvies, compared with that got through by the English gangs. The former took scarcely any meat, preferring to save the wages expended by their comrades in that way. The idea occurred to the contractor of paying the men partly in money and partly in meat; and the result was a marked increase in the amount of work executed, which was brought nearly up to the British average. A mixed diet, with an increase in the proportionate quantity of meat when extra corporeal exertion is required, is the wholesomest, as well as the most economical, for all sorts of manual laborers.

It is absolutely essential that the fleshy machinery for doing work should be continuously replaced by flesh-food as it becomes worn out. Nitrogenous aliment, after a few chemical changes, replaces the lost muscle which has passed away in the excretions, just as the engineer makes ore into steel and renews the corroded boiler-plate or thinned piston. Now, as the renewal of the plate or piston is a "stimulus" to the augmented performances of the engine, so meat is a "stimulus" to augmented muscular action. Taken in a digestible form during exertion, it allows the exertion to be continued longer, with greater ease and less consequent exhaustion. According to the testimony of soldiers experimentally put through forced marches of twenty miles a day, with loads of half a hundredweight each, "meat extract" bears away the palm from the other reputed stimulants commonly compared with it—viz., rum and coffee. "It does not put a spirit into you for a few miles only, but has a lasting

[1] *See* Dr. Pavy on Weston's walk, in *Lancet* of December 23, 1876. The urea excreted when walking bore to that excreted during rest the relation of 17 to 10 ; phosphoric acid, 19 to 10 ; lime, 15 to 10, etc.

effect. If I were ordered for continuous marching, and had my choice, I would certainly take the meat extract," said an unprejudiced sergeant to Dr. Parkes, who was the conductor of the experiments alluded to.[1]

When the continuous repair of the muscular machinery is fully secured, the production of heat and force is most readily provided for by vegetable aliment, by reason of the large proportion of carbon which it contains. In assigning their physiological functions to the several sorts of food, nearly all the business of begetting active force should apparently be ascribed to the solid hydrocarbons, starch and fat, by their conversion into carbonic acid. It is not necessary to be acquainted with every step of the process—which in the body we confessedly are not—to appreciate the argument. It is clearly important that these elements of diet should be furnished in sufficient quantity, and in a digestible form. In additions to diet made in consequence of additional bodily work, not only should the stimulus of animal food be attended to, but the bulk of starch and fat in the rations should be augmented even in larger proportion, for these aliments are the most direct contributors of force.[2]

[1] "On the Issue of a Spirit Ration during the Ashantee Campaign of 1874," by E. A. Parkes, M. D., Professor of Military Hygiene in the Army Medical School, London, 1875.

[2] This is well illustrated by a remarkable feat performed on the Great Western Railway in the summer of 1872. It was necessary to shift the rails from the broad to the narrow gauge on upward of 500 miles of permanent way within a fortnight. The task was enormous, for the Great Western is one of the few English lines whose rails are held down by bolts screwed into nuts. All these had to be unscrewed, and replaced after removing the heavy rail two feet. About 3,000 men were employed, working double time, sometimes from 4 in the morning till 9 at night; and, without one being sick or drunk, they accomplished the work in the prescribed time. The scheme for generating muscular power was this : The men were hutted along the line, so as not to waste their strength by coming and going, and they brought with them bacon, bread, cheese, cocoa, etc., to provide their usual meals at usual times. But they had no beer, nor alcohol in any form. A pound and a half of oatmeal and half a pound of sugar was allowed extra to each man daily, and for every gang of twenty-one a cook was provided. The first thing done in the morning was to breakfast; and then the cook and his caldron started along the line till water was found convenient; a fireplace of stones was built, and the pot boiled. Oatmeal was then sprinkled into it with sugar, and thoroughly well boiled till thin gruel was made. As soon as the "shout for drink" was heard, buckets were filled and carried round, with small pannikins to convey the liquid to the panting mouths. The men liked it exceedingly, and learned by experience the importance of having it well cooked.

The incident may remind the reader of classical medicine of Hippocrates, who considers the culinary preparation of oatmeal ptisan so important, that, in a short treatise "On the Treatment of Acute Disease," he devotes to it the only cookery recipe he has inserted in his works. He describes how it is to be boiled till it can swell no longer (so that it may

Training for athletic sports is based on the principles above enunciated. The usual time allotted to it is six weeks, and the objects to be attained in this period may be described as—

1. The removal of superfluous fat and water.
2. The increase of contractile power in the muscles.
3. Increased endurance.
4. "Wind," that is to say, a power of breathing and circulating the blood steadily, in spite of exertion.

The first is aimed at by considerably adding to the daily amount of nitrogenous and by diminishing farinaceous and liquid food, and providing that it should be so consumed as to be fully digested. The second and third are secured by gradually increasing the demands made upon the muscles, till they have learned to exert at will all the powers of which they are capable, and for as long a period as the natural structure of the individual frame permits. "Wind" is improved by choosing as part of the training an exercise such as running, which can be sustained only when the respiratory and circulating organs do their duty fairly.

As an example, the Oxford system of training for the summer boat-races may be cited. It may be considered a typical regimen for fully developing a young man's corporeal powers to fulfill the demands of an extraordinary exertion—a standard which may be modified according to the circumstances for which the training is required. It is as follows:

A DAY'S TRAINING.[1]

| Rise about 7 A. M. | | |
|---|---|---|
| Exercise..................... | A short walk or run. | Not compulsory. |
| Breakfast at 8.30......... | Of tea..................... | As little as possible. |
| | Meat—beef or mutton........ | Underdone. |
| | Bread or dry toast........... | Crust only recommended. |
| Exercise in forenoon......... | None. | |
| Dinner at 2 P. M........... | Meat—much the same as for breakfast. | |
| | Bread........................ | Crust only recommended. |
| | Vegetables, none............. | Not always adhered to. |
| | Beer, one pint. | |

swell no more in the stomach), how it is to be settled and strained through a coarse colander. He prescribes it, indeed, for sick people, but he would have been the first to agree with our advanced physiologists in the opinion that overstrained muscular effort produces the same effect as continued fever (ες πυρετὸν καθίσταται μακρότερον), its chief dangers lying in rise of temperature and arrested cutaneous action, and that its true antagonist is nutriment capable of rapid absorption, dissolved in that most essential nutriment, water.

[1] See Maclaren's "Training in Theory and Practice," appendix to edition of 1866.

| | |
|---|---|
| Exercise..................... | About 5 o'clock start for the river, and row twice over the course, the speed increasing with the strength of the crew. |
| Supper at 8.30 or 9 P. M...... | Meat, cold. Bread, and perhaps a little jelly or water-cresses. Beer, one pint. |
| Bed about 10. | |

The Cambridge system differs very slightly, and in neither is any exaggerated severity of discipline enforced, while some latitude is permitted to peculiarities and a wish for variety, and plenty of time is left for business and social intercourse. Other plans are objectionable, from involving, without any corresponding advantage, a complete departure from the usual habits of the educated classes. For instance, according to Clasper, dinner is to be at noon, with only a light tea afterward, and no supper. Then a country walk of four or five miles is to be taken before breakfast, and two hours' row afterward, and another hard row between dinner and tea.[1] "Stonehenge," again, requires the time between breakfast and dinner to be spent entirely on billiards, skittles, quoits, rowing, and running, in spite of another hour's row being prescribed at 6 P. M. He also requires the aspirant for athletic honors to sleep between ten and eleven hours.[2] Only professionals will carry out such rules, and even they do not either benefit their health or lengthen their lives by the sacrifice; for it is notorious that "overtraining" leads to a condition of system in which the sufferers describe themselves as "fallen to pieces." The most peculiar symptom is a sudden loss of voluntary power after exertion. It is sometimes called "fainting," but there is no loss of sense, and it is quickly relieved by liquid food. It is to the pathologist a timely warning of that consequence of overstrained muscle which constitutes paralysis scriptorum, turner's palsy, and blacksmith's palsy, and which results in fatty degeneration of the red muscular fibre. To get and to keep its health, a muscle needs a constant alternation of active contraction and rest, and an enforced protraction of either one or the other leads to the loss of vital properties. The limbs of an Indian fakir, voluntarily held in a strained posture, or those of a bed-ridden invalid, are

[1] "Rowing Almanac," 1863.
[2] Article "Boat-Racing," in "British Rural Sports," 1861.

equally apt to become useless.  Over-trained persons are also liable
to a languor and apparent weakness, which is found, on examination,
to depend on an excessive secretion of urea by the kidneys.

Such are not the results, however, of the training adopted at the
universities, by which it would appear that the constitution is
strengthened, the intellect sharpened, and life lengthened.   Dr. John
Morgan ("University Oars," 1873) has collected statistics of the sub-
sequent health of those who have rowed in the university races since
1829, and he finds that, whereas at twenty years of age, according to
Farr's life tables, average expectation of survival is forty years, for
these oarsmen it is forty-two years.   Moreover, in the cases of death,
inquiry into its causes exhibits evidence of good constitutions rather
than the contrary, the causes consisting largely of fevers and acci-
dents, to which the vigorous and active are more exposed than the
sick.   And it is not at the expense of the mind that the body is cultivated, for this roll of athletes is adorned with the names of bishops,
poets, queen's counsel, etc.

Training greatly increases the vital capacity of the chest, so that
much more air can be blown in and out of the lungs, and with greater
force, than previously.   And this vital capacity endures longer than
the other improvements.   It is evidence of the permanent elasticity
of the pulmonary tissue, and an efficient protection against asthma,
emphysema, and other degenerations of the organ of breathing.

Indigestion, sleeplessness, nervous indecision, palpitation of heart,
and irregularity of bowels, disappear under training; but if they
exist, the regimen should be entered on with more than usual caution.

An important modification of training is that which contemplates
the reduction of corpulence which has increased to the extent
of interfering with comfort and preventing active exercise.  If an
exhausting amount of muscular effort is enforced, the digestion of
meat is interfered with, while at the same time there still goes on
the absorption of such fat as is unavoidably present in the victuals,
so that the muscles and nerves lose strength, while the adipose tissue
grows.   Besides this, if by violent means the weight is worked down,
then, to keep it down, those violent means must be persisted in;
and if they be neglected for more interesting occupations, the burden
rapidly increases to a greater degree than ever.   Many uncomfortably
obese persons are very active in mind and body, and could not add
to their muscular exercise without risk of harm.

Regimen, then, is more essentially important to them than to other trainers, and they will probably be more induced to attend to it if they understand the principles on which it is based. This is simply to exclude from the bill of fare all those articles which contain fat, or which, by the chemical actions of the digestive viscera, may be converted into fat.

For the reduction of corpulence, the following rules may be observed for a three weeks' course:

Rise at 7, rub the body well with horse-hair gloves, have a cold bath, and take a short turn in the open air. Breakfast (alone) at 8 or 8.30, on the lean of beef or mutton (cutting off the fat and skin), dry toast, biscuit or oat-cake, a tumbler of claret and water, or tea without milk or sugar, or made in the Russian way, with a slice of lemon. Lunch at 1 on bread or biscuit, Dutch cheese, salad, water-cresses or roasted apples, hung beef or anchovies, or red-herring, or olives, and similar relishes. After eating, drink claret and water, or unsweetened lemonade, or plain water, in moderation. Dine at any convenient hour. Avoid soup, fish, or pastry, but eat plain meat of any sort except pork, rejecting the fat and skin. Spinach, haricots, or any other green vegetable, may be taken, but no potatoes, made dishes, or sweets. A jelly, or a lemon-water-ice, or a roast apple, must suffice in their place. Take claret and water at dinner, and one glass of sherry or Madeira afterward.

Between meals, as a rule, exercise must always be taken to the extent of inducing perspiration. Running, when practicable, is the best form in which to take it.

Seven or eight pounds is as much as it is prudent to lose during the three weeks. If this loss is arrived at sooner, or indeed later, the severe parts of the treatment may be gradually omitted; but it is strongly recommended to modify the general habits in accordance with the principle of taking as small a quantity as possible of fat and sugar, or of substances which form fat and sugar, and sustaining the respiratory function. By this means the weight may be gradually reduced for a few months with safety.

Small quantities of dilute alcoholic liquids taken with meals slightly increase the activity of the renewal of the nitrogenous tissues, mainly muscle; that is to say, there is a more rapid reconstruction of those parts, as is shown by the augmented formation of urea and the sharpened appetite. Life is fuller and more complete, old flesh is removed, and food appropriated as new flesh, somewhat more quickly than when no alcohol is ingested. There appears to be a temporary rise in the digestive powers of the stomach, which is probably the initiative act. The nerve-functions are blunted, and a lessened excretion of phosphorus exhibits a temporary check in the wear and renewal of the nerve-tissue. The "vital capacity" of the lungs, as indicated by the spirometer, is reduced, showing a diminished oxidation of the blood.

The effect on a healthy man of taking with a meal such a quantity of fermented liquor as puts him at ease with himself and the world around, without untoward exhilaration, is to arrest the wear of the nervous system, especially that part employed in emotion and sensation. Just as often, then, as the zest for food is raised to its normal standard by a little wine or beer with a meal, the moderate consumer is as much really better as he feels the better for it. Where the food is as keenly enjoyed without it, the consumption of a stimulant is useless. But alcohol is not a source of force, and its direct action is an arrest of vitality.

*Diet for Mental Work.*—An expression of Büchner's —"No thinking without phosphorus" [1] — has gained an unhappy notoriety. Strictly speaking, it is a groundless assumption, for we cannot say that intellectual being may not exist joined to any form of matter, or quite independent of matter. We certainly do not know enough of the subject to lay down such a negative statement. And if it be held to mean that the amount of phosphorus passing through the body bears a proportion to the intensity of thought, it is simply a misstatement. A captive lion, tiger, leopard, or hare assimilates and parts with a greater amount of phosphorus than a hard-thinking man, while a beaver, noted for its powers of contrivance, excretes so little phosphorus that chemical analysis cannot find it in the excreta. All that the physiologist is justified in asserting is that, for the mind to energize in a living body, that body must be kept living up to a certain standard, and that for the continuous renewal of life a supply of phosphatic salts is required. The same may be said with equal justice of water, fat, nitrogen, chloride of sodium, oxygen, etc. The phosphates are wanted indeed, but wanted by pinches, whereas water is required by pailfuls. A few days without water, or a few

---

[1] "Ohne Phosphor kein Gedanke," "Kraft und Stoff," section 122.

minutes without oxygen, will terminate the train of consciousness. The practical points taught us by physiology are that, for the integrity of thought, integrity of the nervous tissue is requisite; and for the integrity of the nervous tissue, a due quantity of such food as contains digestible phosphatic salts.

The most perfect regimen for the healthy exercise of thought is such as would be advised for a growing boy—viz., frequent small supplies of easily-soluble mixed food, so as to furnish the greatest quantity of nutriment without overloading the stomach, or running the risk of generating morbid half-assimilated products. For it is essential to the intellectual direction of the nervous system that it should not be oppressed by physical impediments. The presence in the stomach or blood of imperfectly assimilated nutriment impedes its functions in close proportion to their amount, so that not only the constituents, but the mode of administering food, must come into the calculation. "*Repletus venter non studet libenter*" is an old proverb, the application of which saves many a brain and many a stomach from being worked against the grain. Rest from brain-work for twenty minutes before meals, entire abstinence from it during meals, and rest again till the weight has passed from the stomach, are essential to the reconcilement of psychical exertion with bodily health.

The physiology of the action of alcohol has a very important bearing on the physical management of the mental functions. Alcohol has the power of curbing, arresting, and suspending all the manifestations of the nervous system, so that we feel its influence on our thoughts sooner than on any other part of the system. Sometimes it brings them more completely under our command, controls and steadies them; more often it confuses or disconnects them, and then breaks off our power over them altogether. When a man has tired himself by intellectual exertion, a moderate quantity of alcoholic stimulant taken with food acts as an anæsthetic, stays the wear of the system which is going on, and allows the nerve-force to be turned to the due digestion of the meal. But it must be followed by rest from toil, and is in essence a part of the same treatment which includes rest—it is an artificial rest. To continue to labor, and at the same time to take an anæsthetic, is a physiological inconsistency. The drug merely blunts the useful feeling of weariness, and prevents it from acting as a warning. There is no habit more fatal to a lit-

16

erary man than that of taking stimulants between meals; the vital powers go on wearing out more and more, without their cry for help being perceived, and in the end break down irrevocably.

As to quantity, the appetite for solid food is the safest guide. If a better dinner or supper is eaten when it is accompanied by a certain amount of fermented liquor, that is the amount most suitable; if a worse, then an excess is committed, however little be taken.

The aim of the diet should be (to quote the words of John Milton) " to preserve the body's health and hardness, to render lightsome, clear, and not lumpish obedience to the mind, to the cause of religion and our country's liberty, when it shall require from hearts in sound bodies to stand and cover their stations."

It is especially when the mind of genius is overshadowed by the dark clouds of threatened insanity, of hypochondriasis, or of hysteria, that a rational mode of life preserves it. Nothing but daily exercise, temperate meals, and a punctual observance of regular hours of rest and study, could have kept burning the flickering reason in poor Cowper.

As regards the proper quantity of alcohol that may be used, the two following questions naturally occur: How is a man to know when he has had enough? and what are the signs of too much? The ancients used to wear dark-red or purple engraved gems, which they considered preservatives against excess, and called them ἀμέθυστοι— " sober-stones," " amethysts." The name is now limited to the violet rock-crystal, but in early times it was applied to several other stones, cut in intaglio, and worn on the fingers at festive gatherings. So long as the wearer could decipher the minute works of art they bore, he had not reached excess. A more delicate test still is the appreciation of temperature by the skin; if a draught does not chill, if a hot room fails to produce the usual discomfort, the wise man knows he has exceeded and must stop at once. In short, the safest rule is that, when there is a consciousness of any psychical effect at all beyond that of satisfaction at the relief of bodily weariness—such a satisfaction as is felt on taking a good meal by a vigorous person— then the limits of moderation have been attained. On ordinary occasions of daily life, and " for the stomach's sake," no more should be taken. Each fresh drop is a step downward to the evil results of alcohol. But to the practiser of daily temperance, festive occasions are safe and may be beneficial. A man may, from time to time, keep up without harm the above-mentioned sense of satisfaction by good and digestible wine in good company, without fear of getting drunk or failure of health, if he makes it a law to himself to stop as soon as he experiences any hurry of ideas or indistinctness of the senses.

*Diet of Mothers.*—During pregnancy as much care should be taken not to get too fat as is taken by an athlete training for a race. The rules for modified training explained above will afford hints on the subject, but it is not desirable to carry the process so far.

There is a temptation at this time to increase the usual allowance of stimulant; alcohol is taken between meals to overcome the nausea and depression incident to the state of body. And by this mistaken expedient the nausea gradually becomes dyspeptic vomiting. On leaving it off, the sickness ceases. A mother should also remember that nearly all the alcohol she consumes mixes with her blood, which now is one with the blood of the fœtus.

During lactation the most suitable drink for a mother is cow's milk, fresh and unskimmed. If it turns sour on the stomach, limewater mixed with it not only corrects the acescence, but also supplies a valuable aid to the growing bones of the infant. In her solid dietary, also, milk may be fairly taken as the type of a due admixture of alimentary principles, because it is not individual growth or the production of muscular force, but the secretion of milk, that is the object of the selection of diet.

Supposing the full diet to consist of three pounds of solid food, that will require six pints extra of uncombined aqueous fluid to make it as fluid as milk; and, to combine the nitrogenous and carbonaceous constituents in due proportion, the three pounds of solid food should consist of

14½ ounces of meat.
13  ounces of fat, butter, and sugar.
20  ounces of farinaceous food and vegetables.
 ½ ounce  of salt, lime, etc.

At first, from the exhaustion consequent on childbed, from the want of exercise and of fresh air, the appetite turns against meat. Let then milk, especially boiled milk, with arrow-root or the like, chicken-broth, or egg-custards, fill up the deficiency.

Any increase in the habitual allowance of alcohol is as unfitting to this period of life as during pregnancy.

*Diet of Old Age.*—It is a remark extant from the rough times, when famine was more frequent than now, that the older a human being is the better deficiency of food is borne. Old men suffer least from abstinence,[1] and benefit therefore most from temperance in eating. Everybody who has passed the age of fifty, or thereabouts, with a fairly unimpaired constitution, will act wisely in diminishing his daily quantity of solid food. There is less demand for the materials of growth, and consequently animal food should bear a smaller proportion than heretofore to vegetable, and it is mainly in that ingredient of the diet that reduction should be effected. Neglect of this rule in declining years is often punished by gout—a disease attributable to excess of nitrogenous aliment, and for this reason common to elderly men.

In the autumn of life, the advantages derived from fermented liquor are more advantageous, and the injuries it can inflict less injurious, to the body than in youth. The effect of alcohol is to check the activity of destructive assimilation, to arrest that rapid flux of the substance of the frame which, in healthy youth, can hardly be excessive, but which, in old age, exhausts the vital force. Loss of appetite is a frequent and a serious symptom in old age. It usually arises from deficient formation of gastric juice, which, in common with other secretions, diminishes with years. It is best treated physiologically rather than by drugs.

*Diet in Sickness.*—In all that has gone before, health has been presupposed. The modifications necessitated by sickness are of three kinds: 1. The avoidance of such articles of consumption as would increase the disease under the special circumstances, although ordinarily wholesome; 2. The maintenance of the functions or parts of the frame which remain normal; 3. The administration, for a special curative purpose, of peculiar food which would not be recommended for general use.

In all *fevers* which are classed together as being apparently due to a poison multiplying itself in the blood, the art of diet consists in giving an almost continuous supply of liquid nutriment, holding very soluble aliments in a dilute form. There is nothing so digestible as water, and we take advantage of this high digestibility to get whatever it can dissolve digested along with it. For the first three or

---

[1] Hippocrates, Aphorism xiii.

even four days, patients, previously strong, should have only farinaceous food, well boiled and cooled to the temperature of the body.
Evidence has been already quoted of the power which oatmeal-gruel
possesses of sustaining force under the trying circumstances of excessive toil. Now, fever closely resembles muscular effort in its arrest
of the digestive functions, at the same moment that it makes an ur-
gent demand for nutriment. With ultra-Egyptian rigor, while straw
is withheld, "the tale of the bricks is doubled," and we know by the
quantity of urea and phosphates in the urine, and by the fœcal excretion, that the muscles and nerves of the bed-ridden sufferer are melt-
ing away as fast as if he were scaling the Alps with nothing to eat.
It is quite reasonable to transfer the experiences derived from health
to sickness, and to feel satisfied that we are not wasting precious op-
portunities when we are giving fever-patients such a time-honored
diet as oatmeal-gruel, care being taken that it is thoroughly well
boiled. After three days, the tissues are beginning to suffer, and it
is advisable to add chicken-broth, meat-jelly, and strong soup. Let
that be supplied which the emaciation shows to be passing away—
nitrogenous tissue.

The administration of alcohol is to be regulated partly by the
temperature and partly by the condition of the nervous system. Usually, if the heat of the blood (as taken at the axilla) is above 103°,
and always if it is above 105°, there is a necessity for it. Again, if
there is great prostration of strength, or tremor of the hands, or
quivering in the voice and respiration, if there is low muttering delirium when the patient is left quiet, it is required.

*Green-sickness*, or anæmia, is characterized by the rapid disappear-
ance of the red particles which float in the blood. To what a strange
extent this goes may be seen by looking at the insides of the lips,
which naturally hold such a quantity of the fluid as to be quite scar-
let, but which now are pale like those of a corpse. It is calculated
that the loss of material in marked cases of green-sickness may
amount to three pounds of this important constituent of the blood.[1]
Yet it is capable of complete renewal by diet. If by dint of remedies, notably iron, the appetite can be so regulated as to enjoy meat
in excess of the immediate wants of the body, that meat is converted
into hæmatine, and the healthy hue returns to the cheeks as quickly

---

[1] Chambers's "Lectures," chiefly Clinical, lect. li.

as it left it. Wine is useful at meals on account of the stimulus it gives to the appetite; it is injurious between meals by spoiling it.

*Acute rheumatism* and *acute gout* are best treated on an opposite principle. A nutrient nitrogenous diet, which the patient assimilates only too readily, retards recovery, and will even bring on a relapse during convalescence. If meat in any form, solid or liquid, be eaten, it seems to turn to acid, which is already in excess in the blood. The power of fully converting it into living flesh is wanting; and, until this power is regained, a semi-conversion into an organic acid takes place. The redder and more muscular the meat is, the more it disagrees.

*Chronic gout* is indubitably due to good cheer indulged in either by the sufferer or his ancestors. When a man, day after day, swallows more nitrogenous food than is wanted for the repair of his tissues, the following results may be expected, with variations dependent upon his original constitution: If the digestive solvents are weak and scanty, the excess passes through the canal in an undigested state, and is partially decomposed there. Thereon ensue all sorts of abdominal derangements, which, however, have the advantage of getting rid of the offending matters. If, on the other hand, the stomach secretes vigorously on being stimulated, then, indeed, the excess is digested and absorbed, and is subject to the future changes consequent on assimilation. An active out-of-door life neutralizes this in some measure by augmenting oxidation; much of the albumen goes to form glycogen, and acts as a fuel for the maintenance of muscular force. The balance is wasted in an unexplained way, and does not necessarily injure a hardy frame. The violent muscular exertion and high training needful for oxidation being inconsistent with the habits of intellectual society, a man in the prime of life who puts too much meat into a good stomach habitually retains in his blood an excess of uric acid, into which the nitrogenous waste converts itself. Uric acid in the blood has been distinctly traced as the essence of gout. Perhaps this imaginary first offender develops the full consequences; and that is the best thing that can happen, inducing greater carefulness in future.

These views can suggest but one line of preventive treatment: The children of gouty families should be brought up to a life of strict abstemiousness and muscular activity. From the earliest years vegetables and "meagre" soups should form a considerable portion of their dietary.

Gouty adults require meat but once in twenty-four hours. The bill of fare should be varied from day to day, but as simple as possible at each meal. Rich sauces are to be eschewed, and a lemon, an infusion of herbs and pepper, bread-sauce, or a *purée* of vegetables, adopted in their place. Sugar, at the end of meals, generates an excess of organic acid, and it is to be avoided. If cheese is eaten, it should be new, and is best toasted and creamed.

Dilute alkaline waters containing soda, such as Apollinaris or the weaker Vichy, are a rational drink during meals; but it is probably best to keep to pure water. Those who live idle lives require no alcohol, and it should not be an habitual accompaniment to meals.

*Red gravel* is evidence of a constitution so closely allied to gout, that nothing need be said further about its appropriate regimen.

In *Bright's disease* of the kidneys, in *contracted liver*, and, in short, in all degenerative lesions, alcohol has a baneful influence. Its action upon the tissues is directly the same as theirs. Moreover, if we agree with its latest expositor, Dr. Sibson, that Bright's disease is closely associated with increased arterial tension, alcohol (whose effect is also to increase tension) must be peculiarly poisonous. [1]

For the cure of these diseases, independent of the nutrition of the rest of the body, a milk diet has been proposed, and it seems to offer a fair prospect, if the patients can be persuaded to persist in it. How safely a milk diet may be adopted in middle life is shown by the example of Dr. Cheyne, a Bath physician of the last century, who, at about fifty-five, restricted himself entirely to milk and biscuits, and yet was able to fulfill the duties of his laborious profession. He took at first of the former six pints, of the latter twelve ounces; but he shortly diminished the quantity to half, and, after sixteen years' experience, found it fully sufficient, and indeed capable of further reduction in quantity. [2]

*Weak and slow digestion* is a condition which enforces an especial care for meat and drink. The cause of the imperfection lies in a deficiency in the supply of nerve-power to the stomach, so that it both secretes its solvent fluid and also rotates its contents too slowly;

---

[1] Sibson's "Harveian Lectures," *British Medical Journal*, February 10, 1877.
[2] "The Natural Method of Curing Diseases of the Body," etc., by George Cheyne, M. D., 1742.

and the more it is loaded the slower it goes. Of the medicinal means of curing such a state, this is not the place to speak; but none of them will avail without the aid of a rational dietary. Time must be given to the oppressed organ wherein to empty itself of every complete meal, and such a period of rest given as will allow of the recovery of force; or, if the meals are frequent, they must be very sparing. The observations of Busch (Virchow's "Archiv," xiv.) show that a period of five hours elapses in the healthy subject before a fully filled stomach can empty itself, and in the dyspeptic the process is still longer. Whenever, therefore, the organ is loaded as healthy people rightly load it, a man should allow at least seven or eight hours to elapse before sitting down to another meal, and he must never eat till the need for food is announced by appetite. Perhaps a more generally applicable and easier-obeyed law is not to make full meals at all, but to stop short at the feeling of repletion, and, when that has gone off, again to take in the supply allowed by circumstances. Three moderate meals are usually sufficient to keep up the strength.

Meat should be once cooked. Mutton, feathered fowl, venison, lamb, and beef are digestible in the order they here are placed in. The more difficult dishes should have the longest time allowed to them. Of the farinaceous articles of diet, bread and biscuits are the most easily penetrated by the gastric juices, and all their preparations are safe. The best bread is the "aërated," which is free from decomposing yeast. Macaroni is good if soaked till quite macerated. Pastry is difficult of solution. Vegetables are very necessary; cauliflowers, Jerusalem artichokes, beet-root, French beans, soft peas, stewed celery, turnip-tops, spinach, are the most readily disposed of.

When the usual mixture of meat and vegetables is found to induce flatulence, it is a good expedient to eat vegetables only at one meal and meat and bread only at another. The principle on which this plan is based is that starchy food is dissolved mainly by the alkaline saliva, whereas meat is dissolved by the acid gastric juice. In a vigorous person both are copious enough to render immaterial their mutual neutralization; but when they are scanty, their separate employment is a physiological economy.

*Consumption* is a disease whose treatment is almost wholly dietetic. The children of a mother whose pedigree exhibits proof of a consumptive tendency may with propriety be put to a healthy wet-nurse immediately on birth, and, on being weaned, be fed from a Channel Island cow. The milk should be boiled and then cooled down to tepidity. A small teaspoonful of " saccharated solution of lime " may be advantageously added to each quart of milk when the coming teeth require the elements of their nutrition to be added to the diet. The rules already given for the healthy management of the young should be adhered to with unusual strictness, and any departure from them should be made only to provide for some peculiar necessity of the case according to medical advice.

In cases of consumption it is difficult to say that drugs are useless, but certainly those that come nearest to aliments have most evidence in their favor, such as iron, cod-liver oil, and the phosphates of lime. Their effect on the appetite must be sedulously watched, and the end must not be sacrificed to the means; that is to say, if they spoil the appetite, they must be left off. The reason for administering oil is to afford an easily assimilated basis of renewed organic growth, to take the place of the abnormal tendency to form tubercular matter. If anything prevents its easy assimilation it is obviously useless. The use of climate in the treatment of phthisis may be tested by its dietetic action; if it improves the appetite it is doing good; if it injures the appetite it is doing harm.

In *chronic jaundice* the function of the liver is best restored by the free use of green vegetables at all meals.

*Diabetes*, when it has once assumed a chronic form, is never really cured, but life may be much prolonged by the employment of a diet from which sugar and starch are excluded as far as practicable, and the patient nourished on animal food. The best fare for diabetic patients is that given by Prof. Bouchardat in his work " Du Diabète sucrée," Paris, 1852.

*In functional nervous diseases*, such as hysteria and hypochondriasis, the appetite, muscular elasticity, and mental powers will often be observed to be deficient in the early part of the day, and to recover their tone in the evening. At this latter time, therefore, it is advisable to make the principal meal.

*Scurvy* is a notable example of a disease of which, more than any other, the prevention depends on the adoption of a suitable diet. Its symptoms so far resemble those of general starvation that, from the earliest time of its appearance in history, it has been suspected that it is due to a dietary defective in some necessary ingredient; and practical observation soon showed that this was fresh vegetables. It was found on every long voyage that the crew suffered from scurvy in proportion to the length of time they were restricted to dry food, and that they recovered rapidly as soon as they got access to a supply of succulent plants. This requisite for health is obviously the most difficult of all things to procure aboard ship, and efforts were made to find a substitute capable of marine transport. From the time of Hawkins [1] (1593) downward the opinion has been expressed, by all the most intelligent travelers, that a substitute is to be found in the juice of fruits of the orange tribe, such as oranges, lemons, etc. But in its natural state this is expensive and troublesome to carry, so that skippers and owners for a couple of centuries found it expedient to be skeptical. The pictures of scurvy as it appeared during the eighteenth century are horrible in the extreme. But the statute of 1795, passed through the exertions of Captain Cook and Sir Gilbert Blane, has enforced the carrying of lime-juice. This invaluable preventive has shown its influence all the more decidedly by the disease still appearing occasionally under strong promoting circumstances, and to a certain extent in spite of the antidote; but it is so modified as to be usually more of the nature of a warning or demonstration than of a serious invasion. Some, indeed, have questioned and even denied altogether the blessings derived from the enforced use of lime-juice. But they make a very scanty show when weighed with those whom they undertake to oppose; and it is superfluous here to enter into the arguments and results of observation constituting the ponderous "Report of the Committee appointed by the Lords Commissioners of the Admiralty to inquire into the Causes of the Outbreak of Scurvy in the Recent Arctic Expedition, etc., and presented to both Houses of Parliament, May 7, 1877," which seems to settle forever the preventive powers against scurvy of the use of lime-juice.

The committee alluded to was appointed in consequence of one of those exceptional outbreaks of scurvy induced by exceptional circumstances. The ships sent on the exploring expedition of 1875 were amply provided with lime-juice, and with printed expositions of its value. During the voyage out and in the long inaction of the

---

[1] Sir Rd. Hawkins's "Voyage," edited by Hakluyt Society, page 60.

winter, the men's health was so well preserved by general attention to hygiene that no cases of even mild scurvy were detected; the pallor and languor and depression of spirits of some among the sailors were attributed to the want of sunlight for 142 days, and it was expected that a few days' sledge traveling in the open air would reinvigorate them. There was plenty of lime-juice aboard; but it seems that it is not the custom to add to the weight of provisions which polar sledging-parties have to propel, by including the preservative among them. Sir George Nares, the commander of the expedition, cites the names of 10 admirals, 10 doctors, and 15 captains, who have conducted land explorations in this fashion without it; and they returned unscathed to any serious extent. But on this recent occasion the crews seem to have been peculiarly predisposed to illnesses of scorbutic nature by the more than ordinary scarcity of fresh meat in their dietary, arising out of the deficiency of game in the extremely high latitude where they wintered. With few exceptions the whole of the crews of the Alert and the Discovery were employed in sledging, and the consequence was, that of the 122 officers and men 59 were more or less incapacitated by scurvy, and four died.

The real reason for not carrying lime-juice in such expeditions is its cumbersomeness. Including bottles, though in truth they are not wanted in a hard frost, it may be said that one pound a week for each man would have to be added to the baggage [1]—a serious item, no doubt. And with a view of remedying the inconvenience, medical men have long sought to discover to what constituent of the complicated mixture afforded by Nature it is that it owes its efficacy. In a contribution to the *Medico-Chirurgical Review* for 1848, Dr. Parkes examined exhaustively the evidence concerning the various deficiencies in ship-food as compared with fresh food, which might be filled up by one or other of the components of lime-juice; and by exclusion he is led to the conclusion that the cause of scurvy is to be found in deficiency of salts whose acids form carbonates in the system, viz., citric, tartaric, acetic, lactic, and malic acids.

Though not so good as when in their natural form, because less digestible and pleasant, yet a supply of citrates, tartrates, lactates, and malates of potash might be packed in small bulk, and, under

---

[1] In merchant-ships lime-juice is used during polar service in a ration of an ounce daily. See "Report" above cited. But the opinions of the officers examined seem to agree that the quantity is not sufficient, and advise half as much again, or more.

circumstances where weight is of importance, might take the place of lime-juice. Or bolo-lozenges might be made of lime-juice freed from its aqueous portion and preserved with sugar. Three or four of these a day might be easily swallowed without stopping work.

Before leaving the subject of maritime scurvy, it may be suggested how useful it would be if those who sail in desolate regions were to carry seeds of antiscorbutic vegetables, which, strewed broadcast in uninhabited places, would form a flora capable of saving the lives of many a wrecked or weather-bound crew.

Scurvy, as landsmen see it in time of peace, amounts to little more than anæmia, with a softening and bleeding condition of the gums; but it indicates the use of exactly the same preventives and remedies as the more severe complaint.

*Starvation* is a disease which it is a platitude to say may be prevented by diet; nevertheless there are connected with it a few peculiarities of scientific and practical interest which may not be unworthy of notice. "Inedia," as it is called in the nomenclature of diseases by the London College of Physicians, is of two kinds, arising from *want of food* and from *want of water*.

When entirely deprived of nutriment the human body is capable of supporting life under ordinary circumstances for little more than a week. In the spring of 1869 this was tried on the person of a "fasting girl" in South Wales. The parents made a show of their child, decking her out like a bride on a bed, and asserting that she had eaten no food for two years. Some reckless enthusiasts for truth set four trustworthy hospital nurses to watch her; the Celtic obstinacy of the parents was roused, and in defense of their imposture they allowed death to take place in eight days. Their trial and conviction for manslaughter may be found in the daily periodicals of the date; but, strange to say, the experimental physiologists and nurses escaped scot-free. There is no doubt that in this instance the unnatural quietude, the grave-like silence, and the dim religious light in which the victim was kept, contributed to defer death.

One thing which remarkably prolongs life is a supply of water. Dogs furnished with as much as they wished to drink were found by M. Chossat ("Sur l'Inanition," Paris, 1843) to live three times as long as those who were deprived of solids and liquids at the same time. Even wetting the skin with sea-water has been found useful by shipwrecked sailors. Four men and a boy of fourteen who got shut in Tynewydd mine, near Porth, in South Wales, in the winter of 1876–'77, for ten days without food, were not only alive when released, but several of them were able to walk, and all subsequently recovered. The thorough saturation of the narrow space with aqueous vapor, and the presence of drain-water in the cutting, were probably their chief preservatives, assisted by the high, even temperature always found in the deeper headings of coal-mines, and by the enormous compression of the confined air. This, doubtless, prevented evaporation, and retarded vital processes dependent upon oxidation. The accumulation of carbonic acid in the breathed air would also have a similar arrestive power over destructive assimilation. These prisoners do not seem to have felt any of the severer pangs of hunger, for they were not tempted to eat their candles. With the instinctive feeling that darkness adds a horror to death, they preferred to use them for light.

It is a paradoxical fact that the supply of the stomach even from the substance of the starving individual's body should tend to prolong life. In April, 1874, a case was recorded of exposure in an open boat for thirty-two days of three men and two boys, with only ten days' provisions, exclusive of old boots and jelly-fish. They had a fight in their delirium, and one was severely wounded. As the blood gushed out he lapped it up; and instead of suffering the fatal weakness which might have been expected from the hemorrhage, he seems to have done well. Experiments have been performed by a French physiologist, M. Anselmier ("Archives Gén. de Médecine," 1860, vol. i., page 169), with the object of trying to preserve the lives of dogs by what he calls "artificial autophagy." He fed them on the blood taken from their own veins daily, depriving them of all other food, and he found that the fatal cooling incident to starvation was thus postponed and existence prolonged. Life lasted till the emaciation had proceeded to six-tenths of the animal's weight, as in Chossat's experiments, extending to the fourteenth day, instead of ending on the tenth day, as was the case with other dogs which were not bled.

These instances of the application of the art of dietetics to the treatment of disease are sufficient to show the principles which should be kept in sight. The pathology of the ailment should be considered first, then its bearing upon the digestive organs, and lastly the bearing of the digestive organs upon it.

And before quitting the subject of health as affected by diet, the common-sense hint may be given to those who are in good sanitary condition, that they cannot do better than let well alone. The most trustworthy security for future health is present health, and there is some risk of overthrowing Nature's work by overcaring.

### PLEASURE AS AN OBJECT OF DIETETICS.

The social importance of gratifying the palate has certainly never been denied in practice by any of the human race. Feasting has been adopted from the earliest times as the most natural expression of joy, and the readiest means of creating joy. If ascetics have seemed to put the pleasure away from them, they have done so in the hope of purchasing by their sacrifice something greater and nobler, and have thus tacitly conceded, if not exaggerated, its real value. Experience shows that its indulgence, unregulated by the laws which govern our progress in civilization, leads to unutterable degradation and meanness, brutalizes the mind, and deadens its perception of the repulsiveness of vice and crime. But that is no cause why this powerful motive power, governed by right reason, should not be made subservient to the highest purposes.

The times of meals must be regulated with a regard to the disposal of the remainder of the day, whether that depends on choice or on necessity. Violent exertion of either mind or body retards digestion; and, therefore, when this is practised, food is not called for so soon as on a day of rest. The heaviest meal should be postponed till the day's work is done; it is then that social home joys give the requisite repose to the body and mind. Light eaters may dine as late as they please, but those of larger appetite should lengthen the interval between their repast and bedtime. After the night's sleep and the long fast which has emptied the digestive canal of its nutritive contents, a breakfast should be taken before any of the real business of life be begun. It is no proof of health or vigor to forego it without inconvenience; but it is a proof of health and vigor to be able to lay in then a solid foundation for the day's labor. Not less than four and not more than six hours should elapse before the store is again replenished. A light, farinaceous lunch, with vegetables and fruit, may be made most appetizing, and is followed by a cheerful afternoon, whereas a ponderous meat and wine meal entails heaviness of spirit.

## DIET IN RELATION TO ECONOMY.

*Due Proportion of Animal and Vegetable Food.*—It has been taken for granted thus far that the mixed fare, which has met the approval of so many generations of men, is that which is most in accordance with reason. But there are physiologists who argue that our teeth resemble those of the vegetable-feeding apes more than those of any other class of animal, and that, therefore, our most appropriate food must be of the fruits of the earth.[1] And if we were devoid of the intelligence which enables us to fit food for digestion by cookery, it is probable no diet would suit us better. But our reason must not be left out of account, and it is surely quite as natural for a man to cook and eat everything that contains in a convenient form starch, fat, albumen, fibre, and phosphorus, as it is for a monkey to eat nuts or an ox grass. The human race is naturally omnivorous.

Moreover, man is able not only to develop his highest faculties and perform all his duties on any form of digestive aliment, but he is able also very much to diminish the requisite quantities by a due admixture. The diet which supplies the demand most accurately will be the most economical in the highest sense; and that this diet is a mixed one can be shown by the following method of calculation: We can measure by experiment the ultimate elements of all that is thrown off from the body as the result of vital decomposition—the ashes, the smoke, and the gases, which the fire of life produces; and thus we can lay down a rule for the minimum quantity of those elements which the daily food must contain to keep up the standard weight. If the diet be such as to make it necessary to eat too much of one element in order to secure a sufficient amount of another, there is a waste, and the digestive viscera are burdened with a useless load. But there is no single article procurable for the food of the adult population which presents the exact proportion of elements required by an adult, and therefore no single article alone can supply human wants without waste.

As an example, apply this reckoning to the elements carbon and nitrogen, which constitute the main bulk of solids in our food and in our bodies. Suppose a gang of 100 healthy prisoners to excrete, in

[1] Milne-Edwards, " Cours de Physiologie," volume vi., page 198.

the shape of breathed air and evacuations, 71½ pounds of carbon and 4¼ pounds of nitrogen (which is pretty nearly the actual amount of those elements in the dried solids of the secreta, as estimated by current physiological works). Both nitrogen and carbon to that extent must of course be supplied in the food. Now, if you fed them on bread only, there would be wanted daily at least 380 pounds of it to sustain them alive long, for it takes that weight to yield the 4¼ pounds of nitrogen daily excreted; while in the 380 pounds of bread there are 128½ pounds of carbon, which is 57 pounds above the needful quantity of that substance.[1]

If, on the other hand, the bread were replaced by a purely animal diet, there would have to be found 354 pounds of lean meat in order to give the 71½ pounds of carbon; and thus there would be wasted 105 pounds of nitrogen contained in the meat, over and above the 4½ pounds really required to prevent emaciation.[2]

In the first case, each man would be eating about 4 pounds of bread, in the second, 3½ pounds of meat, *per diem.* If he ate less, he would lose his strength. The first would carry about with him a quantity of starch, and the last a quantity of albuminous matter, not wanted for nutrition, and would burden the system with a useless mass very liable to decompose and become noxious.

When work is undertaken, much more is actually wanted. According to Mr. Vizetelly, the laborer in a Spanish vineyard consumes daily between 8 and 9 pounds of vegetable food, consisting of bread, onion-porridge, and grapes.[3] And when animal food alone is taken, as in the case of the Esquimaux, 20 pounds of it a day is the usual allowance.

Now, if a mixed dietary be adopted for the gang of 100 prisoners before mentioned, 200 pounds of farinaceous food, with 56 pounds of animal muscle, would fulfill the requirements of the case; 2 pounds

---

[1] Dr. Letheby's analysis gives 8.1 per cent. of nitrogenous matter to bread ("Lectures on Food," page 6). Of this one-seventh is nitrogen, Boussingault's analysis of gluten giving 14.60 per cent. ("Annales de Chim. et Phys.," lxiii., 229). M. Payen makes the proportion of nitrogen to carbon in bread as 1 to 30.

[2] The proportion of nitrogen to carbon in albumen is as 1 to 3¼ (15.5 to 53.5 by Mulder's analysis, quoted in Lehmann, "Phys. Chemie," i., 343). In red meat there is 74 per cent. of water (ditto, iii., 96).

[3] "Facts about Sherry," chapter i., 1876, and Sir John Ross's "Second Voyage for the Discovery of the Northwest Passage," page 413.

of bread and a little more than ½ pound of meat a head would be enough, under ordinary circumstances, for each man's daily food.

200 pounds of bread contains ............................... 60 oɪ carbon, 2 of nitrogen.
60 pounds of meat (including 12½ pounds of fat on it) contains. 12 "     "     2¼ "     "
                                                                   ──          ──
                                                                   72          4¼

*Balance of Food and Work.*—The most important modification to be made in the above estimate arises from the differences of work demanded. Men may exist in inaction on a scale of food-supply which is followed by death from starvation when they are put to hard labor. It is of importance, therefore, to have some measure of the effects of physical exertion. And here mechanical science has contributed to physiology a precision rarely attainable in our dealings with social economy. Mr. Joule, of Manchester, analyzed, about thirty years ago, the relation which the heat, used as a source of power in machinery, bore to the force of motion thus made active. He showed that raising the temperature of 1 pound of water 1° Fahr. was equivalent to raising 772 pounds to the height of 1 foot; and conversely, that the fall of 772 pounds might be so applied as to heat 1 pound of water 1° Fahr. Thus, the mechanical work represented in lifting 772 pounds 1 foot, or 1 pound 772 feet, forms the "dynamic equivalent," the measure of the possible strength of 1° of temperature as marked by the thermometer in 1 pound of water. Physiologists seized eagerly on the opportunity which Joule's demonstration seemed to afford them of estimating in actual numerals the relation of living bodies to the work they have to do. So much earth raised on an embankment represents so much heat developed in the machinery, be it living or dead. The fully digested food, converted through several stages into gaseous, liquid, and solid excretory matters, produces by its chemical changes a definite amount of heat, of which a definite amount escapes, and a definite amount is employed in working the involuntary machinery of the body, and the rest is available for conversion at will into voluntary muscular actions.

It may be reckoned that the daily expenditure of force in working the machinery of the body—in raising the diaphragm about 15 times and contracting the heart about 60 times a minute, in continuously rolling the wave of the intestinal canal, and in various other involuntary movements, without anything to be fairly called

work—it may be reckoned that the expenditure of force in doing
this is equal to that which would raise a man of 10 stone 10,000 feet.

There are several reasons for believing that, in assigning their
physiological functions to the several sorts of food, nearly all the
business of begetting force should be ascribed to the solid hydrocarbons, starch and oil, by their conversion into carbonic acid and
water, just as there are good grounds for thinking that it is the conversion of the solid hydrocarbon of coal into the same substances
which drives a locomotive. To the nitrogenous aliments seems allotted primarily the task of continuously replacing the wear and tear
of the nitrogenous tissues, while any excess of them assists the starch
and oil in keeping up the animal heat.

One of the most cogent of the reasons for this view is that the
chief nitrogenous excretion, the urea, is not increased in amount in
proportion to the work done, as shown by the experiments of Messrs.
Fink and Wiscelenus; whereas the excretion of carbonic acid in a
decided manner follows the amount of muscular exertion. Now, it
is very clear that, if the supply of power to do work depended on
the decomposition and renewal of the muscles by flesh food, the
urea must be exactly proportioned to the exertion, which is not the
case.

To give an example of the mode of working out a problem by
this theory: Prof. Frankland, in a series of experiments made in 1866
at the Royal Institution, and published in the *London Philosophical
Magazine*, vol. xxxii., p. 182, ascertains with the "calorimeter"
(which reckons the *amount* of heat evolved as a thermometer does
its *degree*) the quantity of energy or force evolved under the form of
heat during the oxidation of a given weight of alimentary substance.
It has been explained that heat and mechanical work, being con-
vertible into one another, bear a constant proportion to one another;
so that a definite production of so much heat invariably represents the
potentiality of so much motion, used or wasted according to circumstances. From the reading of the calorimeter, therefore, may be
calculated how many extra pounds ought to be raised a foot high by
a man who has eaten an extra pound of the food in question; how
many steps a foot high he ought to raise a weight of ten stone (say
himself) before he has worked out the value of his victuals. Prof.
Frankland has thus estimated the comparative value of foods as bases
of muscular exertion, and he has made out a table of the weight and

cost of various articles that would require to be consumed daily to enable a man to support life, the equivalent of which has been already reckoned as the muscular force in action which would raise a man of 10 stone 10,000 feet.

| NAME OF FOOD. | Weight in Pounds required. | Price per Pound. | Cost. |
|---|---|---|---|
| | | s. d. | s. d. |
| Cheshire cheese | 1.156 | 0 10 | 0 11½ |
| Potatoes | 5.068 | 0 1 | 0 5½ |
| Apples | 7.815 | 0 1½ | 0 11¾ |
| Oatmeal | 1.281 | 0 2¾ | 0 3½ |
| Flour | 1.311 | 0 2¾ | 0 3⅝ |
| Peameal | 1.335 | 0 3¼ | 0 4⅓ |
| Ground rice | 1.341 | 0 4 | 0 5⅓ |
| Arrow-root | 1.287 | 1 0 | 1 3½ |
| Bread | 2.345 | 0 2 | 0 4¾ |
| Lean beef | 3.532 | 1 0 | 3 6½ |
| Lean veal | 4.300 | 1 0 | 4 8½ |
| Lean ham (boiled) | 3.001 | 1 6 | 4 6 |
| Mackerel | 3.124 | 0 8 | 2 1 |
| Whiting | 6.369 | 1 4 | 9 4 |
| White of egg | 8.745 | 0 6 | 4 4½ |
| Hard-boiled egg | 2.209 | 0 6½ | 1 2½ |
| Isinglass | 1.377 | 16 0 | 22 0½ |
| Milk | 8.021 | 0 2½ | 1 8 |
| Carrots | 9.685 | 0 1½ | 1 2½ |
| Cabbage | 12.020 | 0 1 | 1 0¼ |
| Cocoa-nibs | 0.735 | 1 6 | 1 1¼ |
| Butter | 0.693 | 1 6 | 1 0½ |
| Beef fat | 0.555 | 0 10 | 0 5½ |
| Cod-liver oil | 0.553 | 3 6 | 1 11¼ |
| Lump sugar | 1.505 | 0 6 | 0 9 |
| Commercial grape sugar | 1.537 | 0 3½ | 0 5½ |
| Bass's pale ale (bottled) | 9 bottles. | 0 10 | 7 6 |
| Guinness's stout | 6¾ bottles. | 0 10 | 5 7½ |

After the supply of sufficient albuminoid matters in the food, to provide for the necessary renewal of the tissues, the best materials for the production of internal and external work are non-nitrogenous matters, such as oil, fat, sugar, starch, gum, etc. When the work is increased, not so much extra meat as vegetable food, or its dietetic equivalent, fat, is demanded.

In comparing the cost of a daily sufficiency of the various foods to produce the required force, we must not forget the inconveniences which many of them entail. These inconveniences must be added to the cost. For example, suppose a man to have been living upon potatoes only, just supporting life with 5 pounds a day, and then to get work which enabled him and required him to take a double supply of non-nitrogenous food, he would act unwisely if he were to swallow it in the form of 12 pounds of cabbage. He would be knocked up by the sheer labor of carrying 12 pounds extra in a vessel so ill-adapted to sustain heavy loads as the stomach. A similar objection would lie against milk or veal or apples, however cheap accident might make them; and a more serious objection still would hold against nine bottles of ale, or seven of stout. On the other hand, the over-concentration of cheese, beef dripping, and lump sugar, makes them nauseous when in large quantity or monotonously persisted in, though when introduced as a variety they are appetizing and digestible. There is no saving in using that against which the stomach is set, or which the absorbents refuse to assimilate.

Reverting to the illustration of the gang of 100 prisoners, and supposing it were requisite to put them on hard labor equivalent to half "Frankland's unit" of 10 stone raised 10,000 feet—such, for instance, as carrying up ladders, altogether $1\frac{1}{4}$ mile high, 3 tons of stone daily—calculation would show that to add this amount of labor to the outgoings caused by the functioning of physiological life would involve the addition to their spare diet of at least 117 pounds of bread, or of 58 pounds of bread with 44 pounds of lean meat and 63 pounds of potatoes. The slightest imperfection or indigestion of any of this would cause a loss of bodily weight, and cases of illness would be culpably frequent. Were a draught of milk, or a cup of cocoa and sugar, or some oatmeal porridge and treacle, or even a little dripping or butter or bacon, given, the danger would probably be averted.

The most conspicuous fault in the dietary of the working classes is want of variety. Many of the articles which combine ample nutritiousness with small cost are habitually neglected, because, when used exclusively, they are disagreeable and unwholesome. From never being eaten they become absolutely unknown. There are many sorts of cheap beans, vetches, and peas, unheard of except at gentlemen's tables, of which a complete meal may be made, or which may support the dish of meat; while beet-root, cresses, kail, carrots, and other plants easily grown, are left unused.

*Quantity of Food required.*—The calculations of Dr. Playfair "on the food of man in relation to his useful work"[1] enable us, by another route, to arrive at an estimate of what amount of solid

[1] Lectures delivered at the Royal Institution, London, April 28, 1865.

victuals is required by an adult living by bodily labor to preserve his health under various circumstances. The circumstances which chiefly affect the question can be classified thus: (1) bare existence; (2) moderate exercise; (3) active work; and (4) hard work.

1. The first is calculated from the mean of sundry prison dietaries, of the convalescents' diet at hospitals, that of London needlewomen, and of that supplied during the Lancashire cotton famine, as reported by Mr. Simon. The result is that, in a condition of low health, without activity, 2¼ ounces of nitrogenous food, 1 ounce of fat, 12 ounces of starch, and ¼ of an ounce of mineral matters a day are necessary. The amount of carbon in this is equal to 7.44 ounces. In other words, a man's life will be shortened or burdened by disease in the future, or he will die of gradual starvation, unless his provision for a week is equivalent to three pounds of meat with one pound of fat on it, or with the same quantity of butter or lard, two quartern loaves of bread, and about an ounce of salt and other condiments. If he cannot get meat, he must supply its place with at least two extra quartern loaves, or about a stone and a half of potatoes, or between five and six pounds of oatmeal, unless he is, indeed, so fortunate as to be able to get skim milk, of which five pints a week will replace the meat.

A person reduced to bare existence diet can undertake no habitual toil, mental or bodily, under the penalty of breaking down.

"Bare existence" diet is that which requires to be estimated for administration to certain classes of the community who have a claim on their fellow-countrymen that their lives and health shall be preserved *in statu quo*, but nothing further. Such are prisoners, paupers, or the members of a temporarily famine-stricken community.

It would be obviously unjust to apply the same scale of quantity and quality to all persons under varying circumstances of constitution and outward surroundings; and to attempt to feed in the same way all these people for short or long periods, idle or employed, with light work or hard work, in hot or in cold weather, excited by hope or depressed by failure, involves an error of either excess or defect, or both at once. The dietaries recommended by the Home Office for prisoners very properly take all these circumstances into consideration. They allot "bare existence" diet only to those sentenced for short terms without labor. And they recognize the fact that a man's health is not injured (perhaps sometimes it is improved)

by a few days of such abstinence as would in the long-run be dele-
terious to him. Under a sentence of seven days, a prisoner gets
daily one pound of bread and a quart of gruel containing four ounces
of oatmeal. For more than seven and under twenty-one days, he
has an extra half pound of bread. For longer terms it is advised to
add potatoes and meat.

The nutritive value of the first-named diet is thus calculated by
Dr. Pavy ("Treatise on Food," page 415):

Nitrogenous matter............................................ 1.800 ounce.
Fat......................................................... .480 "
Carbohydrates............................................... 10.712 "

Of the second:

Nitrogenous matter............................................ 2.448 ounces.
Fat......................................................... .608 "
Carbohydrates............................................... 14.792 "

In the convict establishments prisoners are all under long sen-
tences, and are classified for dietetic purposes according to their
occupation.

The sparest of all is called "punishment diet," and is administered
for offenses against the internal discipline of the prison. It is equivalent to corporeal chastisement, being designed to make the stomach
a source of direct pain. It is limited to a period of three days, and
fully answers its purposed end as a deterrent by causing the solar
plexus to experience the greatest amount of distress it is capable of;
for after the expiration of that period sensation becomes blunted.
It consists of one pound of bread and as much water as the prisoner
chooses to drink. This last-named concession is not an unimportant
one; for it has been already remarked that a supply of fluid enables
starvation, and by implication abstinence, to be longer borne. At
the same time, it probably postpones the anæsthesia, and therefore
makes the intended suffering more real. "Punishment diet" contains, in Dr. Pavy's estimate:

Nitrogenous matter............................................ 1.296 ounce.
Carbohydrates............................................... 8.160 "
Fat......................................................... 0.256 "
Mineral matter ............................................. 0.368 "

Total of dry solids..................................... 10.080 "

This is about half of what an average man requires to sustain himself without work, and under its discipline he would probably lose three or four ounces of his weight daily till his bodily substance was reduced by six-tenths, at which period, according to Chossat's experiments, he would die.

"Penal diet" is that which is apportioned for more protracted punishment. It may be continued for three months. It consists of 20 ounces of bread, 8 ounces of oatmeal, 20 ounces of milk, and 16 ounces of potatoes daily. Its chemical constituents are as follows:

| | | |
|---|---:|---|
| Nitrogenous matter | 3.784 | ounces. |
| Carbohydrates | 19.864 | " |
| Fat | 1.580 | " |
| Mineral matter | 0.972 | " |
| Total of dry solids | 26.200 | " |

Upon this diet a fair amount of work may be done. The combustion of the carbohydrates evolves sufficient force to raise a ton 4,193 feet; and thus the effete muscular substance may be worn off by destructive assimilation, making place for new muscle derived from the nitrogenous matter, of which a bare sufficiency, but yet probably a sufficiency, is supplied. A man of strong constitution is usually found at the end of it to be in good health and of normal weight; yet he has never probably experienced the content which arises from a *luxus* consumption of food. It is intended to deny him the normal pleasure of the accumulation of reserve force in the gastric region. This pleasurable sensation under ordinary circumstances much promotes digestion, so that the whole of the ingesta are made the best use of; and therefore in " penal diet," as above quoted, it has been found expedient to introduce the slight excess to be noticed above what is needful to accomplish the required work in "foot-tons" (*see* before). The penalty of the regimen involves a certain degree of waste.

A close imitation of " penal diet " is that which the duty of a responsible government demands should be served out during a temporary famine, that is, one calculated not to last above three months. It is more economical to introduce the elements of variety in the diet than to be too monotonous—that is, to save in the daily issue and to be occasionally liberal, to feast from time to time as a break in the regular fast. The expense of the excess is more than replaced by the diminished habitual ration, and that powerful preservative of life, anticipation of pleasure, is brought into play. A reduction of the allowance below what experience has indicated as " bare existence diet," made during the famine in Madras in the beginning of 1877, was attended with disastrous results.

By dint of mixing and varying his diet, and making it consist of very nutritious articles, such as bread, meat, yolk of eggs, and soup, Signor Cornaro succeeded in reducing the quantity he daily consumed to as little as 12 ounces (Venetian). But then he made the solids go much farther by the addition of 14 ounces of good wine. And the probability is that this gentleman had a peculiar constitution, for, in spite of his many readers, he has had no imitators of the experiment on their own persons.

2. The appropriate food of the second class may be fairly represented by the dietaries of European soldiers in time of peace. The English soldier on home service, according to Dr. Parkes, receives from Government 5¼ pounds of meat and 7 pounds of bread weekly, and buys additional bread, vegetables, milk, and groceries out of his pay. Such a diet is sufficient for anybody under ordinary circumstances of regular light occupation; but should extra demands be made upon mind or body, weight is lost, and, if the demands continue to be made, the health will suffer. Mr. F. Buckland, surgeon in the Guards, remarks (*Society of Arts Journal*, 1863, quoted by Dr. Playfair) that, though the sergeants in the Guards fatten upon their rations, the quantity is not enough for recruits during their drill.

The Prussian soldier during peace gets weekly from his canteen 11 pounds 1 ounce of rye bread and not quite 2½ pounds of meat. This is obviously insufficient, but under the conscription system it is reckoned that he will be able to make up the deficiency out of his own private means, or obtain charitable contributions from his friends. Dr. Hildesheim (" Die Normal-Diät," Berlin, 1856, page 60) states that asthenic diseases are very common in the army, which leads to the inference that the chance assistance on which the authorities lean is not trustworthy. As the legal ration in these two services does not profess to be a man's full food, it is needless to analyze it. In the French infantry of the line, each man during peace gets weekly 15 pounds of bread, 3⅜ pounds of meat, 2½ pounds of haricot beans or other vegetables, with salt and pepper, and 1¾ ounce of brandy. This seems to be enough to support a man under light employment. Its analysis gives:

| | |
|---|---|
| Water | 179.83 ounces. |
| Nitrogenous matter (or albuminates) | 30.17 " |
| Fat | 9.29 " |
| Carbohydrates (or starch) | 126 84 " |
| Total of dry solids | 166.30 " |

An Austrian under the same circumstances receives 13.9 pounds of bread, ½ pound of flour, and 3.3 pounds of meat. The alimentary contents are:

| | |
|---|---|
| Water | 129.50 ounces. |
| Nitrogenous matter | 27.40 " |
| Fat | 8.23 " |
| Carbohydrates | 119.45 " |
| Total of dry solids | 155.08 " |

The Russian conscript is allowed weekly: [1]

| | |
|---|---|
| Black bread | 7 pounds. |
| Meat | 7 pounds. |
| Kawass (beer) | 7.7 quarts. |
| Sour cabbage | 24¼ gills—122¼ ounces. |
| Barley | 24¼ gills—122¼ ounces. |
| Salts | 10¼ ounces. |
| Horse-radish | 28 grains. |
| Pepper | 28 grains. |
| Vinegar | 5¼ gills—26¼ ounces. |

The "moderate exercise" of brain and muscle combined in the above classes is fairly represented in the convict scale by "light labor" (such as oakum picking) and by "industrial employment" (such as tailoring, cobbling, Roman mosaic and mat making, basket weaving, etc.). The dietary for prisoners thus engaged is nearly identical, except that the artisans using their brains are supplied with about an ounce extra daily.

The "industrial employment diet" for a week is thus analyzed by Dr. Pavy:

[1] "Report of Sanitary Commission," 1858, p. 425, quoted by Dr. Parkes.

| WEEKLY ALLOWANCE. | | Nitrogenous Matter. | Carbohy- drates. | Fat. | Mineral Matter. | Total Water- free Matter. |
|---|---|---|---|---|---|---|
| | Ounces. | Ounces. | Ounces. | Ounces. | Ounces. | Ounces. |
| Cocoa................. | 8.500 | 0.560 | 1.540 | 1.295 | 0.105 | 3.500 |
| Oatmeal.............. | 14.000 | 1.764 | 8.932 | 0.784 | 0.420 | 11.900 |
| Milk................. | 28.000 | 1.148 | 1.456 | 1.092 | 0.224 | 3.920 |
| Molasses ............ | 7.000 | ........ | 5.390 | ........ | ........ | 5.390 |
| Salt................. | 3.500 | ........ | ........ | ........ | 3.500 | 3.500 |
| Barley .............. | 1.000 | 0.063 | 0.743 | 0.024 | 0.020 | 0.850 |
| Bread............... | 148.000 | 11.988 | 75.480 | 2.368 | 3.404 | 93.240 |
| Cheese.............. | 4.000 | 1.340 | ........ | 0.972 | 0.216 | 2.528 |
| Flour ........... ... | 8.625 | 0.931 | 6.081 | 0.172 | 0.147 | 7.331 |
| Meat (cooked with- out bone or gravy). | 16.000 | 4.416 | ........ | 2.472 | 0.472 | 7.360 |
| Shins (made into soup). | 8.000 | 1.688 | ........ | 0.320 | 2.072 | 4.080 |
| Suet ................ | 1.500 | ........ | ........ | 1.244 | 0.030 | 1.274 |
| Carrots ............. | 1.000 | 0.013 | 0.145 | 0.002 | 0.010 | 0.170 |
| Onions............... | 3.000 | 0.036 | 0.216 | ........ | 0.018 | 0.270 |
| Turnips.............. | 1.000 | 0.012 | 0.072 | ........ | 0.006 | 0.090 |
| Potatoes ........ .... | 96.000 | 2.016 | 21.120 | 0.192 | 0.672 | 24.000 |
| Total water-free matter...... | | 25.975 | 121.175 | 10.937 | 11.316 | 169.408 |

This is probably a fair model for the most economical dietary on which an artisan or laborer on light work can thrive. It may be observed that the principle of variety is very conspicuous, and in private life it is possible to introduce still more variety by cookery. In the English and Prussian armies the introduction of variety is left to be attained by forcing the soldier to purchase some portion of his food out of his own pocket; in the French scale it is managed by issuing spices and various vegetables, and trusting to the innate genius of the Gaulish warrior for cooking. The issue of an occasional glass of brandy on holidays makes an agreeable change and benefits digestion; but if wine could be obtained it would be better and not extravagant. The Austrian bill of fare is sadly monotonous. The Russian ration may be noticed as particularly liberal of accessory and antiscorbutic food, from which civil as well as military dieticians might take a useful hint. Vinegar and other vegetable acids are too much neglected by our handicraftsmen and soldiers. The Carthaginians are stated by Aristotle to have used vinegar as a substitute for wine during their campaigns; and the recipes given by Cato for flavoring vinegar with fruits show that it was in use among the laboring population in Italy.

3. "Active" laborers are those who get through such an amount of work daily, exclusive of Sundays, as may be represented by a walk

of twenty miles. In this class are soldiers during a campaign, letter-carriers, and engineers employed on field-work or as artisans. These habitually consume on the average about a fifth more nitrogenous food and twice as much fat as the last class, while the quantity of vegetable hydrocarbons is not augmented, except in the Royal Engineers.

The "hard-labor diet" of convict prisons fairly represents what the authorities consider the minimum. It is the same as that already described as "industrial-employment diet," with the following additions: barley, one ounce; bread, twenty ounces; shins for soup, eight ounces; carrots, one ounce; onions, one-half ounce; turnips, one ounce. It contains, however, fourteen ounces less milk and one ounce less "meat."

The nutritive value of the additions may be seen by Dr. Pavy's alimentary analysis, which is as follows:

| WEEKLY ADDITIONS. | | Nitroge-nous Matter. | Carbo-hydrates. | Fat. | Mineral Matter. | Total Water-free Matter. |
|---|---|---|---|---|---|---|
| | Ounces. | | | | | |
| Barley | 1.000 | 0.063 | 0.743 | 0.024 | 0.020 | 0.850 |
| Bread | 20.000 | 1.620 | 10.280 | 0.320 | 0.460 | 12.680 |
| Shins | 8.000 | 1.688 | ...... | 0.320 | 2.072 | 4.080 |
| Carrots | 1.000 | 0.013 | 0.145 | 0.002 | 0.010 | 0.170 |
| Onions | 0.500 | 0.006 | 0.036 | ...... | 0.003 | 0.045 |
| Turnips | 1.000 | 0.012 | 0.072 | ...... | 0.006 | 0.090 |
| Total water-free matter | ...... | 3.402 | 11.276 | 0.666 | 2.571 | 17.915 |

From these totals must be deducted the articles cut off:

| WEEKLY DIMINUTIONS. | | Nitroge-nous Matter. | Carbo-hydrates. | Fat. | Mineral Matter. | Total Water-free Matter. |
|---|---|---|---|---|---|---|
| Milk | 14.000 | 0.574 | 0.728 | 0.546 | 0.112 | 1.960 |
| Meat | 1.000 | 0.276 | ...... | 0.154 | 0.030 | 0.460 |
| Total water-free matter | ...... | 0.850 | 0.728 | 0.700 | 0.142 | 2.420 |

The same food must be given summer and winter, though the demand must be greater to provide for the extra quantity of heat required to be produced in cold weather. But then the amount of work is diminished at the latter season by 1¾ hours, which is equivalent to an augmentation of the diet. The additions are more judicious than those made by the classes above mentioned, who partly furnish their own food; for bread and vegetables constitute a large portion of the convict ration, and the extra quantity of soup replaces the lost milk, without risk of the waste in cooking, common when the uneducated deal with solid meat.

4. "Hard work" is that got through by English navvies, hard-worked weavers, and blacksmiths, etc., which is more earnest and intense than the enforced "hard labor" of the convict. It is difficult to obtain accurate information, but it would appear from Dr. Playfair's estimates that the customary addition to the diet is entirely in nitrogenous constituents. The higher their wages, the more meat the men eat.

The neglect of vegetables by the last two classes is, in a physiological point of view, imprudent, and possibly may be a contributing cause of an inordinate thirst for alcohol which impoverishes and degrades many among them. To satisfy their instinctive craving for a hydrocarbon, they take one convenient, indeed, in some respects, but of which any excess is unwholesome. The discovery already mentioned of the production of force from the assimilation of starch leads to a knowledge, opposed to old prejudices but supported by experience, that the raising of the energies to their full height of usefulness may be effected by vegetable food quite as well as by the more stimulating and more expensive animal nutriment, or by the more rapidly absorbed alcohol.

With regard to the tables quoted above, in which ultimate analyses are used as data for dietetic rules, it must be noticed that their authors deprecate arguments being founded on any but the very broadest characters of the articles analyzed. Specimens, even when of the highest quality, differ strangely from one another. Season, soil, modes of culture, the variations of species, and many other little-known influences, come into play and prevent our taking the market names of eatables as representatives of a definite chemical constitution. And it may be added that ample scope should be allowed for the peculiarities of the individual and of his life-history. In the application of general rules, some one must be trusted to relax or strain them when circumstances require, or failures of a fatal character may occasionally result, and more often a galling perversion of justice.

Estimates for the thrifty management of food-supply have usually reference to the feeding of others rather than to the calculation of a man's own dietary. Enough has been said on that point under the head of the influence of diet upon health; and if a person really wants to bring down the expense of feeding himself to the lowest point, he can readily rate himself under one of the classes enumerated above, and act accordingly. It may, however, be doubted whether it is wise to reduce the diet to the minimum which the work requires. The certain evils of an accidental deficiency, or of a miscalculation, are so serious that the danger outweighs the possible inconvenience of a slight excess. It were an unthrifty thrift, indeed, which imperiled vigor of mind and body to effect a pecuniary saving; for there is no investment so remunerative as high health. A man need not consider that he is wasteful when he spends money upon making his bill of fare palatable and provocative of indulgence to the extent of moderate superfluity. Pleasure and prudence here walk hand in hand.

# LIST OF UTENSILS REQUIRED IN A FIRST-CLASS SCHOOL-KITCHEN.

3 copper stewpans, varying in size from 3 pints to 3 quarts.

3 enameled stewpans, sizes from 1 pint to 2 quarts.

1 copper sauté-pan; 12 iron saucepans, sizes from 1 pint to 2 gallons.

Iron pot for boiling.

Stock-pot, to hold 8 quarts.

Frying-pan.

Iron omelet-pan, tinned.

Fish-kettle, sheet-iron and tin.

Frying basket and pan.

Copper preserving-pan.

2 gridirons.

Tin oven and roasting-jack.

Steamer and saucepan.

Weights and scales, to weigh from ¼ ounce to 14 lbs.

Coffee-mill; 1 marble mortar and hard-wood pestle.

6 kitchen knives; 3 kitchen forks.

12 iron spoons; 6 wooden spoons, various sizes.

1 fish-slice; 1 egg-slice.

3 larding-needles; 1 trussing-needle.

1 set of skewers; 1 corkscrew.

1 flour-dredger; 1 sugar-dredger.

1 pasteboard; 1 chopping-board.

1 rolling-pin; 1 steak-pounder.

1 chopper; 1 saw.

1 box of fluted cutters; 1 box of round cutters.

1 box of vegetable cutters.

1 egg-whisk; 1 grater.

2 flour-tubs, or 1 double bin.

2 cake-tins; 1 coffee-pot (French), to hold 3 pints.

2 block-tin jelly-moulds, sizes 1 pint and 1 quart.

2 white china moulds, sizes 1 pint and 1 quart.

1 iron kettle, to hold 3 quarts; 3 baking-sheets.

2 square pudding-tins, sizes 1 pint and 1 quart.

2 tart-pans, and 12 patty-pans.

2 soufflé-tins, sizes 1 pint and 1 quart.

2 strainers, for gravy, etc.; 1 silk sieve.

2 wire sieves; 4 hair sieves, various sizes.

1 seasoning-box; 1 spice-box.

1 tin colander; toasting-fork.

1 paste-brush; 1 steel.

1 string-box and scissors; 1 basting-ladle.

1 jelly-bag and stand; 1 tammy cloth.

6 pudding-basins, sizes from ½ pint to 3 pints.

12 basins (8 common), sizes from 1 quart to 4 quarts, and 4 lip-basins, from 1 quart to 1 gallon.

6 dishes; 6 pie-dishes, sizes from 1 pint to 2 quarts.

24 plates; 1 salting-plate, to hold 3 or 4 gallons.

1 bread-pan and cover; 1 cheese-pan and cover.

3 iron trivets, various sizes.

1 black-board for lectures, size about 5 feet by 4 feet.

Kitchen-range.

Gas-stove.

Salamander.

Kitchen-paper.

Cost, about £52.

## IN A SECOND-CLASS SCHOOL-KITCHEN.

5 iron saucepans and covers, sizes 1 pint, 1½ pint, 1 quart, 1½ quart, and 4 quarts.
1 iron saucepan and steamer.
1 gridiron.
1 frying-pan.
1 iron kettle.
1 tin colander.
1 square pudding-tin.
1 baking-tin.
1 pasteboard.
1 rolling-pin.
1 tin roasting-oven and ladle.
1 coal-scuttle.
1 coal-shovel.
1 cinder-sieve.
1 set fire-irons.
6 iron spoons.
6 knives and forks.
3 wooden spoons.
6 tea-spoons.
6 basins, various sizes.
3 pudding-basins.
3 pie-dishes.
6 dishes, various sizes.

12 meat-plates.
Seasoning-box.
1 toasting-fork.
1 dust-pan.
1 salt-cellar; 1 pepper-box.
1 mustard-pot and spoon.
1 hand-bowl.
1 steel.
1 dish-tub.
2 brown pans.
3 jugs.
1 meat-saw.
1 chopper.
Scales and weights.
1 corkscrew.
1 grater.
1 coffee-pot; 1 tea-pot.
1 cake-tin.
1 flour-tub.
Black-board for lectures, size about 5 feet by 4 feet.
Small range.

               Cost, about £12.

## LIST OF MATERIALS AND UTENSILS REQUIRED FOR CLEANING.

1 pail, wooden.
Scrubbing-brush.
Set of black-lead brushes.
Sweep's brush.
Flue-brush (supplied with range).
Sink-brush.
Sieve-brush.
Dust-pan and brush.
Broom (hair).
2 tubs.
1 hearthstone.
1 box of black-lead.
Whitening.
Rotten-stone.
Bath brick-dust.

½ quire emery-cloth.
6 lbs. of soda.
1 bar of scrubbing-soap.
Sand.
Salt.
White chalk.
1 yard of house flannel.
1 leather.
1 pair of gloves.
1 coal-shovel.
1 cinder-sifter.
1 dust-pan and coal-hammer.
1 coal-scuttle.
1 set of fire-irons.

               Cost, about £3.

# INDEX.

# 378 INDEX.

THE END.

# LESSONS IN COOKERY:

Hand-book of the National Training-School for Cookery, South Kensington, London. To which is added the Principles of Diet in Health and Disease, by Thomas K. Chambers, M. D. Edited by Eliza A. Youmans. In one vol., 12mo, 382 pages bound in cloth. Price, $1.50.

---

THIS is an important work for such American housekeepers as are interested in the principles of good cookery; but it differs so much from ordinary cook-books that, to prevent misunderstanding, it is needful to call attention to its special features. Emanating from a school, and that school a working kitchen, the manual is beyond comparison the most thoroughly practical cook-book for general use that has ever been made.

The novelty and merit of the work are in the method by which it secures *successful* practice. Its lessons, the plainest, easiest, and fullest, anywhere to be found, have grown out of a long and painstaking experience in finding out the best plan of teaching beginners and ignorant persons how to cook well. They were perfected through the stupidities, blunders, mistakes, questionings, and difficulties, of hundreds of pupils, of all ages, grades, and capacities, under the careful direction of intelligent, practical teachers.

A cook-book's highest test is, Does it actually teach the art of cookery, or will it make good practical cooks? Thus judged, this volume is without a rival. It is not a mere compilation, nor the work of any one person. The managers of the training-school found that there was no cook-book suitable for their purposes, and that they must make one. The proof of its success is that, by following its simple directions, many hundred women have become qualified to fill responsible situations as cooks, or to instruct their daughters or servants in cookery, or to go out and establish other cooking-schools themselves.

Ordinary cook-books boast of the rarity, novelty, or great extent, of their receipts. The "Lessons in Cookery" makes no claim of this kind. Those who look in it for the last touches in oysters, terrapin, cake, or ice-cream, will be disappointed. There are thousands of English receipts that will not be found in it, and, of course, it does not treat of the dishes that are special to this country. The receipts of the work are *lessons in practice*, and these occupy so much space that a great multitude could not be furnished.

The volume, however, covers sufficient ground for a liberal and varied diet. It contains upward of 200 lessons in the preparation of a wide range of dishes—soups, fish, meats, poultry, game, vegetables, entrées, soufflés, puddings, jellies, creams, rolls, biscuit, bread, and a variety of suitable dishes for the sick. The wants of well-to-do families as well as those of more moderate means are thus amply provided for.

The chief advantage of the book consists in its efficient method of improving the quality of common cookery. In this respect it is strong where other books are defective. It will be useful in cooking-schools, cooking-classes, and cooking-clubs; but it will be still more useful in private kitchens. Many American women know how to cook well, but they are not so successful in teaching what they know to others. By the aid of these simple lessons they may turn their kitchens into little domestic cooking-schools, and thus elevate an important branch of household economy, now too much neglected.

---

D. APPLETON & CO., 549 & 551 BROADWAY, NEW YORK.

# D. APPLETON & CO.'S RECENT PUBLICATIONS.

### I.

**ALL AROUND THE HOUSE;** or, How to make Homes Happy. By Mrs. HENRY WARD BEECHER, author of "Motherly Talks," etc. 1 vol., 12mo. Cloth. Price, $1.50.

This volume, as its title implies, consists of papers upon topics concerning the ordering and well-being of the household. It contains, in addition to a large number of receipts for cooking, and rules for marketing, numerous hints for the management of servants, directions as to furnishing, repairing, cleansing, etc., and information on all the innumerable things on which housekeepers need information, while, in addition to its usefulness as a guide to practical knowledge, it is eminently interesting and suggestive to every one concerned in the welfare and happiness of home.

### II.

**ENGLISH LITERATURE,** from 596 to 1832. By T. ARNOLD. Reprinted from the "Encyclopædia Britannica." Forming No. 20 of Appletons' "New Handy-Volume Series." Paper cover, price, 25 cents.

### III.

**THE GREAT GERMAN COMPOSERS.** Comprising Biographical and Anecdotical Sketches of Bach, Handel, Gluck, Haydn, Mozart, Beethoven, Schubert, Schumann, Franz, Chopin, Weber, Mendelssohn, und Wagner. Forming No. 16 of Appletons' "New Handy-Volume Series." Price, 30 cents.

### IV.

**IN PARADISE.** From the German of PAUL HEYSE. Forming No. 14 of Appletons' "Collection of Foreign Authors." In two volumes. Price, in paper cover, 60 cents per vol.; in cloth, $1.00 per vol.

" 'IN PARADISE' *is a book which from the freshness of its theme, the great variety and individuality of its characters, the strength of its plot, and its happy execution, will command unusual admiration.*"—THE INDEPENDENT.

### V.

**REMORSE.** A Novel. From the French of TH. BENTZON. Forming No. 13 of Appletons' "Collection of Foreign Authors." 16mo. Paper, 50 cents; cloth, 75 cents.

"Remorse," which appeared recently in the *Revue des Deux Mondes*, is a novel of great power. The author, who writes under the name of "Th. Bentzon," is Madame Blanc, "a woman," says a writer in *Lippincott's Magazine*, "of great intelligence and the highest character."

### VI.

**JEAN TETEROL'S IDEA.** A Novel. From the French of VICTOR CHERBULIEZ, author of "Samuel Brohl and Company," "Meta Holdenis," etc., etc. 16mo, 320 pages. Paper cover, 60 cents; cloth, $1.00.

"The raciest and most entertaining Paris novel of the season."

"Jean Têterol's Idea" forms No. 14 of Appletons' "Collection of Foreign Authors."

# WORKS ON COOKERY

AND

## HOUSEHOLD MANAGEMENT.

---

I.

*Haskell's Housekeeper's Encyclopædia ;*

Or, Useful Information in Cooking and Housekeeping. 1 vol., small 8vo. Cloth, $1.75.

II.

*Blot's (P.) Hand-book of Practical Cookery,*

For Ladies and Professional Cooks. Containing the Whole Science and Art of preparing Human Food. By PIERRE BLOT, Professor of Gastronomy and Founder of the New York Cooking Academy. 1 vol., 12mo. Cloth, $1.75.

III.

*Beeton's (Isabella) Every-day Cookery and Housekeeping Book;*

Comprising Instructions for Mistress and Servants, and a Collection of over 1,500 Practical Receipts, with 104 Colored Plates, showing the Proper Mode of sending Dishes to Table, and numerous additional Illustrations. 1 vol., 12mo. Half roan, $1.50.

IV.

*Beeton's (Isabella) Book of Household Management.*

Being a History of the Origin, Properties, and Uses, of All Things connected with Home Life and Comfort. Also, Sanitary, Medical, and Legal Memoranda. 12mo. 1,140 pages, with Colored Illustrations. 1 vol., 12mo. $3.00.

V.

*Eassie's (W.) Healthy Houses.*

A Hand-book to the History, Defects, and Remedies of Drainage, Ventilation, Warming, and Kindred Subjects. With Estimates for the Best Systems in Use, and upward of 300 Illustrations. By WILLIAM EASSIE, C. E., F. L. S., F. G. S., etc., etc., late Assistant Engineer to Renkioi Hospital during the Crimean War. 1 vol., 12mo. Cloth, $1.00.

VI.

*Scott's (Frank J.) Suburban Home Grounds,*

And the Best Modes of laying out, planting, and keeping Decorated Grounds. Illustrated by upward of 200 Plates and Engravings of Plans for Residences and their Grounds, of Trees and Shrubs and Garden Embellishments. With Descriptions of the Beautiful and Hardy Trees and Shrubs grown in the United States. 1 vol., large 8vo. Cloth, extra, $8.00.

D. APPLETON & CO., 549 & 551 *Broadway, New York.*

---

## APPLETONS'

# NEW HANDY-VOLUME SERIES.

*Brilliant Novelettes; Romance, Adventure, Travel, Humor;*

*Historic, Literary, and Society Monographs.*

### I.

JET: Her Face or her Fortune? By Mrs. ANNIE EDWARDES, author of "Archie Lovell," "Ought we to visit Her?" etc. 30 cents.

"'Jet' is a thoroughly good book. It is pure in purpose, fresh and attractive in style, and fully justifies all the 'great expectations' based upon the reputation Mrs. Edwardes has gained for herself."—*Boston Post.*

### II.

A STRUGGLE. By BARNET PHILLIPS. 25 cents.

"A charming novelette of the Franco-German War, told in a pleasant and interesting manner that absorbs the mind until the story is finished."—*Philadelphia Times.*

### III.

MISERICORDIA. By ETHEL LYNN LINTON. 20 cents.

"We are not sure that we like anything by Mrs. Linton better than this."—*New York Evening Post.*

### IV.

GORDON BALDWIN, and THE PHILOSOPHER'S PENDULUM. By RUDOLPH LINDAU. 25 cents.

"Both tales are full of dramatic interest, and both are told with admirable skill."—*New York Evening Post.*

"We recommend to readers of fiction these two remarkable stories."—*New York Times.*

### V.

THE FISHERMAN OF AUGE. By KATHARINE S. MACQUOID. 20 cents.

"A particularly good bit of work by Katharine S. Macquoid. The story has a strong plot, and some of its scenes are fine bits of dramatic writing."—*New York Evening Post.*

### VI.

ESSAYS OF ELIA. First Series. By CHARLES LAMB. 30 cents.

"The quaintness of thought and expression, the originality and humor and exquisite elaboration of the papers, have made them as much a standard as any of the writings of Addison and Steele, and far more agreeable."—*Philadelphia North American.*

### VII.

THE BIRD OF PASSAGE. By J. SHERIDAN LE FANU, author of "Uncle Silas," etc. 25 cents.

"The heroine is a pleasant relief from the crowd of conventional beauties that one knows by heart. The scenes of the book are as odd as the characters."—*Boston Courier.*

### VIII.

THE HOUSE OF THE TWO BARBELS. By ANDRÉ THEURIET, author of "Gérard's Marriage," "The Godson of a Marquis," etc. 20 cents.

"The tale is pretty, and so naïvely and charmingly told, with such delicate yet artistic characterization, that it leaves a most delightful impression on the reader's mind."—*New York Express.*

"A delightful little romance, exquisite in its conception and perfect in its style." —*Philadelphia Record.*

"The character of Germain Lafrogne is one of the best in modern fiction."—*Baltimore Sun.*

### IX.

LIGHTS OF THE OLD ENGLISH STAGE. Biographical and Anecdotical Sketches of Famous Actors of the Old English Stage. Reprinted from *Temple Bar.* 30 cents.

"The book treats of Richard Burbage and other 'originals' of Shakespeare's characters, the Cibbers, Garrick, Charles Macklin, 'Peg' Woffington and George Anne Bellamy, John Kemble and Mrs. Siddons, Cooke, Edmund Kean, Charles Young, Dora Jordan, and Mrs. Robinson. A more interesting group of persons it would be hard to find."—*New York World.*

### X.

IMPRESSIONS OF AMERICA. From the *Nineteenth Century.* By R.
W. DALE. I. Society. II. Politics. III. and IV. Popular Education. 30 cents.

"Mr. Dale's chapter upon American politics shows a greater degree of fairness and
a better understanding of the spirit of our institutions than are exhibited by most
English writers. In speaking of our social characteristics, he says that during the
whole of his stay, and in all parts of the country, East and West, he was struck 'with
the extreme gentleness of American manners,' and gives several instances which came
under his observation."—*Boston Evening Transcript.*

"The book shows how our society, politics, and systems of popular education, strike
an intelligent, observing, fair-minded foreigner. The style of the book is pleasant, and
the writer notices our republican ways with a mingling of surprise, admiration, and
amusement, that is refreshing to read about."—*Louisville Courier-Journal.*

### XI.

THE GOLDSMITH'S WIFE. By Madame CHARLES REYBAUD. 25 cents.

"No one but a woman could have sounded the depths of the nature of this goldsmith's wife, and portrayed so clearly her exquisite purity and the hard struggles she
underwent."—*New York Mail.*

"The simplicity and delicacy of this little story render it as unique as it is exquisite."—*Albany Argus.*

### XII.

A SUMMER IDYL. By CHRISTIAN REID, author of "Bonny Kate,"
"Valerie Aylmer," etc. 30 cents.

"A Summer Idyl" is a charming summer sketch, the scene of which is on the
French Broad, in North Carolina. It is eminently entertaining as a story, as well as a
delightful idyllic rural picture.

"We consider it one of Christian Reid's best efforts. It is full of spirit and adventure, relieved by an exquisite love-episode."—*Philadelphia Item.*

### XIII.

THE ARAB WIFE. A Romance of the Polynesian Seas. 25 cents.

"The Arab Wife" is a picturesque and romantic story, of a kind to recall to many
readers those brilliant books of thirty years ago—Melville's "Typee" and "Omoo."

### XIV.

MRS. GAINSBOROUGH'S DIAMONDS. By JULIAN HAWTHORNE, author of "Bressant," "Garth," etc. 20 cents.

"This interesting little story fully sustains the reputation of Julian Hawthorne.
In him, at least, we have one more proof of the 'heredity of genius.'"

## XV.

LIQUIDATED, and THE SEER. By RUDOLPH LINDAU, author of "Gordon Baldwin" and "The Philosopher's Pendulum." 25 cents.

"Rudolph Lindau is a young German author, rising rapidly to fame, whose stories have principally Americans and Englishmen for their *dramatis personæ*, and are remarkable for dramatic directness and force, insight into character, and freshness of motive and incident."

## XVI.

THE GREAT GERMAN COMPOSERS. Comprising Biographical and Anecdotical Sketches of Bach, Handel, Gluck, Haydn, Mozart, Beethoven, Schubert, Schumann, Franz, Chopin, Weber, Mendelssohn, and Wagner. 30 cents.

## XVII.

ANTOINETTE. A Story. By ANDRÉ THEURIET. 20 cents.

"Theuriet is the envied author of several graceful novelettes, artistic and charming, of which 'Antoinette' is not the least delightful."—*Boston Post.*

## XVIII.

JOHN-A-DREAMS. A Tale. 30 cents.

"A capital little story; spirited in the telling, bright in style, and clever in construction."—*Boston Gazette.*

## XIX.

MRS. JACK. A Story. By FRANCES ELEANOR TROLLOPE. 20 cents.

"It is a well-written story, and will generally be voted too short. The characters are vividly imagined and clearly realized, while the author has a sense of humor which lightens the work."—*Philadelphia Inquirer.*

## XX.

ENGLISH LITERATURE, from 596 to 1832. By T. ARNOLD. Reprinted from the "Encyclopædia Britannica." 25 cents.

"Emphatically a history of intellectual ideas rather than a tedious catalogue of books and authors. Scarcely any notable book or author is omitted."—*N. Y. Even'g Express.*

## XXI.

RAYMONDE. A Tale. By ANDRÉ THEURIET, author of "Gérard's Marriage," etc. 30 cents.

"A story well planned, well written, and not long. It is bright, readable, and unexceptionable in its tone and inculcations."—*Worcester Spy.*

## XXII.

BEACONSFIELD. A Sketch of the Literary and Political Career of Benjamin Disraeli, now Earl of Beaconsfield. With Two Portraits. By GEORGE M. TOWLE. 25 cents.

---

*∗∗∗ Any volume mailed, post-paid, to any address within the United States, on receipt of the price.*

D. APPLETON & CO., PUBLISHERS, 549 & 551 BROADWAY, NEW YORK.

# WORKS

## OF

# WILLIAM CULLEN BRYANT.

**Illustrated 8vo Edition of Bryant's Poetical Works.** 100 Engravings by Birket Foster, Harry Fenn, Alfred Fredericks, and other Artists. 1 vol., 8vo. Cloth, gilt side and edge, $4.00; half calf, marble edge, $6.00; full morocco, antique, $8.00; tree calf, $10.00.

**Household Edition.** 1 vol., 12mo. Cloth, $2.00; half calf, $4.00; morocco, $5.00; tree calf, $5.00.

**Red Line Edition.** With 24 Illustrations, and Portrait of Bryant, on Steel. Printed on tinted paper, with red line. Square 12mo. Cloth, extra, $3.00; half calf, $5.00; morocco, $7.00; tree calf, $8.00.

**Blue and Gold Edition.** 18mo. Cloth, gilt edge, $1.50; tree calf, marble edge, $3.00; morocco, gilt edge, $4.00.

---

**Letters from Spain and other Countries.** 1 vol., 12mo. Price, $1.25.

**The Song of the Sower.** Illustrated with 42 Engravings on Wood, from Original Designs by Hennessy, Fenn, Winslow Homer, Hows, Griswold, Nehlig, and Perkins; engraved in the most perfect manner by our best Artists. Elegantly printed and bound. Cloth, extra gilt, $5.00; morocco, antique, $9.00.

**The Story of the Fountain.** With 42 Illustrations by Harry Fenn, Alfred Fredericks, John A. Hows, Winslow Homer, and others. In one handsome quarto volume. Printed in the most perfect manner, on heavy calendered paper. Uniform with "The Song of the Sower." 8vo. Square cloth, extra gilt, $5.00; morocco, antique, $9.00.

**The Little People of the Snow.** Illustrated with exquisite Engravings, printed in Tints, from Designs by Alfred Fredericks. Cloth, $5.00; morocco, $9.00.

---

D. APPLETON & CO., 549 & 551 BROADWAY, NEW YORK.

CPSIA information can be obtained
at www.ICGtesting.com
Printed in the USA
LVHW110325170622
721523LV00004B/22